THE SCIENCE AND ART OF RIDING IN LIGHTNESS:
Understanding training-induced problems, their avoidance, and remedies.
English Translation of
Medizinische Reitlehre

By ROBERT STODULKA, D.V.M.

© Xenophon Press 2015

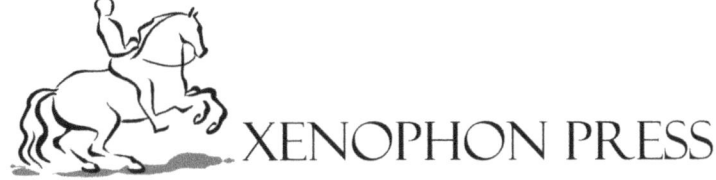

I dedicate this book to my parents Karl-Erhard and Gerlinde who, through their continual support, have allowed me to become what I am today.

German edition Copyright © 2006 by Parey in MVS Medizinverlage Stuttgart GmbH & Co. KG Oswald-Hess-Str. 50 70469 Stuttgart, Germany

German Language Edition ISBN: 9783830441670

Title: *The Science and Art of Riding in Lightness*

Copyright © 2015 by Xenophon Press LLC

Translated by Desiree Dupisanie

Edited by Richard F. Williams and Frances A. Williams M.D.

All rights reserved. No part of this work may be reproduced or transmitted in any form or by any means, electronic or mechanical, including photocopying, or by any information storage or retrieval system except by a written permission from the publisher.

Published by Xenophon Press LLC

7518 Bayside Road, Franktown, Virginia 23354-2106, U.S.A.

XenophonPress@gmail.com
Available at www.XenophonPress.com

Print book edition	ISBN-10:	093331647X
	ISBN-13:	9780933316478
E-book edition	ISBN-13:	9780933316478

Cover photo by Gabrielle Metz

From the Publisher

In researching biomechanics, I came across the book of Robert Stodulka D.V.M. entitled *Medizinische Reitlehre: Trainingsbedingte Probleme verstehen, vermeiden* loosely translated as *Medical Equestrian Studies: training-related issues to understand and avoid.* I contacted Dr. Stodulka and asked him to consider translating his work into English in order to reach and benefit a worldwide audience of riders. His unique expertise as vet, osteopath, holistic thinker, trainer and master rider uniquely qualify him to present this material. Four years later, we are delighted to present the expanded edition of the work originally presented in the German language. We owe a huge debt of gratitude to Frances A. Williams M.D. for her tireless editing and verification of medical terminology. Without this expert editing, this English edition would not have been possible.

Dr. Robert Stodulka's holistic approach combines the necessary knowledge of biomechanics, rehabilitative training and the equestrian art in lightness. His approach helps maintain healthy, sound horses and will undoubtedly help injured horses recover to daily work and competition. His primary goal is to find an individual training program for each horse, focusing on lightness and biomechanically correct movement in balance.

The individuality of each horse compels us to learn in each and every training session.

With great success internationally, Robert Stodulka has used his knowledge of the old French masters and has applied it alongside modern scientifically-proven biomechanics. Dr. Stodulka's system helps every horse improve in wellness while supporting the progression of training. His technique improves horses' behavior by restoring lightness and balance under the weight of the rider. It also prevents tension and resolves stiffness through the holistic approach of mobilization work and the osteopathic method of his teacher, Dominque Giniaux D.V.M., author of *Healing Hands* and *Equine Osteopathy: What the horses have told me*, both Xenophon Press titles.

This book is a powerful tool to help maintain your horse's health and to develop his desire to work. *The Science and Art of Riding in Lightness* is emerging as an effective multifaceted means of maintaining and improving your horse's abilities by transforming him into a willing partner. I hope that many riders and veterinarians will have the opportunity to benefit from Dr. Stodulka's training system.

Richard F. Williams
Xenophon Press

Xenophon Press Library

Xenophon Press is dedicated to the preservation of classical equestrian literature. We bring both new and old works to English-speaking riders Available at www.XenophonPress.com

30 Years with Master Nuno Oliveira, Henriquet 2011
A New Method to Dress Horses, Cavendish 2015
A Rider's Survival from Tyranny, de Kunffy 2012
Another Horsemanship, Racinet 1994
Art of the Lusitano, Yglesias de Oliveira 2012
Austrian Art of Riding, Poscharnigg 2015
Breaking and Riding, Fillis 2015
Baucher and His School, Decarpentry 2011
Dressage in the French Tradition, Diogo de Bragança 2011
Dressage Principles Illuminated Expanded Ed. de Kunffy 2015
École de Cavalerie Part II, Robichon de la Guérinière 1992, 2015
Equine Osteopathy: What the Horses Have Told Me, Ginaux 2014
François Baucher: The Man and His Method, Baucher/Nelson 2013
Great Horsewomen of the 19th Century in the Circus, Nelson 2015
Gymnastic Exercises for Horses Volume II, Russell 2013
H. Dv. 12 Cavalry Manual of Horsemanship, Reinhold 2014
Handbook of Jumping Essentials, Lemaire de Ruffieu 1997
Handbook of Riding Essentials, Lemaire de Ruffieu 2015
Healing Hands, Giniaux, DVM 1998
Horse Training: Outdoors and High School, Beudant 2014
Legacy of Master Nuno Oliveira, Millham 2013
Manege Moderne, D'Eisenberg 2105
Methodical Dressage of the Riding Horse, Faverot de Kerbrech 2010
Racinet Explains Baucher, Racinet 1997
Science and Art of Riding in Lightness, Stodulka 2015
The Art and Science of Riding in Lightness, Stodulka 2014
The Art of Traditional Dressage, Volume I DVD, de Kunffy 2013
The Ethics and Passions of Dressage Expanded Ed., de Kunffy 2013
The Gymnasium of the Horse, Steinbrecht 2011
The Italian Tradition of Equestrian Art, Tomassini 2014
The Maneige Royal, de Pluvinel 2010
The Portuguese School of Equestrian Art, de Oliveira/da Costa 2012
The Spanish Riding School & Piaffe and Passage, Decarpentry 2013
To Amaze the People with Pleasure and Delight, Walker 2015
Total Horsemanship, Racinet 1999
Wisdom of Master Nuno Oliveira, de Coux 2012

Foreword

It is a special stroke of luck when a highly qualified veterinarian, physical therapist and rehabilitation consultant, adept in alternative medicine, and a rider himself, finds the time to share his vast experience in the form of a book. This author currently practices in two European Union countries, both connected through hundreds of years of riding culture and breeding of world famous horses. In addition, he has assumed an advisory position at the University of Vienna.

What is new and unique to this masterwork is not only the detailed information dedicated to transmitting the art of riding, since the training and formation of the horse is a given; but most notably, the attention paid to the faults that the rider could make that have an immediate impact on the health and well-being of the horse. This point of view is directly in the spotlight.

Horse and rider are two living creatures that are implicitly dependent upon each other. The rider is the one that the horse bestows his full trust upon. The rider must channel the activities of this highly sensitive being under him and carries the responsibility of the horse's potential capability, his well-being and general health.

This unique book will appeal to a large audience of riders, horse owners, veterinarians, students of veterinary medicine and animal sciences, and everyone who loves horses in general.

May this work have an extensive circulation for the greater good of horse and rider.

Prof. Dr. Med. Vet. Dr. Horst Erich König
Professor of Anatomy, Veterinary University of Vienna

Foreword

I have read many teachings of riding. This health-giving route to riding is one of the best and easiest to understand for young and old, professional or amateur. It should be compulsory reading for veterinarians and horse lovers. Both the horse and the rider should be in a position, physically and mentally, to understand what is demanded of them. Dr. Robert Stodulka has understood this, and managed to immortalize his knowledge and experience in one book. A big thank you and lots of success with this book.

Greetings from a rider,
Arthur Kottas-Heldenberg
Chief Rider of the Spanish Riding School in Vienna (retired)

Foreword

The Science and Art of Riding in Lightness offers information to those interested in horses in two broad areas closely associated with each other, inextricably linked to the classical art of riding. Like the Euphrates and the Tigris: the art of riding and the biomechanics of movement flow closely together and build a synergistic whole where one cannot exist without the other.

Whereas there have been many scientific critiques penned over hundreds of years about the art of riding. The biomechanical connection, with its necessary and academic format, has only really been included in the last few centuries. Presently this serves as the science-based foundation for a meaningful and health-preserving training system.

Understanding the problems of the horse during training and profound knowledge in both areas—the art of riding and the anatomy of the horse—are absolute necessities; one flows into the other. Even so, the method of resolution, finding the so-called "riding-problem" in the horse's biomechanics is a very modern one and is not commonly found. However, with the advanced development of modern horse training and the exact knowledge of horse psychology, it is consistently more welcome and meaningful. The art of riding without harmony would be unimaginable and therefore also far removed from art itself.

Everything the old masters of riding said has been written down, but unfortunately read too little, often misinterpreted and therefore frequently executed falsely. It is nevertheless critical to strive for the correct method in order to maintain the horse's health as the most important commodity. Today, thanks to the development of scientific advancement, we can choose from various therapies in order to keep the horse sound in body and mind in order to demand the desired athletic performance, even at the highest level.

Proper training conditions, management, riders, trainers, farriers, and ultimately, veterinary care, all constitute a team that is the base on which athletic achievement rests.

However, nothing is as important as the influence of the rider on the horse. Both must be in a harmonious and trusting relationship with each other in order for the rider to motivate, relax, and understand the horse.

The rider preserves the cadence, rhythm, symmetry of the movement, balance, and the much sought after lightness, solely through tactfulness and feeling. The rider must take in all of this information to become one with the horse. In this way, it is then necessary to obtain detailed information on the mechanical principles of the "living machine"—the horse—to learn *how* the horse moves and especially *which* anatomical parts move. One should always remember that the horse, as our living sports partner, *transforms us* into riders.

I am convinced that the new generation of riders, trainers and horse people will be worthy successors to the "old" generation and perhaps even exceed them, but only with a substantial dose of humility and love for the horse, combined with an enormous and unceasing attempt to gain perfection through effort, diligence and daily sacrifice. Comprehension of biomechanics and the principles of riding in the development of the art must be present. The rider who knows biomechanics will understand the main player: the horse.

D. Francisco Reina Osuna
Director, Real Escuela Andaluza del Arte Ecuestre,
Royal Andalusian Riding School in Jerez de la Frontera

Acknowledgments

I would like to thank my friend and chief rider in the Royal Andalusian Riding School (REAAE) in Jerez de la Frontera, D. Juan Rubio Martinez, and D. José Maria Sanchez Cobos; the technical director of the aforementioned establishment, and the director, D. Francisco Manuel Reina Osuna, for the dynamic manner in which they provided me with advice on questions relevant to the art of riding.

In the same way I would like thank the head of the Horse Clinic of the REAAE, Joachin Cantos Leyba, for his veterinary collaboration. A special word of thanks go to Master Arthur Kottas-Heldenberg for the outstanding technical guidance. I am grateful to the horses, always my best teachers.

I am indebted to Prof. Dr. Horst König and his management-committee from the Anatomy faculty at the Veterinary University of Vienna for the excellent specialist assistance and revision on the anatomical aspects.

Following this I would like to thank my dear colleague Dr. Gabriela Wagner for the beautiful illustrations in this book that she managed to provide despite being pressed for time.

Lastly, I would like to thank my English publisher, Richard Williams for believing in the importance of this work and for pushing to have it completed and translated accurately into the international language.

Robert Stodulka, D.V.M.

Contents

From the Publisher	iii
Foreword by Dr. Horst Erich König	v
Foreword by Arthur Kottas-Heldenberg	v
Foreword by D. Francisco Reina Osuna	vi
Acknowledgements	viii
Preface by Robert Stodulka D.V.M.	1

I FUNDAMENTAL PRINCIPLES AND BASIC KNOWLEDGE	**3**
1. History of riding—The most important points in perspective	3
2. Glossary of Riding Terms	9
3. Why dressage and suppling exercises—Only art for the sake of art?	21
4. The search for lightness—What is *Legerité*?	25
5. Biomechanical principles as the foundation for successful training	27
5.1. The "good" horse—anatomy, physiology and biomechanics	27
5.1.1. The skeleton	28
5.1.2. Muscles, tendons and ligaments	31
Types of muscles	32
Head and neck region	35
The teeth	38
The Poll	39
The Cervical Spine	40
The nuchal ligament	46
The neck muscles	46
The back—thoracic vertebrae, lumbar vertebrae and thorax	48
Diseases of the back muscles	56
Thoracic muscles	57
The forelimbs	59
The haunches	67
5.2. The "good" rider—The correct aids	73
5.2.1. The aids	74
Voice	75
Rein Aids	76
Leg Aids	81
The Rider's Weight Aid	83

II TRAINING AND PREVENTING PROBLEMS   **85**

6. The schooling of the horse   85
6.1. The question of the riding technique
      —French, Spanish or German?   85
6.2. Riding Disciplines and their Specific Problems   87
6.2.1. Dressage   87
6.2.2. Jumping   89
6.2.3. *Doma vaquera*, Western (reining)   90
6.2.4. Eventing   93
6.2.5. Leisure horses   95
6.2.6. Racehorses   96
     Flat racing   97
     Trotters   98
6.2.7. Carriage horses   101
6.2.8. Gaited horses   101
6.3. The green horse, the young horse, the school horse   102

7. Equipment for the horse   104
7.1. The Saddle fitting   104
7.1.1. The English saddle   104
7.1.2. Full shifting panel saddle   107
7.1.3. Western saddles   110
7.1.4. Iberian saddles   111
7.1.5. Icelandic pony saddles   113
7.1.6. Panels, elastic trees, broken trees   114
7.1.7. Saddle influence on the Shu-points of the horse   117
7.2. The appropriately fitting bridle   119
7.2.1. Basics of fitting a bridle   119
7.2.2. Criteria for choosing the correct bit   121
     Curb bit   124
     Pelham   126
     Bit-less bridle   127
7.2.3 Influence of the bit on movement disorders
     of the horse and the rider's hands   129
7.2.4. The teeth of the horse and the bit   131
7.2.5. Nose-bands and their effects on acupressure points
     on the horses head   132

8. Developing the Training   136
8.1. Prevention and Fitness   136

8.2. Basic Training Fundamentals	137
8.3. Correct warm-up and cool down of the horse	138
9. Lungeing	139
9.1 General Advice	139
9.2. Equipment	141
9.3. Use of training aids	144
9.4. Round pen	147
9.5. Communication with the horse on the lunge	148
9.6. Starting the green horse—problems and their solutions	149
9.7. Lunge work and the ridden horse	152
9.8. Double lunge	153
10. The training scale	155
10.1. Rhythm—the quality of the gaits	160
10.1.1 The walk	162
10.1.2. The trot	164
10.1.3. The canter	167
10.2. Relaxation	170
10.2.1. Inner freedom from constraint—mental relaxation	171
10.2.2. The stretched position—forward and downwards	171
10.3. Contact	175
10.3.1. On the bit	176
10.4. Impulsion	176
10.4.1. Controlled forward impulsion vs. speed	178
10.4.2. Trot extension—a special case?	179
10.5. Straightness	181
10.5.1. Natural asymmetry	182
10.5.2. Paths to straightness	183
10.5.3. Riding with bend—limits and possibilities of bending the rib cage	184
10.6. Collection	187
10.6.1. Rein-back	189
11. Use and benefits of counter position and lateral exercises	191
11.1. Riding in counter position	191
11.2. Lateral work	192
11.2.1 Shoulder-in—counter shoulder-in	197
11.2.2. Haunches-in (Travers)	200
11.2.3. Haunches-out (Renvers)	202
11.2.4. Half-pass	203

11.2.5. Leg-yield	205
12. Application and benefits of high school exercises in classical dressage	206
12.1. Piaffe	207
12.2. Passage	211
12.3. Canter pirouette	213
12.4. Flying change	215
12.5. Spanish walk—*Paso Espanol*	216
13. Cavaletti work	218
14. Mobilization exercises in-hand	220
14.1. Mobilization according to François Baucher	220
14.2. Physiotherapeutic mobilization techniques to improve maneuverability	226
14.2.1. Neck	227
14.2.2. Front legs	229
14.2.3. Hind legs	231
14.2.4. Back and sacra-iliac joint	233
14.3. Spanish work in-hand	236
14.4. Work in-hand according to the Spanish Riding School in Vienna	238
15. Long reins	239

III PROBLEM SOLVING AND SPECIAL PHYSIOTHERAPY — 245

16. Course of examination	245
16.1. Case history	245
16.2. Examination at the halt and in motion	246
16.2.1. At rest	247
16.2.2. Presenting the horse in-hand	247
16.2.3. Presenting the horse on the lunge	249
16.2.4. Presenting the horse under saddle	249
16.3. Movement-palpation-analysis	250
16.3.1. Head and neck	250
16.3.2. Forehand	252
16.3.3. Hindquarters	253
16.3.4. Vertebrae	254
16.4. Thermography	254
17. Movement therapy—Rehabilitation and training	259

17.1. The difference compared to normal training	260
17.2. Lunge work	260
17.2.1. Correcting badly-trained horses	260
17.2.2. The rehab patient on the lunge	262
17.3. Use of training aids and their importance in rehabilitation and training	264
18. Complimentary physiotherapeutic methods at a glance	266
18.1. Manual therapies	266
18.1.1. Stretching and mobilization	266
18.1.2. Osteopathy and chiropractic	267
18.1.3. Massage	268
Effleurage (stroking)	269
Petrissage (kneading)	270
Friction	270
Vibration	271
Tapotement (percussion)	271
Lymph drainage	272
Connective tissue massage	272
18.2. Device Therapies	272
18.2.1. Trans electrical nerve stimulator (TENS)	273
18.2.2. Soft laser	274
18.2.3. Magnetic field therapy	275
18.2.4. Therapeutic Ultrasound	276
18.2.5. Ionthoporesis	277
18.3. Cold and its uses—Cryotherapy	277
18.4. Heat therapy	278
18.5. Acupuncture	279
18.5.1. Combining acupuncture and mobilization therapy	281
18.6. Neural therapy (trigger points)	282
19. Rehabilitation—course of action with particular symptoms	284
19.1 Problems caused by the rider	284
19.2. Temporary loss of rhythm, bridle lameness, faulty gaits	284
19.1.2. Over-bending and the "broken" neck	287
19.1.3. Problems with contact, the mouth and tongue	289
19.2. Back problems	290
19.2.1. General treatment proposals	291
19.2.2. Kissing spine syndrome	294
19.2.3. Tension, vertebrae and joint blockage	296
19.3. Head shaking	298

19.4 Tendon damage	299
19.5. Arthritis	301
19.6. Orthopedic shoeing	303
In closing	307

Preface

Horseback riding as a favored sport is becoming more popular than ever. The number of horse lovers is on the increase. Alongside the ambitious competition rider, there is a multitude of riders that see a correctly trained horse as a goal without premature wear and tear on the equine partner. Interest in "complimentary" riding technique is vigorously growing, thus pushing the trend towards appropriate training and especially biomechanically correct training.

My long standing friend, trainer and mentor for this work, D. Juan Rubio Martinez has taught me the gymnastic properties of riding in all its complexity through his unending endeavors. Night-long discussions that went on for hours allowed us to find a system that has been tried and tested by him, a system that can only be provided by understanding the anatomy and biomechanics of the horse. This allows us to teach this noble animal without the danger of wearing it down over the course of its training.

Based on the fundamental principles of exercise physiology and the tactfulness of the riding master, it is possible to provide a general intelligible idea to the interested rider and the veterinarian attending the young horse right through to the so-called problem horse. Since it is comprehensible to the horse, it is therefore easily accepted by the horse.

It is for this reason that it is advisable and sensible for riders of all disciplines to orient themselves to the guiding principles of the classical art of riding, to make allowances for the anatomical and biomechanical conditions of the horse, and to avoid any unpleasant resistance.

This book builds a bridge between understanding the anatomy and biomechanics of horse training. *The Science and Art of Riding in Lightness* clarifies the art of riding for the non-riding veterinarian, and can help the rider with no prior medical background to spare the horse any uncalled-for suffering.

In this spirit, I wish you and your horse good luck.

Fall 2014
Robert Stodulka, D.V.M.
Specialist in Physiotherapy and Rehabilitation

PART I:
FUNDAMENTAL PRINCIPLES AND BASIC KNOWLEDGE

1. History of Riding:
The most important points in perspective

Domestication of the horse brought a change from the animal being a source of food and changing our relationship with the species to alter the history of man. In ancient Greece, 400+ years BC, the horse was tamed, ridden and used in warfare. There are certainly earlier examples of domestication of the horse.

The philosophical and scientifically advanced civilization of ancient Greece allowed Xenophon (430 B.C.), with his knowledge of movement and training of horses, to write an early book on horsemanship. He was preoccupied with the independent seat, for there were no stirrups at this time. Xenophon was also a scholar of Socrates, and through this philosophical background he absorbed himself in the concept of unity of horse-man-body-soul. This is often reflected in his description of handling the horse. He recognized that a horse should never be punished in anger and that force will never accomplish harmony. He established the basis for tranquility though collected work with a horse. He also appreciated that the sensitive mouth of the horse should be preserved through the use of kinder snaffle bits and that a collected horse is more easily maneuverable in warfare. The trot was used only as a transitional gait to the canter.

In the Middle Ages, (V-VI century A.D. to around the XIV century) the classical art of riding came to an abrupt end as a result of different techniques used in warfare from using heavier horses in battle. The knight in heavy armor, rendered immobile, was hauled upon his horse and deposited on a platform saddle with his pelvis locked forward. The only chance he had to influence his mount was through the use of long shanks on a curb bit and sharp spurs. Stabbing with a lance, as practiced in competitions by the aristocrats in order to prepare themselves for battle, only demanded a brave horse going straight, and the deployment of bodily force in order to topple their opponents from the saddle. In the middle ages as the horse was mostly thought of as a raised platform for battle; only a limited capacity for its suffering was acknowledged. This way of riding became known as *a la brida*. More or less in the same time, in the Iberian Peninsula, another style of riding was developed from the technique of the Moors who defended themselves skillfully wielding bow and arrow using shorter stirrups on their short and agile horses. This way of riding, mainly in use in Spain, Portugal and in the south of Italy, known as *a la gineta*, became the basic technique for bullfighting on horseback This new way of riding—*a la gineta*—also describes the particular horse in use at the time (Berber, Arabian), called *jennets* (Purebred Iberian or native horses of old type).

In the time of the Renaissance, Frederico Grisone, the most famous master of the Neapolitan tradition of horsemanship wrote and published *Ordini di cavalcare*, the widely distributed equestrian treatise on the basic principles of the art of riding. In this work, the handling of the horse, bridle wear and training is described in detail. Grisone was the first to implement technical terminology, for example volte and capriole, in order to standardize the language of riding and he described the aids in great detail.

The aim of his treatise was to explain how to train a horse for warfare. The use of extremely padded saddles caused the riders to adopt an extremely straight, almost standing position in the saddle. He explained that the rider should follow the movement of the horse in order not to disturb the animal. Grisone also utilized the trot as a working gait, to strengthen the hindquarters and to attain more articulation in the haunches and therefore, collection, an admirably modern concept.

He tried to correct resistances and lack of understanding by the use of repression and punishment. He advocated that the horse must, above all, have respect for the rider in order to obey without reserve.

The "Italian school" influenced the German way of riding with the riding master Löhneysen (1552-1622) who wrote a substantial manual on the art of riding. Löhneysen devoted himself to the question of bits and described hundreds of different varieties in his book "Della Cavalleria." He began schooling young horses from the age of 5 years and consequently realized that working and mobilizing the hindquarters are indispensable preoccupations for training horses. He also realized that the outside leg aid to keep the bend is a necessity. A well-placed outside leg prevents the horse's hindquarters from falling out when riding on a volte. Although Löhneysen was a great advocate of Grisone's school, he recognized that praising the horse also had value in the training process, albeit only a small value in comparison to the value of punishment. He advocated the fork seat and emphasized the use of a soft hand—more than necessary given the sharp curb bits that were the order of the day.

The Neapolitan master, Giovanni Batista Pignatelli produced two very important masters of riding in the seventeenth century: Antoine de Pluvinel (1601-1643)[*The Maneige Royal*, Xenophon Press 2010] and Salomon de la Broue (1553-1610) [*Des Préceptes du Cavalerice françois*. 1593]. The latter was the first author to write an equestrian treatise in French and was the first text to explain the use of the *volte carré* (square volte) to approach the canter pirouette. More modern was the development of the system of riding by Pluvinel, who realized that the horse should enjoy his work and that gracefulness and perfection can never be obtained through force. Of utmost importance to him was the obedience of the horse. He viewed praise as highly important and was of the opinion that punishment should follow immediately and be regulated according to the resistance in order to be understood by the horse. Pluvinel also compared the "good" with the "well-seated" rider, which was viewed everywhere as modern.

Pluvinel was seen as the inventor of the pillars. He saw the high school movements as cultivated, natural movements of the horse. Interestingly, he prescribed the fork seat and denoted the modern "three-point-seat" as flawed.

The Duke of Newcastle's school developed in England at around the same time. He is credited as the inventor of the "head in volte" (shoulder-in on a small circle) that can be viewed as the precursor of the shoulder-in. He dismissed Pluvinel's work in the pillars as a matter of principle and recognized the usefulness of mobile hindquarters and the shifting of the weight of the horse towards the hind end in order to make him more collectible. He describes riding on the inside rein as the "quintessence of riding," which goes against most modern doctrine. Although he was on a side-track of the art of riding, even with this assumption, he realized the horse must move with his hind legs stepping relatively close to each other for collection.

In 1733, the master work by François Robichon de la Guérinière, *École de Cavalerie* [Xenophon Press, 1992, 2015], was released and is still vastly significant to this day. The training concept of this great master is based in the first instance on scientific and biomechanical findings, where the horse must, through systematic work, become calm, agile, obedient and comfortable to ride. He was the first to describe piaffe and the counter canter. He furthermore modified the "head in volte" to a straight line, thereby creating the pivotal exercise of the art of riding that we know today as shoulder-in. As a consequence, the haunches can be activated and the horse released. By the same token, he means that the horse should jump in the pirouette with his hind legs and not merely throw himself around the hindquarters with his forehand. Interestingly, he regarded the three-beat canter as a fault and utilized a four-beat school canter [for the pirouette]. He was the first to promote the path from heavy to light and to change the seat of the rider to the modern three point seat through modifying high French style saddles into a flatter saddle. His general training maxim was freedom of movement, suppleness, obedience and collection which largely conforms to the significant training tree currently in use. What's more he advocated the snaffle bridle in the basic training and always encouraged the leg aids to be dominant before the soft hand aids and described the action and importance of the outside rein in the work towards collection. His work is still hailed as the foundation of modern dressage today and serves as the basis upon which the Spanish Riding School in Vienna acts.

In the nineteenth century, as a result of the strong military influence on riding and the introduction of the English Thoroughbred, a complete reformation of the traditional riding systems came about. The speed and rectangular shape of the horses, together with the classical training system where empathy is required, could not be employed to the full extent in the course of a standardized military training. The paramount rule of conduct was to produce recruits and horses that were fit for military service in as short a time as possible, where survival was key and the artistic aspect was disregarded.

The German, Ernst Friedrich Seidler (1798-1865) invented the dropped nose-band, was in favor of cross-country training for green horses, and mentioned the word gymnastic for the first time in riding literature. He mistakenly tried, through isolated actions, to replace the living rider by substituting him with a special gadget, for example the "Spanish jockey," to "speed up" the training of the horse in an attempt to achieve a manageable equilibrium quicker. Thankfully he saw the "soul of riding" in the leg aids, thereby confirming the future coined slogan of Gustav Steinbrecht: "ride your horse forward and make him straight." [*Gymnasium of the Horse*, Steinbrecht, Xenophon Press 1994] (Straight means that the horse is equally bendable in both directions).

The genius, François Baucher, who was unfortunately misinterpreted over and over again, born in France, lived from 1796 to1873. By virtue of both his special equine sensitivity and empathy, it was possible for Baucher to ride newly conceived exercises like tempi flying changes, backwards canter etc Apparently it was not granted to him to write about this talent of his to the less talented amongst us. But the impression arose time and time again that his horses moved mechanically. Baucher tried to find the ever important equilibrium, that is so sought after in the art of riding, first through flexion exercises in-hand on the ground, in order to have better influence afterward in the saddle. Furthermore he discovered that the joint of the jaw and the poll play pivotal roles in the hindquarters, which today would be regarded as contrary to what we find in the training tree. However, he was right. The jaw joint must move freely in order to obtain lightness and be able to influence the horse without any tension on the horse's part. Only a contently chewing horse is able to relax his poll and yield in the process. Baucher was also correct when he said that all tension in the horse must be eliminated before it is ridden, thereby avoiding any resistances. This was the first attempt at equine osteopathy—to eliminate blocked vertebrae with the use of mobilization in-hand. The argument that resistances can often be caused by organic reasons or tensions, is still the basis of today's equine osteopathy therapy.

James Fillis (1834-1913)[*Breaking and Riding*, Xenophon Press 2016] criticized Baucher's system because of his static work with the horse and reformed Baucher's system bu riding forward briskly in order to arrive at impulsion, so essential in riding. In exactly the same way as Baucher, he invented many artificial gaits, for example canter on three legs and backwards—a canter that did not win him any acclaim from German classical riding experts of the day. Fillis expanded the training system with reference to cross country riding and jumping and tried to have his horses always carrying their polls as the highest point through active elevation—also in the extended gaits, which depend on the expansion of the rectangular frame. Nevertheless, the riding of Fillis still influences riding today, even the Russian way of riding dressage, for he was the main riding teacher of some of the Tsars.

The last important major riding master of the nineteenth century was Gustav Steinbrecht (1808-1885). Today he is called the classic master of modern day dressage. In his work, *Gymnasium of the Horse* [Xenophon Press, 1994], Steinbrecht uses his central idea: to ride a horse forward and to straighten him, as a rule of conduct in all training. A controlled forward impulsion, which should not be confused with hurried movement, but should also be present in the collected gaits and in the rein-back. Furthermore, impulsion is enhanced in the straightening of the longitudinally engaged hindquarters, where the activity of dynamic pushing power is first transformed into carrying power and then into elastic power. In one sentence, the complete training scale was explained as the foundation of any meaningful gymnastic training of the horse. Steinbrecht also correctly realized that all movement should commence from the hindquarters and all endeavors to flex or balance the horse from a standstill might go awry, for the art of riding is a dynamic process. The horse itself must also be released from tension through movement. Steinbrecht repeatedly emphasizes the necessity of "shoulder-fore" to make the hindquarters, that is the inside hind leg, compliant.

In the twentieth century, the Italian master, Federico Caprilli introduced the modern jumping seat. We still see the lasting benefits of his work today—that the horse's back can be freed over the jumps.

In 1912, with the collaboration of the cavalry school in Hanover and in due consideration of the German dressage and Italian jumping industry, *The H. Dv. 12, The German Cavalry Manual on the Training of Horse & Rider* (Service regulations 12) [Xenophon Press, 2014] was developed between von Heydebreck, Redwitz, Bürker and Lauffer. This was the mandatory training manual for horse and rider in the German cavalry school. The significance of this manual is to allow for longterm maintenance of good health of the young horse by ensuring correct training and riding to render him serviceable. These rules for training are still used today by the German Riding Association, embodied by the training tree. They describe the foundation of systematic schooling of young horses up to Grand Prix.

2. Glossary of Riding Terms

In this Chapter the terminology of riding will be addressed. Riding has its own vocabulary, and in order to avoid communication problems, it is appropriate to explain the professional terms.

Above the bit: Contact fault due to lack of suppleness and indelicate hands. The horse has its nose way ahead of the vertical and resists the influence of the rider by hollowing the back.

Action: The degree of lifting the legs. A high action is the result of a short forearm and a long metacarpal bone. The opposite is evident when a horse does not lift his carpal joint very high. The stride length can be big when the shoulder is slanted and the upper arm is long, whereas a steep shoulder angle has the opposite effect.

Against the bit: A defense on the part of the horse due to roughness of the rider's hand. The horse tries to pull the reins from the rider in order to avoid the contact.

Aids: Possibilities to influence the horse: voice, weight, legs, reins. Should be used sparingly, but as correctly as possible. The aids can only be effective when they stem from an independent seat. The rider must be able to give the aids independently from each other in a controlled fashion.

Arrêt: A strong, sudden and very painful jerk with the rein.

The art of riding: Systematic schooling that culminates in perfect harmony between rider and horse.

Ballotade: This is a jump of the classical high school where the horse jumps in the air with all four legs and pulls the hind legs under its body whilst airborne, without kicking backwards, as is the case with the capriole.

Barring: Unfair ways to demand performance of horses when they are not physically capable of attaining certain targets in training.

Bascule: The ability of the horse to round its back when jumping, which leads to an improved jumping technique, also applies to a rounded posture in flat-work.

Bearing rein: This is a gadget that should prevent the horse from raising its head. The rein is connected to the lunge roller with a pulley at the poll. This fully prevents an arching of the topline.

Behind the bit: Faulty head position due to strong influence of the rider's hand where the nose of the horse is behind the vertical, half-halts do not reach the hind legs and the horse evades the influence of the rider.

Bend of the haunches: Basis of collection. By decreasing the angle between the major joints in the haunches and developing a longer stance phase, the horse acquires a deeper, more elastic gait. The action of the forehand becomes more free in the process. (Fig. 5.19)

Bit: Mouthpiece that is placed in the mouth to gain control over the horse. Bits are grouped into snaffles, curbs and Pelhams.

Board neck: An underdeveloped and flat neck due poor conformation. It often goes with difficult poll and inadequate length, difficult to flex.

Bolt: Uncontrolled running away of a horse, mainly due to a panic reaction.

Breaking: Starting to ride the green horse.

Bridle lame: Temporary loss of rhythm that only occurs when riding. Mainly due to tension in the back, neck or croup. Caused by strong influence of the hand, where the rider lacks an independent seat.

Broken neck: Faulty head position from too strong an influence of the hand, or a too-strong neck (stallions), where the third vertebrae, not the poll is the highest point. (Fig. 2.3) It is often accompanied by a nose behind the vertical, where half-halts do not reach the hind legs and a serious lack of suppleness can be observed.

Brushing boots: Leg protection made from leather or artificial material, that can also have a supporting effect on the fetlock and ligaments.

Cadence: Increase in the moment of suspension, making the horse seem more majestic, with bigger gaits; for example, in the passage.

Capriole: School jump in classical dressage, developing from the *piaffe* and the *terre a terre*. The horse jumps in the air with all four feet and kicks out to the back.

Catching of the curb: A vice. The horse catches the shank of the curb with the lips rendering it ineffective. Using a lip strap threaded through the loose ring in the curb chain can resolve this problem. S-curved shanks can also solve this problem.

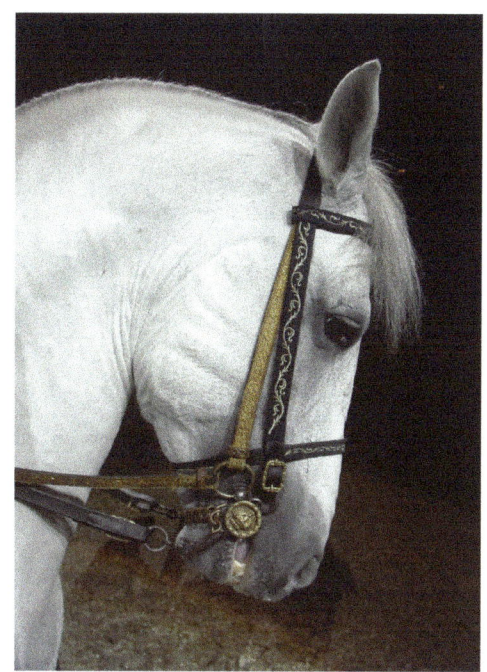

*Fig 2.3.
In a broken neck the third vertebrae is the highest point and not the poll. Stallions with a big neck and many Iberian horses often have a broken neck in spite of correct training. One must distinguish the structural cause of a "broken neck" from one caused by insufficient push from the hindquarters due to a hard hand and a back that does not function properly.*

Cavaletti: Versatile adjustable poles supported on x-shaped holders so the horses cannot hurt themselves when stepping upon them. They are well-suited for back and abdominal gymnastics, jumping and getting spoiled horses used to jumping.

Cavesson: Headpiece with a piece of iron on the nose-band and 3 rings, for lungeing and starting to ride a young horse (fig.9.1) The pressure on the nose forces the horse to relax in the poll whilst keeping the mouth unharmed and sensitive.

Chambon: Training aid that goes from the bit to between the front legs via a pulley system. When the horse lifts its head high, pressure will be exerted on the bars of the mouth until the horse relaxes into the forward and down stretched position.

Classical: Harmonious, perfect in itself.

Climb: Training on a mountain to strengthen the hindquarters and improve the coordination and sure-footedness of the horse.

Collection: The goal and final stage of the correct training scale. To increasingly load the hindquarters of the horse and relieve the front legs, which naturally carry more weight due to the anatomy the horse. The center of gravity is moved backwards. Collected horses are easier to maneuver. Greater freedom of the shoulder is achieved. The horses has an "uphill" tendency. Prerequisites: the horse is perfectly balanced, flexible, and can execute all required movements with the greatest of ease.

Contact: A light, uniform, but flexible connection with the mouth of the horse. The third step in the training scale, that will develop from rhythm (step 1) and relaxation (step 2).

Cooperative horse: The mental and physical characteristic of a well-trained, supple horse, with improved co-ordination, that easily accepts the aids of the rider and is pleasant to ride.

Courbette: an air above the ground in which the horse begins in a terre-a-terre, cantering in place, then jumps up and forward in several bounds on his hind legs. (see fig. 2.2)

Curb: Bit with shanks and port that puts pressure on the poll, bars of the mouth, palate and curb groove with the aid of a chin chain. In dressage tests it is prescribed from basic level as finer aids are required. It can be used alone (with 2 reins) or with a bridoon (with 4 reins).

Diastema: The toothless part of the horse's mouth where the bit lies.

Draw reins: Training aid. Passes from the girth through the reins of the bit to the hands of the rider in order to aid the horse in the forward and down stretch. A lot of damage can be done when misused!

Dressage: Systematic and purposeful training of a horse with the goal to improve the physiological and psychological skills and to improve the balance of the horse that has been disturbed by the rider. The horse becomes more agile, experiencing less wear and stays healthy for longer.

Elevation: The head and neck positioned in a beautiful circular arch, the result of systematic training where the hindquarters

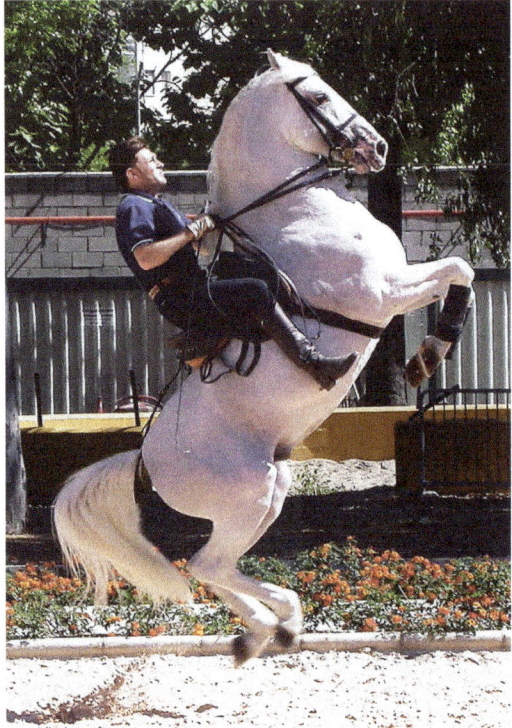

Fig 2.2. Courbette

are capable of carrying more of the horse's weight. This is also known as relative elevation. The horse should strive to search for the contact with the hand of the rider through the forward and down stretched position. The active influence of the rider's hand to elevate the head of the horse will obstruct the movement of the horse's back. This will give the impression that the horse's neck has an "S"-form, which is the result of lacking activity in the back.

Ewe-necked: Incorrect neck shape that is made worse if the back is not properly strengthened and the M. Brachiocephalicus over-develops causing difficulty in coming on the bit and making the horse difficult to influence. A problem caused mainly by incorrect riding where the horse resists the hand of the rider.

Extension: Controlled development of suspension that increases the length of stride without changing the rhythm of the gait.

Flexed at the poll: Direct yielding of the neck at the poll so the nose is in front of the vertical and the poll remains the highest point. This should be the result of correct contact and should not be confused with collection.

Flying change of lead: The changing of leads at canter from one lead to the other without breaking gait, during the moment of suspension.

Four beat canter: Faulty canter rhythm where the diagonal phase is split and the three beat becomes a four beat rhythm. Mainly caused by strong hand influence and tension in the back of the horse.

Grinding the teeth: Sign of immense tension, lacking relaxation.

Hackamore: A bit-less bridle that works on leverage on the nasal bone, used in western riding and jumping. When used incorrectly, it can negatively influence breathing.

Half-halt: The most important form of communication between the horse and rider. A light pulse on the outside rein works directly on the outside hind leg, which will improve the bend of the haunches. This is indispensable for riding at different speeds, transitions and as preparation for halt.

Half-pass: A lateral gait that develops from the travers.

Half-pirouette: Lesson at the walk, the horse executes a turn on the haunches without the loss of rhythm in the walk.

Halt: Reducing the gait to a standstill.

Haunches: The big joints of the hindquarters: hip, knee and hock.

Head tilt: Crooked position of the head at the poll due to uneven hand influence. One ear is higher than the other.

High school: Highest form of riding, demanding perfect accordance from horse and rider to become one in the movement. High school movements include *piaffe*, *passage*, Spanish walk, pirouettes, flying changes and the airs above the ground; namely, *levade*, *pesade*, *courbette* and *capriole*. This art of riding is still practiced in the Spanish Riding School in Vienna and the Royal Andalusian School of Equestrian Art in Jerez de la Frontera.

Hippology: The study of horses (Greek).

Impulsion: A forward impulse controlled by rhythm, relaxation and contact, whereby the horse shows more charisma when the rider drives with the aids. It is the basis for cadence and collection. Should not be confused with running or hurrying.

Lançade: The horse goes into pesade and then executes a single courbette like jump up and continues forward.

Lateral bend: Continuous, as even as possible, sideways curvature of the spine, starting at the atlas and ending at the last bone in the tail. Ultimately, the use of bend is to straighten the horse by [alternately] asking each inside hind leg to step more under the body. Anatomically, "bending in the ribcage" in the inflexible thorax area, in conjunction with the width of the ribs, is almost impossible.

Leg-yield: Lateral movement without bend. Should help the horse understand the sideways driving leg, is part of the basic training of green horses.

Lesson: A single exercise in dressage.

Levade: From the classical school, the horse sits down in the piaffe and raises the forehand up off the ground and holds a 40 degree angle. When the angle is greater, it is called a pesade. (fig.2.5)

Loosening up: Process during the warm-up where the horse stretches forward and down in good contact, round in the topline to enhance activity of the back.

Loss of rhythm: Irregularities in rhythm, resulting from incorrect influence from the rider, has a negative influence on the quality of the gait.

Lunge line: A 8-12 meter long rein to move the horse around the trainer.

Lungeing: Moving the horse on a lunge line in a circle around the trainer to improve rhythm, contact, impulsion.

Lungeing surcingle: A girth-like accessory for lungeing with many rings where training aids can be attached, and to get the horse used to a saddle.

Martingale: A strap with 2 rings where the reins pass through, to stop the horse from striking with its head. Often used in jumping.

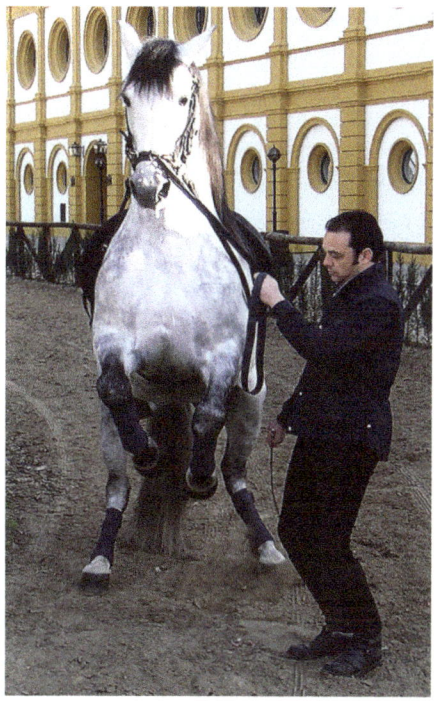

Fig. 2.5. Levade

Mezair: A classical school jump. Levade with a jump. After each lift of the forehand, the horse lowers it, jumps forward slightly and lifts into the levade again.

Mouthing the bit: Formation of saliva in the horse's mouth, resulting from a relaxed chewing on the bit. The horse is on the aids in a correct manner. (Fig. 2.1)

Narrow jowl: The horse has difficulty to relax in the poll because there is too little space between the lower jaw and the wing of the atlas. The parotid gland is

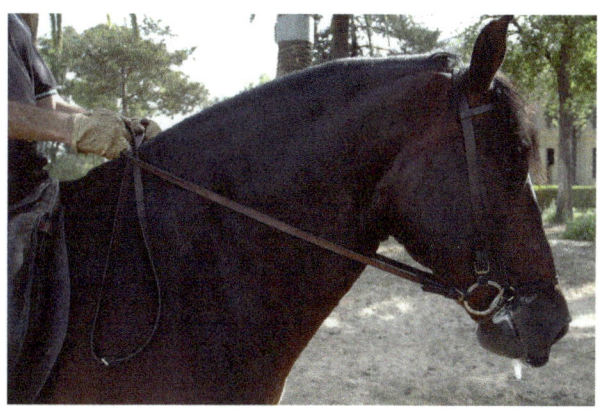

Fig. 2.1. Mouthing the bit is a sign that the horse is relaxed and releasing the mandible. Please note the straight line from the lower arm of the rider to the horse's mouth.

squashed every time the horse attempts to come onto the bit.

Natural crookedness: Inherent one-sidedness of the horse due to the position in the womb. The horse steps with the hind feet slightly to one side of the track of the front feet.

Over-track: The ability of the horse to step with his hind feet in front of the track of the front feet.

Passage: Floating trot, developed from the piaffe. The moment of suspension is prolonged so the horse moves with high knee action and extremely bent haunches from one stride to the other, without achieving much length of stride.

Pelham: A bit that intends to combine the effect of the snaffle and the curb. The shanks are similar to the curb and are moving. It has extra rings on the mouthpiece for a second pair of reins. This bit is suitable for horses with a short mouth.

Piaffe: Trot on the spot. The highest degree of collection in which the horse seems shorter with the croup lower. The hind legs continue to step actively without losing the trot rhythm.

Pirouette: The turn on the hindquarters in the canter. The hind legs describe a small circle, the longitudinal bend is kept as is the rhythm of the canter. In order to perform this, the horse needs well-muscled, supple and collected hindquarters.

On the bit: The correct position of the horse's head, where the poll is the highest point and the nose is slightly in front of the vertical. The horse is in light contact with the hand of the rider.

On the forehand: The tendency of the horse to resist taking weight on the hindquarters and thus leaning on the rein aids. The horse fakes the "uphill" tendency, has the nose behind the vertical and is difficult to maneuver.

Over-check: A thin bit that gets strapped with the normal snaffle in the mouths of trotters in order for them to keep their heads in an unusually high position and thereby reduce the risk of breaking into a canter.

Paddling: Abnormal movement of the front limbs, where the carpal bone swings in a strong circular movement when the foot lifts, can lead to early wear of the carpal joint. Often seen in gaited horses (Paso Fino) and Iberian horses from old-fashioned breeding stock.

Position (of horse): This is the degree of inclination the horse has to the track of the school, where no lateral bend is required (for example leg-yielding). Not to be confused with bend.

Push off: The state where the horse wants to stretch into the receiving hand of the rider due to the forward movement of the hindquarters

Rassembler: The concentration of forces of the horse in its center, accompanied by tilting in the lumbar region and raising of the neck and head in longitudinal flexion. It is the essential quality allowing the rider to have controlled access and use of the power of the horse, independent of the degree of bend in the joints of the haunches.

Re-balance: Communication between horse and rider in the form of light vibration on the rein and at the same time leg and weight aids. One gets half-halts as well as full halts, the half-halts will lead to change in tempo and transitions between gaits.

Rein-back: Diagonal movement backwards, to verify obedience and submissiveness.

Relaxed snorting: This is induced by free moving and forward strides, allowing the diaphragm of the horse to swing with the movement.

***Renvers*: [Haunches-out]** A lateral movement with the horse bent in the direction of the movement, moving on four tracks; the hindquarters on the track are bent toward the arena wall (instead of away from it as is the case in haunches-in) and the head is towards the middle of the school.

Rising trot: The opposite of sitting trot. The rider rises every second stride to relieve the horse's back.(Fig. 2.4)

Rollback: This comes from Western riding. A speedy turn on the hindquarters in the gallop, a 180 degree change of direction.

Rhythm: The regular, measured movements in a gait. The first element on the training scale. Rhythm, suppleness and contact, with the driving aids result in impulsion. A rhythmic horse must not move with speed.

Rubbing of the penis in the sheath: A sign of tension. A vacuum is formed in the sheath when the M. retractor penis tenses, makes a rhythmic noise. Only present in male animals.

Rushing: Moving too fast, associated with high frequency footfalls and shortened steps. One has the impression the horse hurries in order not to fall over.

School horse: A horse that has been taught all the lessons of classical riding.

Shoulder-in: Lateral gait on three tracks, the horse is bent in the direction of movement and the head is in the direction of the middle of the school. It is the basis for straightness and collection, as the inner hind leg is activated and the outside shoulder becomes more free.

Side reins: A training aid that is attached to the bit on both sides to aid the horse in coming on the bit; a lungeing aid.

Sidesaddle seat: The rider, normally a lady, sits with both legs to one side, and uses a riding crop as the leg aid on the opposite side.

Sitting trot: Staying seated in the trot. At rising trot the rider only sits every second stride and relieves the back of the horse.

To Supple: Warming the horse up before commencing the actual work.

Sticky: A vice, the horse does not want to leave the herd, tries to buck, rear, becomes nappy when asked to remove itself from the situation.

Straightening: The fifth stage of the training scale which results from working on flexibility and correcting the natural crookedness. A horse is required to move forward in a rhythmic, relaxed manner full of impulsion with good contact. Through increased bend and shoulder-fore the shoulders are aligned with the pelvis, and the inside hind leg is motivated to step under the body more. In this way the horse will stretch into the outside supporting rein, which also regulates the size of the gait. All of this is essentially done to achieve a degree of collection, as pushing power can be transformed into carrying power and then the mobility of the shoulders can be improved.

Suppleness: An acquired skill of the horse to react immediately to fine aids of the rider, to transform this into performance without delay. This ability is only possible through the systematic application of the training scale and never by forceful aids. Second stage in the training scale and is a prerequisite for meaningful training. A relaxed horse moves in a satisfied, rhythmic and purposeful manner and seeks forward and down stretch. One can often hear snorting in canter and an even muscle play in the loin section. Supple horses are never stressed or tense and always look happy and motivated. Noise of the sheath in male horses or pinched and crooked tails are signs of a lack of suppleness.

School gaits: Highest degree of collection in all three gaits. School walk, school trot and school canter distinguishes itself with little forward movement, but the steps are more majestic with the most powerful bend of the haunches.

Sliding stop: Western, the horse skids to a halt on the hindquarters from a full gallop, whilst the front legs continue to move to support the hind legs.

Spanish walk: A walk whereby the horse alternately elevates his front legs, the hind legs stepping under the body on the same side should give the movement a majestic air. (Fig. 12.5.a) Improves the freedom of the shoulders and the action of the front legs.

Spin: Western, a movement where the horse turns several times very fast around the hindquarters.

Tail swishing: A statement of displeasure with the leg of the rider and a sign of lack of suppleness, leads to tension as the horse cannot relax.

Take up the slack: Shortening the gait in order to get the horse more collected, or shortening the reins.

Teeth baring: Sticking the tongue out due to faulty influence of the hand of the rider, tooth problems, or an ill-fitting bit.

Three beat canter: The rhythm of a correct and even canter.

Tongue problems: The horse either puts the tongue over the bit or lets it hang out to the side. Can develop from too-strong hand or incorrectly fitted bit.
Touch: Energetically influencing the horse with the leg and back aids.

Tour: Circle with different diameters (20m, 10m, 8m, 6m)

Track: An enclosed, mostly rectangular area of either 20 x 40 meter or 20 x 60 meter. A race track or oval track has oval connections as opposed to square corners.

Training scale: Systematic set of rules to train a horse correctly without wear, based on anatomical and psychological requirements. The steps are consecutive and not interchangeable:
    1. Rhythm
    2. Suppleness
    3. Contact
    4. Impulsion
    5. Straightness
    6. Collection

Travers: **[Haunches-in]** A lateral movement on four tracks [sometimes three], the horse is bent in the direction of movement, the head towards the wall, the movement is sideways and forward. It activates the outside hind leg and frees the inside shoulder. When it is performed across the diagonal it becomes the half-pass, with the shoulder leading slightly.

Turn on the haunches: Rhythmic turn around the hindquarters, achieved from the standstill. The hindquarters should remain active and move in as small a circle as possible while the forehand, bent in the direction of movement, should move in a bigger circle around the hindquarters. This has an effect of collection as the horse must bend in the haunches.

Turn on the forehand: Loosening exercise where the horse moves with the hindquarters around the front. This teaches the horse to accept the sideways driving leg aid.

Volte: Smallest possible circle a horse can perform. The *Barockvolte or Karree* is a small square with rounded corners that can strongly increase the collection of the hind legs.

Working posture: The posture a green horse should adopt when moving freely forward, in clean rhythm and in a relaxed manner with a good contact with the reins. The horse seems to be more rectangular because the topline is stretched and there is no real elevation of the forehand.

Working tempo: This is the basic tempo in which the horse should step rhythmically, relaxed and with impulsion. From this tempo, collected and extended gaits can be developed.

3. Why Dressage and Suppling Exercises: Only Art for the Sake of Art?

When one examines the anatomy or the spinal column of the horse, it becomes clear that it is subjected to enormous static and biomechanical forces due to its shape. The spinal column connects the hind legs to the front end in the form of a bridge, the top being connected by the nuchal and spinous ligaments and the bottom braced by the sinewy Linea alba, thus forming the circle of muscles whereby the horse is elastically "positioned." Through the gravitational weight of the innards of the horse, a continual downward pull is generated on the spinal column, thus bringing the dorsal vertebral processes closer together. A reflex contraction of the muscles of the belly work against this force. Furthermore, a horse living free in nature spends at least twenty hours a day grazing whereby the nuchal ligament is always under tension as the head of the horse remains mainly in a lowered position. The lever action of the lowered head while grazing raises the withers and the thoracic vertebrae up to the middle of the thorax, giving stability to the spinous processes. In this way the downward pull of gravity on the spinal column is physiologically counteracted. The weight of the rider increases this pull. Damage occurs to the horse when he attempts to carry a rider unless there is additional muscle training and lifting of the back.

When one watches a green horse on the lunge, it becomes very clear that a young, unbalanced horse finds it hard, if not impossible to bend and move evenly on a circle. The young horse will look to the outside, fall in on the circle with the shoulder and the hindquarters will often float to the outside, which is a sign of lack of pushing and carrying ability and especially lack of balance. (Fig. 3.1 and 9.4a)

Here, it is worth mentioning "natural crookedness." This is a phenomenon present in all four-legged animals, yet it brings with it a specific challenge to the training of the riding horse, since the riding horse should be able to work equally on both reins.

Definition: "Natural crookedness" is a congenital one-sidedness, that is explained, on the one hand, by the way the foal lies in the uterus and, on the other hand, by its "triangular form."

This "triangular form" implies wide, powerfully driving hindquarters that attach to the forehand which becomes narrower towards the head. In the young horse, the lack of coordination and balance in the beginning causes the driving force to be transmitted in a crooked way and not in a straight

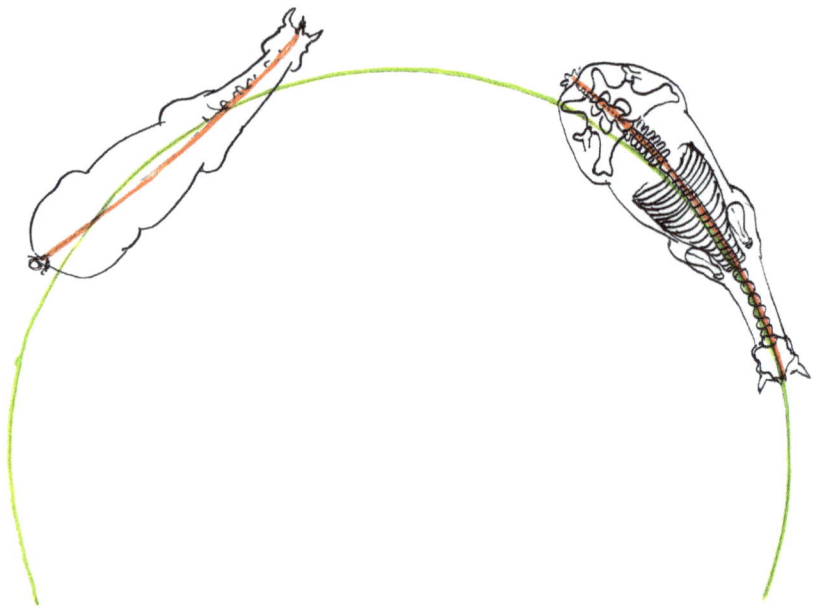

Fig. 3.1. A lack of auto-equilibration (shown at left) in the young horse makes him unable to follow the circle line with his spine; instead the horse takes on an outward curve and use his neck and head as "balance-pole" to navigate the circle. Despite careful gymnastic exercising and straightening, the complete maintenance of a circular bend through the entire horse's spine is anatomically impossible (due to the fact that his forehand is narrower than his haunches); nevertheless, the horse should be flexible to both sides. Thus he can be relatively parallel with the circle his is on (shown at right).

line through the spinal column. Because of this, the horse will not track up evenly with the two hind legs. Instead, he will prefer working in one direction more than the other. In this way muscle shortening is developed and creates the apparently easier or hollow or concave side; the "stiff" side is much more difficult to bend.

Consequently, one of the goals of correct use of gymnastic exercises must be the consistent and symmetrical training of both sides of the body, in order for the horse to perform all the lessons effectively in both directions. In the event of an obstructed vertebra or osteopathic lesion, it is of vital importance to have this adjusted before the training of the horse so that the central mobility of the spinal column is recuperated. Otherwise the reflex posture the horse adapts to prevent damage will cause more tension and resistance.

The second goal of gymnastic exercises should be to establish the horse's balance under the rider. Once the horse has managed to reach the stage of automatically balancing himself through the correct lungeing by the rider,

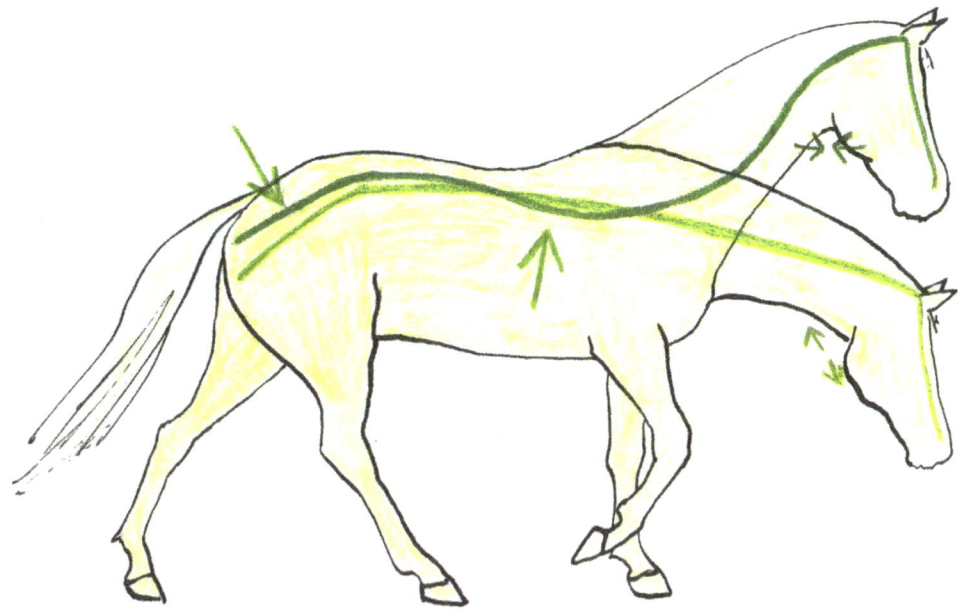

Fig. 3.2. With correct forward and downward movement of the neck, the withers elevate slightly and support the rider's weight. Due to the elongation of the neck, the horse is able to lengthen the stride. After stretching, when he is collected and in self-carriage, the strides should become shorter without disturbing the engaged movement of his back.

without the use of accessory training aids, and he can move on a big circle (20 meter) with regular, rhythmic and cadenced steps, one should attempt to ask for contact by attaching long side reins. The neck of the horse is essential for finding balance and to keep this balance. Thus the side rein should not be attached too early and never too tightly, as one will then run the risk of destroying the forward movement, building up tensions in the back and neck, and bad behavior will be preconditioned.

Following this phase the horse should be able to bend and stretch lightly to the inside as he follows the line of the circle when the side reins are attached at the same length.

Seeing that we are only addressing the first three steps of the training tree (regularity, freedom, contact), one cannot ask for true bend, due to the fact that the horse is not yet capable of straightness.

It would be a big mistake to shorten the inside rein in order to coerce the horse into the inside bend. The only thing that will happen is that the horse will progressively get more tension in his neck and lose his balance. Finding the contact through carefully directed stretching that starts from the hindquarters will be more difficult if the head is fixed to the inside.

Once the horse succeeds in finding his balance on the line of the circle, the rider should gently sit on the horse, with an independent seat, and attempt not to disturb the horse's balance. Trying to get the horse on the bit at this early stage will make any reasonable activity of the back impossible and suppress the development of impulsion and regular steps.

> **Note:** *The horse should search for the contact due to the rounding of the back on the basis of the engaged hind legs and not because the rider wants to enforce a certain shape.*

This is one of the underlying faults often repeated in the training of a horse. The horse must, in this stage of his training (perhaps even in a round pen) be able to find his balance under the rider with a freely moving neck. Once he has managed to do this, the contact is a result thereof. The horse will also discover, as long as the rider praises him every time he shows some signs of the stretching, that carrying a rider with a rounded back is much easier than with a hollow back. (Fig. 3.2)

It is assumed that the horse does not fall into muscle fatigue at this junction. For this reason, short riding bursts of ten minutes are sufficient in the beginning.

In the course of systematic training, the horse develops and strengthens the important muscles of the back, hindquarters, abdomen and neck. All of that enables the horse to carry us without difficulty.

One must never forget that a rider sits mainly on the thoracic-lumbar intersection, which has very little bony support, yet it is furnished with greater mobility. It is for this reason that this area is very susceptible to tension and osteopathic lesions and thus rendered more fragile. When the gymnastic development of the young horse is disregarded, it is not possible for the horse to show good quality in the basic gaits. This will lead, through the absence of suppleness in the horse's back, to the back being "split in two." The push from the hindquarters will break down in the middle of the thoracic vertebrae due to the hollow back. No collection will be possible under these circumstances. The rest of the impulsion will be transferred to the more or less rigid front end of the horse, and the joints and ligaments will be exposed to a reinforced burden. On account of the extra burden on the front end, the locomotive muscle chains will cause tension in the neck vertebrae and, in turn, lead to difficulty with contact and cooperation. Hence the importance of gymnastic work for horses in all age groups, for only a body that works in perfect harmony is capable of excellent athletic performance.

4. The Search for Lightness: What is "*Legerité*"?

When one compares horses in the same exercises of classical equitation from different countries, one notices that in the countries of the south (Spain, Portugal, France) the horses move with a balletic lightness in the movements of the piaffe, passage and pirouette. This is something that one seldom sees in the competition arenas of the northern regions. Nevertheless, horses perform these exercises correctly, rhythmically, balanced and with the appropriate degree of collection.

> **Definition:** *Lightness is a state of balance in which the horse becomes able to respond instantly without tension to the slightest hint of the rider's leg, seat and hand. The horse 'in position' [ramener] allows the impulsion from the hindquarters to flow through a supple and mobile back, filtered by the hand, forward to the mouth. The horse answers this impulse with a gentle, rhythmic lifting and dropping of the bits in the his mouth. All horses become equally light in the contact once they work in this state of balance, since the connection to the horse's mouth is limited to the mere weight of the leather reins.*

This type of riding, on almost loose reins in the highest degree of collection, is the result of years of preparation on the assumption of preserving the horse's charisma and character and not breaking it.

To arrive at this goal is not necessarily dependent on a certain type of horse; but rather, regulated by the systematic development of the training. Many horses are proficient in certain exercises, but are marked down in competitions because their charisma and character have been "ridden out of them." The robotic performance of exercises without mutually meaningful development for the horse, leads to mechanical competition machines but never to the creation of art.

"*Legerité*" can never be reached by force from the outside, nor by the use of training aids or strong bits. It is produced from within via mental freedom, through which the horse demonstrates his willingness to collaborate with the rider, so that his individual character can come to the fore.

In the same way, the term "*mise en main*" plays a role in this context, for it describes nothing more than the lowering and release of the rider's hand. Thereby the horse should be given the possibility to carry himself spontaneously in such a manner until the rider asks for the next exercise from him. A horse that is finely adjusted to light aids and strongly focused on the rider will cope with this request easily. Tension in the neck and back are often the result of too strong action from the hands. "*Mise en main*" relieves this back

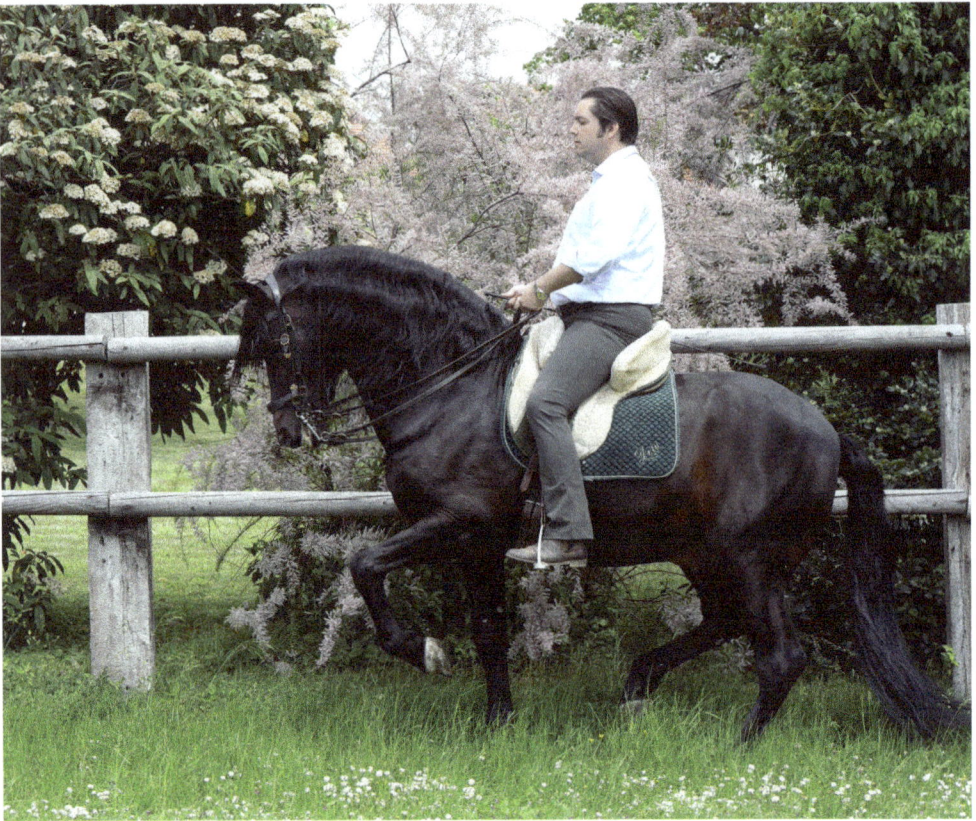

Fig. 4.1. When the balance in the piaffe is perfect, and the activity in this movement is fluid you can also try to ride the piaffe backwards. without the use of the hand—it should be done only by the rider's seat.

tension. This lightness of the hand is produced by the active hindquarters that unite the rounded topline with collection.

Note: *"Repeat often, be happy with little, praise generously."* - Étienne Beudant

[Horse Training: Outdoors and High School, *Xenophon Press 2014*]

5. Biomechanical Principles as the Foundation for Successful Training

5.1. The "Good" Horse—Anatomy, physiology and biomechanics.

In the last few centuries, the breeding of sport horses has developed in such a way that one can believe, based on the predisposition of this superior breeding product, that the systematic training of the horse becomes unnecessary. But upon closer inspection one realizes that this is a fallacy. Time and again the question is posed as to the specifications of the so-called "good" horse. A quiet, even-tempered, well-behaved horse for hacking out is possibly the best animal for the not-so-ambitious rider. The ambiguous Olympic dressage ace that certainly had the better training is of no use to this rider, as the rider's lack of experience and will not be sufficient to handle this extremely specialized animal. On the other hand, the horse with the best predisposition and movement could be extremely difficult to train as a riding horse in the absence of an appropriate work ethic, which brings us back to the question: Is this, indeed, a "good" horse? However, one invariably sees horses that have not, by nature, been endowed with talent, that have, despite incorrect conformation, become worthwhile sporting comrades mainly due to sensible training and a militant work ethic of their riders.

Nevertheless, there are fundamental biomechanical considerations as far as the functionality of the horse goes. These are already important when one examines the exterior of the horse in order to draw conclusions regarding aptitudes for collection or the possible wear and tear that seems to be an unavoidable risk in the use of the sport horse. Training a horse demands time, money and nerves of steel. In the end this should be worth everyone's (also the horse's) time. One will not easily find the "perfect" horse. Just the same, there are some conformational faults that one can live with, and others that will not make sense when one has a specific use of the horse in mind. These faults will always put the horse in some form of stress when intensive training brings him into trouble with his own faulty exterior. This does not mean that these horses cannot be stimulated within the possibilities of their individual framework. The road may be a bit longer and the degree of collection may not always be satisfactory. However, one should be responsive to the distinct uses of specific types of horses in sports.

The dressage horse should be a big, harmoniously built horse in a rectangular form, with a high neck and freedom in the jowl, in order for the horse to go "on the bit" easily. The shoulder should be long and sloped so he can develop the necessary length of stride. The back should be large enough to easily fit the saddle and end in strong loins that can permit a great degree of collection. The croup should be slightly inclined and well-muscled in order to carry more weight. The joints must be wide and powerful and the axis of the joint must preferably be as straight as possible, as every deviance from the ideal line will have an influence on the gait of the horse. The horse should be even-tempered with enough fire to develop a controlled display of power in an elegant and cadenced way. The free, ground-covering walk is the most important gait because it can easily be influenced in a negative way through bad training and can very seldom be corrected. The same applies for the basic quality of the canter.

The jumping horse should have a powerful forehand and a compact back in order to manage the landing phase. The neck should be set deep to simplify the bascule over the jump. A long, slanting shoulder will benefit the mechanics of the forehand and should be completed by a powerful, inclined croup that can be slightly higher. The canter must be ground-covering and elastic in order to execute a jump correctly.

5.1.1. The skeleton

The skeleton of the horse not only constitutes the foundation for biomechanical action, it is also an important component as a reference to the bony orientation points for physiotherapy and rehabilitation practice, as a means to locate tension and find the origin and insertion sites of the muscles.

It is only possible for a person who knows how a healthy organism moves (within an appropriate range of motion) to learn through palpation and mobilization techniques, how to rehabilitate and to help rectify incorrect or deficient patterns of movement.

The skeleton consists of 205 bones and fulfills various functions. On one hand, through its construction (skull, vertebral canal), it has the ability to protect important organs from impact from the outside. When two bones form a joint, that joint contributes to locomotion of the horse. The physical limits of any required exercise can be clearly explained by joint structure and function.

Longitudinal growth of the bones occurs in the growth plate, which is at the ends of every round bone. The longitudinal growth and accordingly the closure of the last growth plate is completed when the horse is in its fifth year. The closing of the growth plates in the distal limbs have already been completed by the time a horse is six. This factor has a big influence on the favorite idea of starting the auction horse too early. These young horses cannot show realistically developed extensions, due to the lack of adequate adaptation (finding its balance under the weight of the rider) and building of muscle without damage. By the same token, the back of the growing horse can only be expected to carry weight for a relatively short time (a few minutes), given that the untrained back muscles will tire quickly and the weight of the rider will then be carried by the spinal column alone. The outcome of this can be the progressive change in the bony structure and the development of kissing-spine-syndrome, all because the youngster was cooperative and easy to handle. (see Chapter 19.2.2) It is for a good reason that the service regulations of the cavalry school of Hanover differentiates between the younger (4-5 years) and the older green horse (5-6 years) where an order exists for the rider to dismount the horse and lead it for 5 minutes as soon as he feels any resistance due to muscle fatigue, in order to avoid the consequent damage that may occur on a mental and physical level. The same point of view can and should be taken with racehorses, as some of them are already in training as early as yearlings or as one-and-a-half-year olds. Fusion of the transverse processes of the last lumbar vertebrae is not uncommon in these cases. Stress linked fractures and arthritic appearances can appear in the inter-vertabral joints as the still growing, constantly changing bones are overtaxed by the extra burden. Thus young horse can easily be damaged.

The change in the hormone balance (deficiency of testosterone) after a stallion has been castrated induces prolonged growth in the long bones and geldings can therefore add a few centimeters to their height. Stallions that have been castrated at an older age, that already have pronounced male characteristics, do not continue their growth, but develop more settled characters and might lose some of their expression and show-off posturing.

The last growth plate that closes is the OS sacrum and the cartilaginous covers over the spinous processes of the withers. The young horse that is not muscled yet, through the course of his training will develop different, rounder muscles and wear saddles of different sizes. Once the last growth plates have closed and the shape of the wither and shoulder have been fashioned, it is of utmost importance to determine the correct size of the saddle for the horse. A badly fitting saddle can have a detrimental effect on the ability of the horse to be ridden.

The sacrum, as the bony component of the sacra-iliac joint, where the closing of the growth plate is between 5 and 6 years, gives us a time limit as to the age where one could commence with collected work without overloading or deforming the bones. Massive overloading (such as with jumping or racing) in the early years can lead to changes in these areas. Early overloading will immensely impact the movement and performance of the horse. With reference to this growth physiology, the performance requirements for stallion approval should be fundamentally reconsidered. It is exactly for this reason that the consistent progression and application of the principles of the training tree gains increased significance.

Bones are ever-changing organs and they react to marginal changes in burden (training, relaxation) by changing growth patterns. This means that inactivity for as little as fourteen days can decrease the thickness of the bone by half, and this will play a significant role in the post-operative maintenance of a convalescent patient with any kind of fracture. Therefore, it is necessary, in order to reach the resilient bone thickness in a healthy horse, that the only training methods considered should be the ones where the compaction of the bones are stimulated by the direct placing of the foot on the ground, stimulating the osteoblasts and consequently thickening the bone. Water training, like swimming, will strengthen the heart, circulation and muscles, but cannot give the bones adequate stimulation, and the stronger muscles then outmatch the weaker bone structure and spontaneous fractures can occur more easily, compared with horses that are trained in the more conventional way.

The condition of the footing must also not be too deep, (more than 10cm = 3.9 inches). Deep footing allows extra sinking of the fetlock causing the ligamental and suspensory apparatus to be overtaxed. Positive proof of overtaxing young horses causes the formation of wind galls. These horses may not actually go lame or develop a change in their gaits, but can show a build-up of liquid in the area of their fetlocks and in the bursae of the flexor tendons; this might be decreased by prompt and adequate cooling and bandaging directly after training. Hard footing that is not springy does not absorb shock, causes each step to be absorbed by the delicate cartilage of the joints. The perfect type of floor would be a 5-6 centimeter deep (2-2.4 inch) mix of sawdust and beach sand, that has enough grip and give at the same time. This is especially critical for young horses that have conformation problems that are not corrected, considering that the rate of loading changes with increasing hoof length. It is for this reason that regular trimming of the hooves (6-7 weeks apart) is of vital importance.

Cartilage, like bone, reacts to training and must also adapt. The latest research from New Zealand has shown that the production of synovial tissue and the development of cartilage in foals was most favorable when the foals were allowed to roam free in paddocks with their mothers, as opposed to the control group that was intensely trained or kept in stables. The latter group revealed massive shortcomings in the formation of cartilage and the quality of the synovial tissue. This research led to the conclusion that the initial training of an undeveloped individual should be properly regulated and well-considered in order to allow the young horse a good start in his sports career instead of ruining his chances through excessive demands made early on. It was for this reason that the old masters of the classical art (de Pluvinel, de la Guérinière) only started to ride young horses at the age of five years.

By the same reasoning, the excessive demands of over-training a growing, and not-yet-sufficiently resilient organism can manifest itself as "bucked shins," an increase in the thickness of the bones as a result of micro fissures on the dorsal side of the cannon bones that can lead to lameness. This is often seen in young racehorses in intensive training. Micro fractures are seen just as often at the site of origin of the suspensory ligament in the course of over-training, especially polo horses and jumpers where the extremely powerful, fleeting moment of loading and torque with full body weight can lead to tears in the cannon bone and subsequent calcification, which will, in turn, affect the suspensory ligament.

Owing to this biological responsiveness, it remains the endeavor of the bones to build a structure as strong as possible through the use of pressure and pulling influences, but, on a structure that is not too massive and therefore too heavy to carry. In the same breath, one should not feed the young horse too much either. Apart from the danger of laminitis, which the baroque type horse shows a tendency towards, it can also lead to the formation of chips. The disparity between the applied load and the loading capacity of the cartilage leads to localized malnutrition and subsequent detachment of the damaged fragment of the cartilage, which, depending on the location and the size of the chip, can influence the functional course of the movement in many different ways.

Sufficient allowance for movement (spacious paddocks with uneven terrain and slopes) is therefore essential for optimal development of the cartilage and bone development of the young horse. This will inevitably have a positive influence on the sporting demands and longevity of the horse. The different surfaces that the young horse walks on and the resulting improved proprioception can, on the one hand, be employed in the adaptation phase of training, and on the other hand, during the recovery in the process of rehabilitation.

5.1.2. Muscles, tendons and ligaments.

The muscles, tendons and ligaments are of primary importance to movement, given that the tendons and ligaments keep the skeleton together and the muscles move the skeleton.

A horse has 504 muscles, but here, we will limit ourselves to those which are important for us and especially to the superficial layer that we can palpate and those which we can influence with therapeutic and rehabilitative riding procedures. (Ill. 5.1)

Deeper muscles will only be dealt with when it is necessary for better understanding the biomechanics of movement.

Types of muscles

There are three basic types of muscles:
- smooth muscle
- striped or skeletal muscle
- heart muscle

Smooth muscles, that are predominantly found in the intestines and blood vessels, have slow, involuntary contractions in order to function most favorably at rest and sleep periods and during digestion etc. They are influenced by the autonomic nervous system. Stress due to the lack of physical and psychological relaxation will often lead to gastritis, ulcers and colic; whereas a calm working atmosphere seems to be essential to induce the best possible results in the training, and to protect the horse from performance difficulties.

The striped or skeletal muscles are under voluntary control and are responsible for sudden energetic action (flight, jumping over jumps). They have the highest activity and need the most energy in the form of adenosine triphosphate (ATP) and oxygen. In order to reach full utilization of their powers, these muscles must have the ability to relax to their maximum capacity and then contract to their maximum capacity. The foundation for physiologically training a quiet, rhythmically forward moving horse depends on incorporating short and regular periods of rest. The horse must be able to arrive at an internal state of calm in order to allow complete relaxation of his muscles, through which the muscles can be most favorably supplied with energy and oxygen to aid in their development. The contraction of the muscle will pump lactic acid and waste products out of the muscle and the relaxation will allow the necessary supply of nutrients to flow in.

A horse that is under mental stress, whose body is already in a higher state of muscle tension, cannot achieve effective use of his muscles since continually tense muscles can only insufficiently generate success in this biological feat. The delayed removal of lactic acid will first induce hyper-acidity in the muscle, that will lead to vaso-constriction and local malnutrition as a consequence. It is for this reason that a relaxed trot, where the neck is deep and stretched, is highly recommended at the end of the training session as this will ensure that the session for the next day will commence in a relaxed manner and the supple horse can, with this method, only be improved upon. If this is neglected, tension in the neck and back of the horse can prolong the warming up phase substantially. Repeated short repetitions followed by short periods of rest are the most efficient way to stimulate the growth of muscles. The development of muscles will, with regular and systematic daily training, take about three months. In order to maintain the muscles, four working sessions a week or light work on the lunge or riding out is adequate. Exercises that the horse already knows should be required as a warm-up or as a preservation of elastic ability and not repeated dozens of times as; besides being tiring and boring, they are of no further use in the horse's training. Over-repetition will merely provoke wear and tear of the joints plus a negative attitude towards the work.

It is of great importance to do at least 10 minutes of walk as a warm-up as muscles need to be warm before demands can be made on them. First, this operating efficiency is enhanced by the distribution of synovial fluid in the joints and secondly, by the stimulation of the circulatory system to transport more oxygen and blood to the muscles.

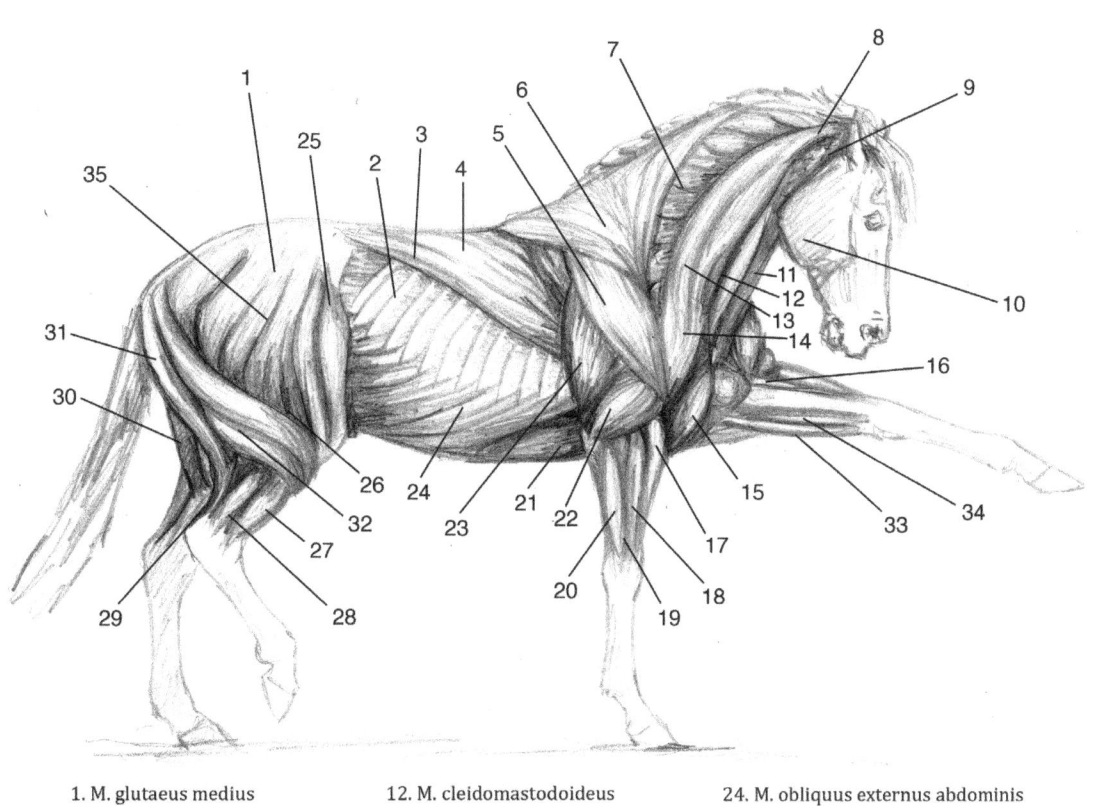

1. M. glutaeus medius
2. Mm. intercostales externi
3. M. serratus dorsalis caudalis
4. M. latissimus dorsi
5. M. deltoideus
6. M. trapezius
7. M. splenius
8. Sehne des M. longissimus capitis
9. Glandula parotis
10. M. masseter
11. M. sternomandibularis
12. M. cleidomastodoideus
13. M. omotransversarius
14. M. cleidobrachialis
15. M. pectoralis descendens
16. M. biceps brachii
17. M. extensor carpi radialis
18. M. extensor digitais communis
19. M. extensor digitalis lateralis
20. M. extensor carpi ulnaris
21. M. pectoralis profundus
22. Caput laterale
23. Caput longum
24. M. obliquus externus abdominis
25. M. tensor fasciae latae
26. M. quadriceps femoris
27. M. extensor digitalis longus
28. M. extensor digitalis lateralis
29. M. gastrocnemius
30. M. semimembranosus
31. M. semitendinosus
32. M. biceps femoris
33. M. flexor carpi ulnaris
34. M. flexor carpi radialis
35. M. glutaeus superficialis

Fig. 5.1 The superficial, palpable muscles of the horse (12 + 14 are also collectively known as M. brachiocephalicus).

Muscles can be further sub-divided into "slow twitch" muscle fibers and "fast twitch" muscle fibers, where the first kind, based on its slow contractile ability and longer working period, functions with successful oxygen utilization but cannot function for long without oxygen supply. This type of fiber is typically found in long distance horses.

Fast twitch muscle fibers are then differentiated between high and low oxidative fibers. Due to their higher myoglobin[1] content, high oxidative fibers can absorb increased amounts of oxygen and are responsible for powerful, sustained performance. These fibers are often found in three-day-eventers, who need power, stamina and speed.

Slow oxidative fibers have less myoglobin, therefore have a whiter appearance and are predestined for fast energy release; for example, in quarterhorses (the fastest horses at a quarter mile) and racehorses. They can rapidly generate high performance, but are not capable of sustaining this kind of performance over the long run.

Interestingly, with appropriate training measures, it is possible to change a fast twitch fiber into a slow twitch fiber, but not the other way round. This means that a sprinter can become a good marathon runner, but not vice versa, as the genetic disposition is responsible for that predisposition.

Every muscle consists of a belly that has an inherent collective ability to contract that takes place in the biggest part of the muscle where the greatest blood circulation is. It is for this reason that one should decide which line of work the horse should eventually pursue when his training has been concluded or even before starting his training, if, only by virtue of the particular specifics of the breed with regard to conformation and restrictions in training circumstances and through the particular response of specific groups of muscles, to be more subjected to power or endurance training.

The origins [ends] of the muscles [or tendons] are always of a sinewy nature; only 4% of their length is expandable and they are poorly supplied with blood. Because of this, tendons have a much higher susceptibility to injury and a relatively drawn-out recovery period. Therefore, when a muscle becomes tired, damage to the tendons can be induced on the grounds of lost elasticity.

In order to function properly, every muscle needs an opponent (antagonist) without which the movement would be impossible.
The most important connective tissues of the axial skeleton are the nuchal and supra-spinous ligament and the Linea alba, as they form the upper and lower support for the skeletal framework.

---

1 A single-chain, iron-containing protein found in muscle fibers, structurally similar to a single subunit of hemoglobin and having a higher affinity for oxygen than the hemoglobin of the blood.

Before we move on to the individual "perfect" body parts, one should always be sure which discipline of riding one wishes to participate in when choosing a horse. Specific breed characteristics, and with it, specific conformational differences will determine the relevant use of the horse during its training. A large German warm-blood with a rectangular form and extravagant movement will experience as much difficulty in a reining competition as a Haflinger would in an eventing competition for big horses. Baroque horses are, on the grounds of their square dimensions, less adapted for jumping, and the compact, croup-high Quarter Horse are not really adapted for so-called classical collection. All of these points should be considered beforehand, given that the anatomical limitations and therefore the athletic use is preprogrammed to a certain degree. Faulty and less than ideal body parts can indeed be improved upon with correct and patient training, but the shortcoming can never be eliminated completely.

Subsequently, we will shed light on the relevant biomechanical connections in order to better understand the implications of schooling.

Head and neck region

The skull of the horse is made up of various flat bones; together with other bones they form part of the cranial cavity and eye sockets. The fissures ossify as the horse becomes older and are of particular importance in cranial-sacral osteopathy, as the mobilization of these "blocked" elements (skull bones) can have a positive influence on the whole organism.

The upper jaw can be felt on both sides by the prominent ridges of the facial crest, where the masseter muscle has its origin. The masseter muscle is the largest muscle for chewing, but is also of great importance to riding since tension and contact problems can always be conspicuously felt along the facial crest as trigger points and are often sensitive to pressure.

***In practice:** Distinct contraction of the chewing muscle is visible when a horse suffers from mental stress due to excessive demands or great bodily effort. The fibers of the masseter muscle become visible, the horse starts to nervously rattle his incisor teeth, provided that this is possible and the horse does not wear a nose-band that is too tight that causes even more stress. When the masseter muscle is tense, it will simultaneously lead to constricted mobility in the temporal-mandibler joint. One always aspires to an elastic and slightly open temporal-mandibular joint in riding, otherwise the rein aids cannot travel through the body of the horse and arrive at the corresponding hind leg. One can often palpate a trigger point under this joint that is characterized by pain and is an unmistakable sign of tension in the horse. This limited chewing activity will result in producing less saliva and the stress resistance comes in the form of* "escaping behind the bit." This will, in turn, tighten the M. brachiocephalicus, the muscles of the hyoid bone, the hyoid bone itself. In turn, the movement possible with regard to extending the front legs will be severely restrained. Grinding of the teeth is also a form of coping with stress for the horse, brought about by tension in the M. masseter and will cause a deduction of marks in a dressage test.

Note: The mouthpiece of a broken snaffle should not protrude more than 0.5cm on each side of the mouth, as it will then pinch the lips and bars of the mouth.

Just a little caudal-dorsal, on both sides there is a depression made up of the zygomatic and the mandibular arch. Often overlooked—but very important for riding—the temporal-mandibular joint is located here. Although a very small, this joint has a huge impact on the rest of the organism.

Baucher already stated that the temporal-mandibular joint constitutes the key to the horse. This means that all the efforts of the rider will be of no avail when there is tension in the horse. T.M.J. is the first sign that the horse becomes heavy in the hand or starts to lean on the bit, twists his head or does not accept the rein aids anymore. This is the result of lacking calmness together with inadequate activity of the hindquarters, where the haunches do not engage but only develop propulsive force. It is a fact that a well-trained horse that is supple will transfer forward impulsion evenly and in a straight line from the hindquarters via the sacra-iliac joint onto the vertebrae, where it will flow over the atlanto-occpital junction across the temporal-mandibular joint onto the bit. Visible signs of powerfully active hindquarters with correct contact and relative elevation is a horse that foams when he chews the bit, a contented expression, ears that point slightly backward attentive to the rider, and a desire to stretch forward onto the bit. The mastication is prompted by the parasympathetic nervous system when the horse is relaxed and can only take place when the temporal-mandibular joint is freely mobile and the root of the tongue and the hyoid muscles are relaxed. Even horses that are ridden bit-less have the ability to achieve this foam formation in the mouth although there is no impulse from a bit that can animate the horse to chew.

The lower jaw is formed by two branches of the mandibular bone that meet in the middle.

The so-called diastema is the space between the canine teeth and the first premolar and is a tooth free area. On average, the space between the two branches of the mandible in this area is about 4 centimeters. This anatomical particularity was compiled in the veterinary faculty of the University of Hanover in the course of research and puts a new facet on the width of bits. According to these findings, most of the 14.5 centimeter bits were too big, even for big warmbloods.

When one examines a skull in cross section, one easily becomes aware that there is actually no more space left for an additional bit in the horse's mouth when the anatomical structures are taken into consideration (tongue, bars of the mouth, lips, roof of the mouth, bones). Every kind of bit can only come into operation when more or reduced pressure is exerted on the tongue, because this takes up most of the space in the diastema. This, then puts the term "mouth-friendly" bits into a different perspective. Furthermore this condition should make allowance for the effect that the nose-band must *never* be fastened too tight, so the horse can at least open his mouth slightly when the pressure on the tongue becomes too great.

By the same token, this anatomical specification should be considered for allowing room for the tongue when a curb bit is chosen, as this bit can easily pinch or bruise the tongue when the space is too big or too small. If the room for the tongue is too big, the mouthpiece is too unstable in the mouth and the lower arch can pinch the sensitive side of the tongue against the bars of the mouth and this can cause defensive reactions against the pain. The horse can tilt and/or start to shake his head.

In the same way, too little room for the tongue can cause pain on the middle of the tongue and then lead to tongue problems. The branches of the lower jaw are lined with a thin mucous membrane and affords the space for the bit. This forms an essential foundation for the choice of a bit for both the riding and driving horse, together with the width of the bit, the thickness of the tongue and the height of the roof of the mouth.

The palate, or roof of the mouth, can similarly be of importance in the choice of a bit, especially when a horse has a palate condition caused by weak connective tissue that forms a "suspended" palate. This means the roof of the mouth does not form an arch in the dorsal direction. But rather, the soft palate hangs down into the mouth cavity. If the palate is filled with blood, this will cause contact difficulties as it is unpleasant for horses to seek contact with the bit. In these cases, surgery is the only solution where a slit incision can successfully accomplish the draining of the accumulated liquid. The border of the wound can be sprinkled with salt which causes he mucous membrane not to seal too soon and the effect of the operation would last longer. The horse can be bridled as usual a few days later.

A horse with thin lips and thin, sharp bars of the mouth can be provided with a thicker, softer bit than a horse with more fleshy bars.

More important than the choice of the individual bit for every horse, is the lightness of the contact on the reins and the correct training of the back, for this will make the horse light and pleasant in the hand by his own choice.

The teeth

The upper and lower jaw both have 6 incisors, 2 canines (often only in male horses), 6 premolars and 6 molars. Sometimes one will find an atavistic tooth, the so-called wolf tooth, in the upper jaw, just in front of the first premolar and this will often cause problems in the search for the correct bit. It is for this reason that wolf teeth should be extracted in all horses as a matter of routine, as this little rudimentary tooth can complicate the shaping of the "bit seat," where the first premolar is rounded at a slanting angle in both the top and the lower jaw. Time and again these "bit seats" are the reason for controversial professional discussion. Many horses take a better contact when the premolar has been prepared in this way. Wolf teeth seem to disturb, as they are pressed against the bit when the reins are taken. These little teeth are embedded only in the mucous membrane and have limited movement possibilities and can therefore lead to unpleasant sensations of pain, where horses shake their heads, hold on to the bit or refuse to be bridled. When these contact difficulties are caused by wolf teeth. They immediately disappear after the extraction of the teeth and the horse can work again after a few days.

Hooks on teeth can also bring about massive complications in contact and acceptance of the bit. These hooks on the teeth can be sharp as razors, and a nose-band (drop or flash type) adjusted too tightly, in combination with the impact of the bit, can bring about painful mucous injuries that can eventually lead to ulcers.

> **Note:** *It is necessary to have regular, annual checks from a dentist to correct the flaws in the teeth.*

The horse starts to shed his milk teeth at 2.5 years and all permanent teeth are in at 4.5 years. It is especially important to inspect the young horse's teeth regularly as the grounds for resistance can often be found in the mouth when the horse goes through painful stages in shedding the teeth. These kinds of problems are predictable and the thinking trainer will be able to interpret the reactions of his horses.

Painful processes in the mouth create tension in the poll and thus have repercussions through the whole back of the horse including the hindquarters. Elasticity, relaxation and cooperation will suffer as a result. Misinterpreted resistances can generally lead to avoidable conflicts. The horse suffers enormous loss of confidence as he cannot deliver a good performance when he has pain. The old saying: "every resistance has a cause" is valid in this case.

The poll

The old masters of the classical schools already knew the importance of a free moving poll and devoted a fair amount of time to keeping it so.

When one touches the horse behind the ears and along in the direction of the tail, one will feel the external occipital protuberances and directly thereafter the foramen magnum and the wings of the atlas (fig. 5.2.)

These anatomical giants are of vital importance to the riding horse, as the nuchal ligament inserts on the occipital protuberance and just after this insertion, there is an important bursae over the body of the atlas that will serve as a sliding support. Inflammation or bruising of these bursae will often induce great difficulty to relax in the poll and problems with the contact, given that there are also crucial neural outlets in this area, which is why too tight browbands or pressure forming poll pieces can have accordingly painful implications. These can cause "head shaker syndrome." The lateral muscles, such as the M. splenius, M. rectuscapitis are significantly involved in the sideways stabilization and rotation of the poll. Muscle inflammation due to abrupt backwards pulling, getting caught on the head collar or alternatively hitting the head on the frame of the window can also lead to difficulty in getting the horse to relax in the poll. In these cases, horses will tend to twist their heads and the nose will point away from the painful side. Local triggers and defense reactions when putting the bridle on or on palpation, are common indications of problems in this area.

When a horse is selected for the sport of dressage, the degree with which the horse is prepared to accept the aids and to relax the jaw is very important as it is precisely in this riding discipline where the outward show is fundamental. The atlas, due to its shape, is essentially responsible for the release of the poll. Osteopathic injuries in this area will regularly give rise to twisting of the head or difficulty in flexing the poll to one side. The distance between the wing of the atlas and the jowl should be at least 2 fingers wide, otherwise difficulty in relaxing the jaw can be experienced, as the parotid gland, that lies in this area, can be bruised and this pain can lead to resistance. Horses with short, thick necks and heavy polls are not very suited as dressage horses as stretching onto the bit will always be more difficult for them. On the other hand, too long and thin necks or swan necks are equally unsuitable due to their lack of stability. These horses will time and again show the tendency to evade an even contact by the snake-like twisting of their necks. What is more, these horses are inclined to be over bent and go behind the bit, which makes it more difficult to maneuver them. Correcting this defect can only be attempted by vigorous forward riding, where the first 4 levels of the scales of training are of primary importance, so that the horse can be ridden from the back onto the bit and develop stability in this manner.

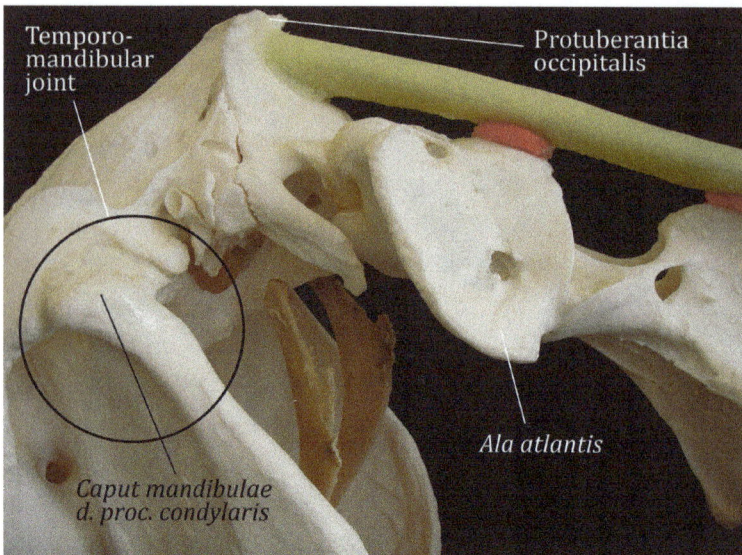

Fig.5.2 The bony landmarks in the poll area are the protuberantia occipitalis and the atlae atlantis (wings of the atlas)

By the same token, in the use of a too heavy hand (up to more than 50 kg/hand), there will be immense pressure on this sensitive area, on account of the length of the horse's head (lever action of 40cm). The improper use of running reins can cause pressure peaks of up to 1000kg on this area. Problems with the origin of the ligament, calcification and bursitis can all be the painful results of improper demands made in this region.

The cervical spine

The cervical spine consists of seven linked bones in the form of an "S" that can be felt in the center of the horse's neck. Ideally the neck of the horse should be set well on the trunk, whereby it yields a good dorsal quadrant curvature (fig.5.3). When a horse has a well-proportioned neck, the changeover from the upper curve into the lower curve of the "S" should take place in an almost perpendicular fourth vertebrae. This will guarantee that the horse can achieve adequate elevation which is very important for the freedom of the shoulder and the action of the forehand.

The spinous process of the axis can be felt in very thin horses. This is also the point of origin for many neck muscles as well as the nuchal lamina.

The remaining five neck vertebrae are relatively uniform and from the outside there are only few differences to be seen. They all have a body and short spinous and transverse processes and are connected with each other through multiple joints (Fig.5.4)

Between every neck vertebra, in the foramen intvertebrate, lies a nerve and, in the case of a blockage, this can cause some constriction in the movement or even ataxia. Positioning and bending difficulties can result from tension in this area and can lead to so-called bridle lameness. In the changeover from the neck to the thoracic vertebrae one also finds the brachial plexus next to the first rib, and this can be aggravated in the event of tension of the M. scaleni and brachiocephalici. When the horse has a fall that causes an osteopathic lesion of the first rib, this sensitive nervous plexus can be irritated in such a manner that every attempt to bend can jar the neck. A break in the rhythm of the trot can occur, but this is not apparent when the horse is moving freely without a rider. An insensitive and unsteady hand can cause massive faults in the rhythm that becomes even more evident when any lengthening of stride is required. Shortened walk steps, bobbing of the head and other balance adjustments are often the result of the rider not having an independent seat, where the rider attempts to balance himself by holding on to the reins.

The actual position of the neck comes from a lateral flexion with mild outside rotation of the rest of the neck vertebrae and not owing to the bend asked in the jowl through the atlas or axis.

The cervical spine is the most mobile part of the spinal column as there is no lateral restriction (e.g. ribs).The neck is furthermore of great importance in maintaining balance and is typically used by the young horse who lacks co-ordination skills, as a "fifth leg" when he tries to reconcile his balance with that of the rider. This balancing pole function can successfully be used with young horses to round their backs and thus carry the weight of the rider with greater ease. The biomechanical function of the nuchal ligament plays a fundamental role in this. This elastic ligament has an important stabilizing function: on one hand, the horse is able to keep his head in the horizontal position without muscular strength. When the horse drops his head, the development of pull on this ligament goes by way of the spinous processes up to the middle of the lumbar vertebrae. Through this action, the lower neck muscles (M. brachiocephalicus, M. sternocleidomastoideus, M. sternohyoideus) relax and the topline, with the M. trapezius, M. serratus cervicis, M. semispinalis and the M. longissimus cervicis and M. splenius, rhythmically contracts and relaxes. This process is of prime importance for finding and achieving contact, for this is the only way the horse can use his back correctly, freely and rhythmically.

As a flight animal, a horse always has the tendency to quickly lift his head in dangerous situations, if for no other reason but to get a better view. This lifting of the head will simultaneously contract the M. longissimus and the M. iliocostalis in order to achieve adequate stability in the breast vertebra should a sudden sprint be needed in the flight sequence. The trainer of young horses therefore still must deal with this primary instinct when he starts his horses, since they will, due to lack of strength, first arch their backs and then hollow their backs as they get tired. This will, in turn, inevitably lead to bracing and shortening of the back. If this continues, the horse will never be able to build his back muscles, as he will always only try to protect the spine. When

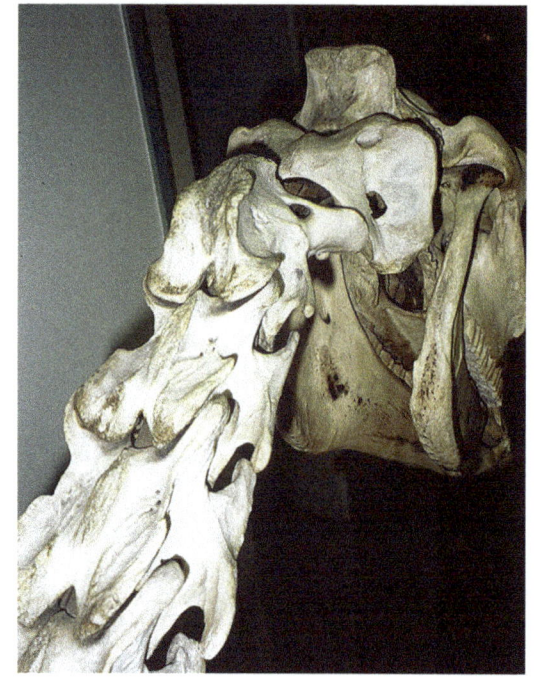

Fig.5.3 The neck vertebrae from the rider's viewpoint. Notice the distance between the mandible and the wing of the atlas (important for getting the horse on the bit) as well as the position of the multiple joints of each particular vertebra.

the horse lifts his head too high, he will only push out the lower neck, the M. brachiocephalicus, in a cranial direction and this will tire the muscle and it will start to tighten. If the horse is worked in this manner for a longer period of time, it will cause hypertrophy of the muscle (fig.5.5). Given that this muscle constitutes a connection between the poll and the forearm, it becomes clear that all kinds of tension in this area will greatly influence the forward strides and with it, extension of the front legs. These horses are not able to keep an even, rhythmic and sweeping gait, but rather are inclined to prance with shortened, tight steps. These horses often look as if they have been split in two. Trigger points in the poll and shoulder joints can frequently be found in such horses. Trust in the rider's hand and methodical forward and down riding is indispensable to correcting this grave fault.

Horses tend to be heavier in the front due to the weight of the head and neck, the only exception being in the levade, when the entire body weight is on both hind legs for a short period of time. The weight of the horse is distributed as follows: 55% on the forehand and 45% on the hindquarters.

Nevertheless, one aspires to improve the collection capability by increasingly moving the center of gravity towards the hindquarters with progressive training. That is to say, the more the hind legs can step under the body, the more the upper body appears to be arching upwards, at the same time the neck is carried higher and in a more proud manner, making the horse seem shorter. The center of gravity appears to be displaced more towards the hindquarters, all because of the higher head and neck position. (Fig. 5.6)

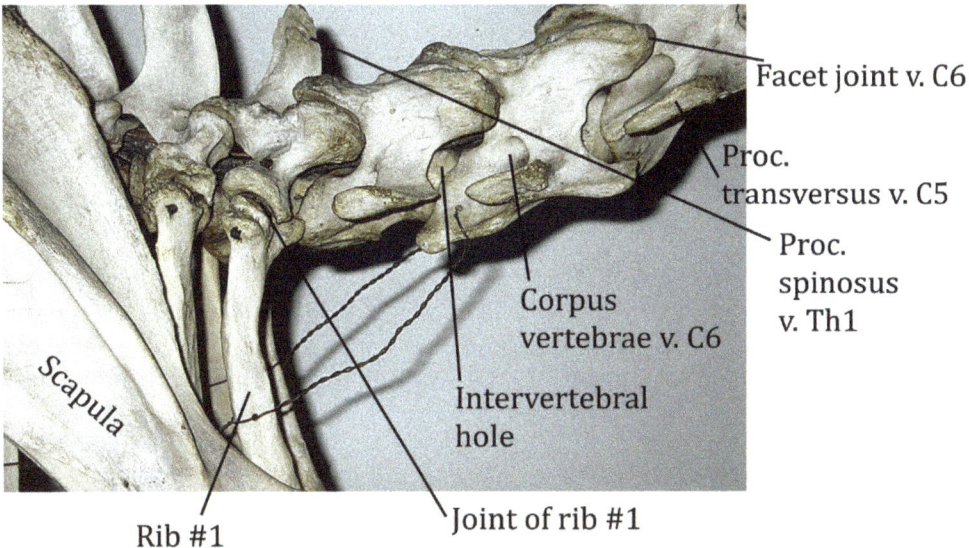

Fig:5.4 The cervicothoracic intersection, due to its anatomical and biomechanic situation, is prone to osteopathic lesions, followed by problems with bending and the quality of the horse that makes him cooperative and easy to handle.

Secondary to the atlas, the axis constitutes an essential foundation for getting the horse on the bit and in a certain position. It is possible for the horse to perform rotational movements by means of the dens axis. Turning and positioning of the head is made possible through this area.

Riding in position[2] will be discussed in detail in Chapter 10.5, as it describes the background for straightening the horse. The slight sideways deviation of the horse's neck from the mid-line, where the rider can only see the glint of the horse's inside eye, is described as "position." This preliminary stage of straightening the horse is only possible when all parts of the neck vertebrae, including the neck muscles on the outside, in particular the M. brachiocephalicus, M. spinalis and the M. longus cervicis are relaxed, making it possible for the hollow side to contract. The horse will then, in combination with the inside leg, stretch into the regulating and rhythm-transmitting outside rein. At this point, the poll should be the highest point.

The demand to see the poll as the highest point, is often not possible in strongly developed stallion necks, especially in the baroque breeds, due to morphological grounds, even if the horse works in the correct position of collection. In this context it is much more important to have an overall picture of the suppleness and the ability to be ridden with the animal in question, rather than to focus only on the neck. Every horse is able to reach a certain degree of elevation, given his

2   *In Stellung*

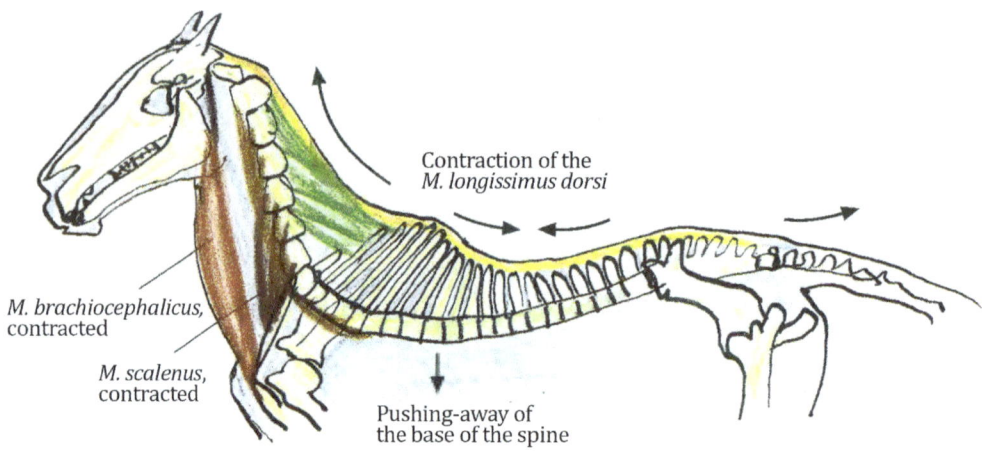

Fig. 5.5 a. Hypertrophy of the M. brachiocephalicus—Schematic diagram

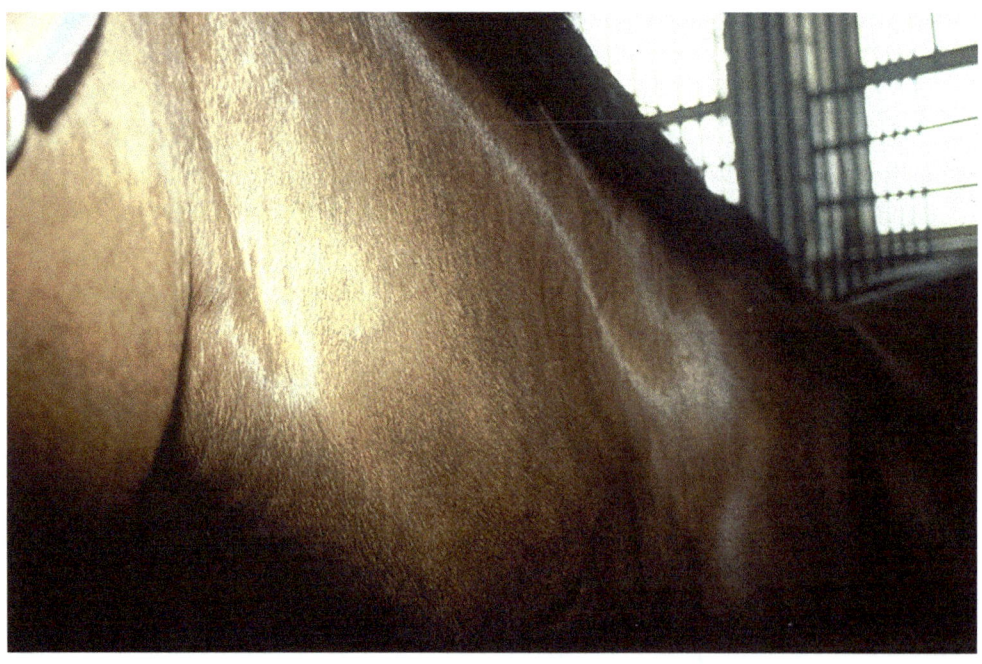

Fig. 5.5 b. Hypertrophy of the M. brachiocephalicus—Formation of a muscular lower neck

anatomy and after passing through the training scale and working efficiently within his body's capabilities. Horses with thick necks and too narrow jowels will by reason of their, non-rectifiable problem of lack of space between the lower jaw and the atlas—never fit this bill and the trainer must just accept this.

However, this does not mean that the broken neck due to too strong a hand should be seen as correct. This is where the horse with ample space between the jaw and the atlas has the third neck vertebra higher than the poll. This faulty method of training shows a clear deficit of suppleness because a horse that is so far behind the bit is incapable of understanding the aids and will, as a result, be less manageable. Consistent forward and down riding with a soft and agreeable hand is the only possibility to correct this fault.

When one is unsure if this fault is caused by incorrect riding or by anatomical problems, the best way to test it is to advance both hands forward at the same time. When the horse stays in the same rhythm and seeks contact in a deeper position, one can assume that the horse has been worked as defined by the training scale and that the position does not originate from the influence of the rider's hand.

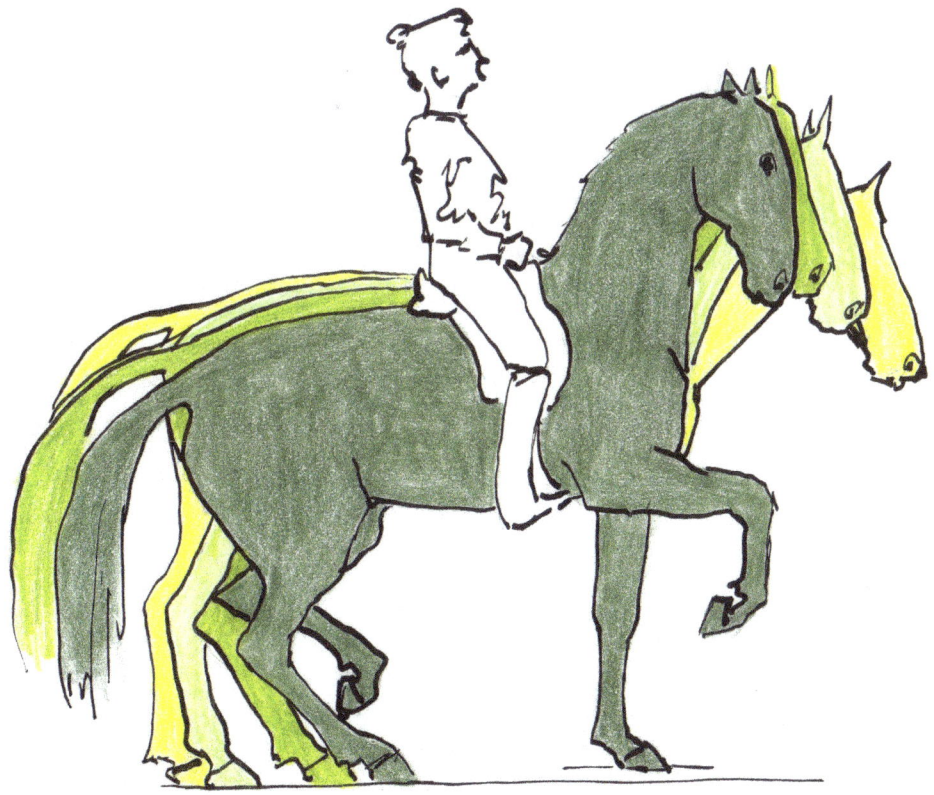

Fig.5.6. A collected horse steps under his body more with the hind legs, displacing his center of gravity backwards and frees the forehand, thus follows an arching of the topline and increased elevation.

The muscles of specific regions will subsequently be dealt with according to the origin (O), insertion (I), function (F) and characteristic (C)

The neck muscles

M. splenius
O: T3-T5 and the nuchal ligament
I: The first part on the occiput and C1, the second part C3-C5
F: Elevates, stretching and sideways tilt of the head and neck

M. scalenus
O: First rib
I: Transverse process of C4-C7
F: With bilateral contraction it flexes the neck, aids in inspiration, sideways movement of the neck

M. semispinalis capitis
O: Fascia spinocostotransversalis, C2-C7 and T3-T7
I: External occipital protuberance
C. Is directly next to the nuchal laminae
F: Elevates, sideways tilt of the head and neck, extends neck

M. brahiocephalicus
O: Crest of the humerus
I: Mastoid process
C: Made up of 3 muscles, the most important muscle under the neck, very obvious in incorrectly worked horses where there is no action in the back, often very tense and sensitive to pressure in the proximal and distal section.
F: Moves forelimb, inclines head & neck when limb is fixed, extends shoulder

M. longissimus cervicis
O: Transverse process of T1-T2, C2-C7
I: Mastoid process and C1
F: Elevates and flexes the head and neck section, extends the neck

M. serratus ventralis cervicis
O: C4-C7
I: Scapular cartilage
C: Together with the M. serratus ventralis thoracis, it is the most important connection between the front limbs and the body
F: Elevates the neck when the limb is fixed

The nuchal ligament

Definition: *The nuchal ligament includes the laminar portion and the funicular portion, and the supraspinous ligament.*

The funicular portion begins at the occipital crest and extends over the spinous processes of the thoracic and lumbar vertebrae in a caudal direction and subsequently inserts on the sacrum as the supraspinous ligament. The laminar portion is found deep in the neck and is not palpable, the origin being on the dorsal surfaces of C2-C7 and inserts on the spinous processes of T3-T5 (Fig.5.7)

The function of the nuchal ligament enables the horse to have his neck in an almost horizontal position without particular effort on the part of the muscles. It is the upper elastic opponent of the Linea alba that runs ventral and medial between the breastbone and the pubic bone.

When the back muscles are shortened, the reflex will be a shortening of the nuchal ligament as well, bringing the spinous processes closer to each other and makes it very difficult for the horse to round his back.

Many horses with back problems have a thickening of the supraspinous ligament as a reaction to excessive pressure from saddles and harnesses.

Directly behind the occiput and on top of the atlas, one finds a bursa that can provoke restriction in the movement when it is thickened through pathological circumstances. (fig.5.8) One also finds a bursa in the area of the withers, that can be damaged when a saddle or harness does not fit properly.

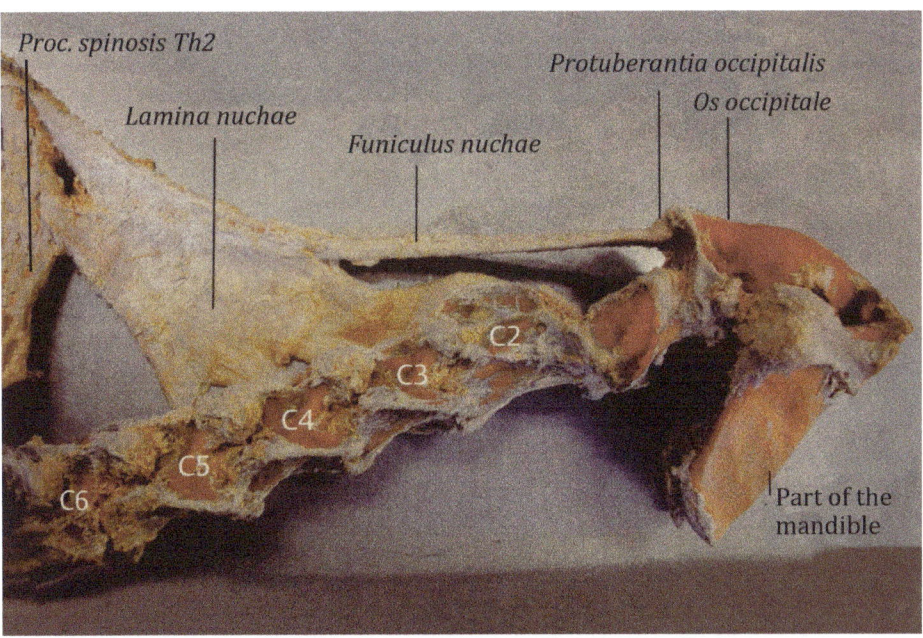

Fig 5.7. Nuchal ligament, made up of a funicular portion and a laminar portion. The funicular portion originates at the occipital protuberance and runs to the spinous processes of T3 or T4. In the caudal third it fuses with the laminar portion, that originates at the spinous processes of C2-C7.

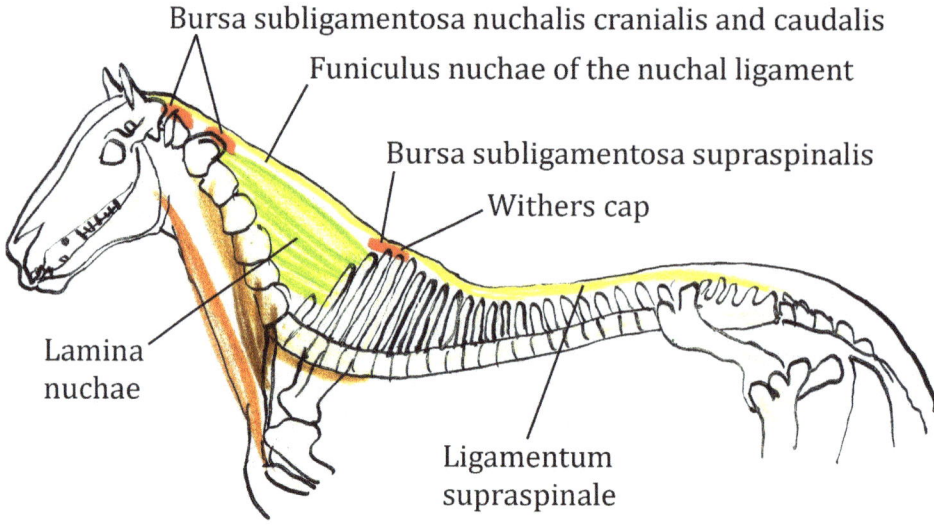

Fig.5.8. Diagram of the nuchal ligament with the bursae

The inter-vertebral ligament can be found between the spinal processes. It is arranged in such a way as to allow all movement in the spinal cord without constriction.

The Back—thoracic vertebrae, lumbar vertebrae and thorax

The spinal column builds the bridge-like connection between the "pillars" of the front limbs and the hind limbs, in which the action of the intestines can cause a downwards pull of up to 280 kg in a horse of about 480kg.

Spinal nerves exit between each vertebra at the foramen intervertebralia and corresponds with organs and muscles. It is for this reason that osteopathic lesions have a direct implication on the surrounding muscles, where the muscles can out of reflex tense up and cause flexion and collection problems. The horses tense up unilaterally, do not want to step under their bodies. They lose contact, which is why they appear to be heavy in the rider's hand.

The spinal nerves also provide the morphological substrate of the Shu-points of acupuncture and with it the foundation for neuro-vegetative reflexes. (See Chapter 7.17)

In riding, the back of the horse takes center stage, not only because it carries the rider, but in the course of the reaction from the horse, it serves as a corridor for transmission of information. The forward impulsion from the hind legs directly and uniformly gets carried on to the back, and a correctly working back will then convey a pleasant feeling to sit on for the rider. Training deficiencies, for example, in horses that are difficult to sit and especially horses that bounce the rider out of the saddle in the extended trot, become obvious. In these cases, it is best to work on rhythm and relaxation before higher lessons are attempted.

The thoracic spinal cord is made up of 18 thoracic vertebrae that are endowed with articular processes to join the ribs. The first eight ribs are directly connected to the sternum and from a biomechanical point of view have a considerably static function and form the perfect position for the girth, about one hand's width behind the elbow. The first nine thoracic vertebrae form the anatomically known withers, can be up to 30cm long in a fully grown warm-blood horse and are aligned to point caudally (fig.5.9).

The spinous processes of the first nine thoracic vertebrae are so long that the nuchal ligament can be put under tension by this long lever when the horse lowers his head to graze and have an antagonistic counteraction on the pull of gravity.

The subsequent thoracic vertebrae have shorter spinous processes, where they point caudal up to T15, then change direction and have a more cranial direction. This area creates the basis for the position of the saddle and includes the first and respectively second lumbar vertebra. This area is incorrectly looked upon as *the* back by lay persons. The alignment of the thoracic spinous processes in a caudal direction, the lumbar spinous processes in a cranial direction and then the caudal direction of the sacrum, is purely for static reasons. By means of the first two directions, the supraspinous ligament will execute a pull on the nuchal ligament as it extends when drawn down and pull the spinous processes forward. The outcome is that the wither gets raised, which allows all of the ventral neck muscles to relax. The maximum raise in the thoracic area can be found approximately in the middle of the saddle area. The

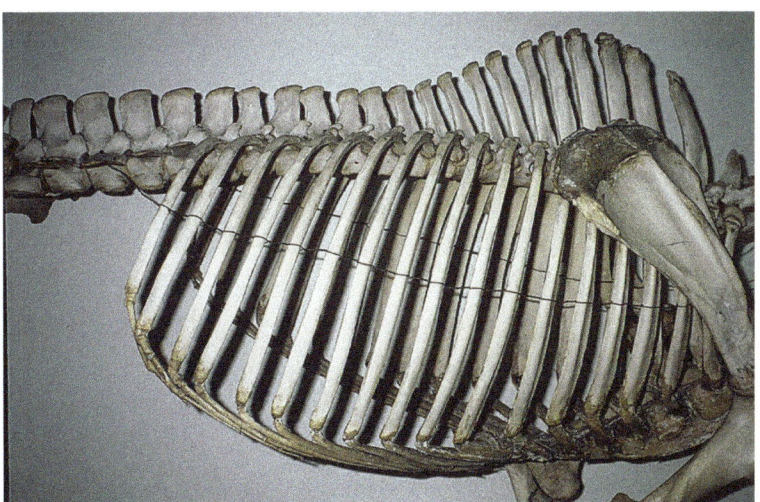

Fig. 5.9. Thorax, thoracic and lumbar vertebrae

caudal direction of the sacrum functions as a counter bearing, as this is where the supraspinous ligament attaches. In the event of the lowering of the pelvis with the use of the M. psoas, direct flexion of the sacroiliac joint and simultaneous lifting of the lumbar area is the outcome. Impulsion (stepping under the body) will thereby stretch the supraspinous ligament backwards, which would not be possible through only lowering the head and neck. Now one can see clearly why sufficient activity in the back and contact can never be obtained through only dealing with the head and neck.

The first eight ribs, known as the true ribs are more or less joined fixedly with the sternum and serve as areas of insertion for the serratus muscle, affording the front limbs a muscular connection to the thorax. This serratus attachment takes on a special act, namely that of shock absorber, especially when landing after a jump. The serratus muscles spread out like a fan and are split up between a cervical and a thoracic part, and besides sideways flexion of the neck, also influence the horse's breathing. In cases of strains or tears of this muscle, horses show lameness that is difficult to pinpoint. Shortened gaits and grunting sounds are signs, as the horse holds his breath out of fear of the oncoming pain when he has to land after a jump and then the weight of the horse emits the grunt when he lands.

The other ten ribs, the so-called breathing ribs, are attached to the breastbone with the help of cartilaginous connections and have a very important role to play in breathing. They allow the expansion of the thorax during in- and exhalation.

The rib joints allow a small amount of dorsoventral and craniocaudal movement to pass through the ribs that has a big impact on the expansion of the thorax when the horse breathes. The dorsal arches of the ribs shape the bearing surface of the saddle and also offer a shock absorbing action, due to the loose-jointed connection with the relatively rigid spinal column. This allows the rider to sit comfortably whilst the back muscles can work unhindered.

When the horse is saddled too far back, this shock absorbing action is lost and the immobile transverse processes of the lumbar vertebrae have to bear weight. This makes the back really hard because of the handicapped activity of the back muscles and the rider will bounce more in the saddle. This causes tense gaits and irregular trot rhythms. At this stage, collection will no longer be possible.

Any kind of blockage in the ribs can cause respiratory problems as the diaphragm is attached under the last third of the thoracic vertebrae, and a reflex caused by failed nervous transmissions can hinder it from expanding sufficiently. Under these circumstances "Poor performance syndrome" can result when insufficient oxygen is supplied to the horse.

The lateral flexion of the thoracic vertebral column is restricted by the joints of the ribs and accordingly the width of the ribs. The maximum "flexion of the ribcage" is thereby limited to a few centimeters, on the one hand because of the distance between the ribs that is on average 3-4cm, and on the other hand because of the width of the ribs (4-5cm) and the intracostal muscles on the opposite side that have to stretch.

> **Note:** *The term flexion in the ribs, so often used in riding, in fact, is anatomically impossible. The bend that often impresses in the lateral movements, is a rotation and simultaneous upwards curve of the thoracolumbar intersection, as there are no limiting ventral portions in this area.*

The real bending in the horse takes place in the thoracolumbar intersection by means of an upwards curve and rotation of the spinal cord in this area. Through this movement it seems as if the horse is bending his ribs around the inside leg of the rider. (Fig.5.10)

There are 5 or 6 lumbar vertebrae, depending on the breed of the horse. Andalusian and Arabian horses, due their square shapes, often have

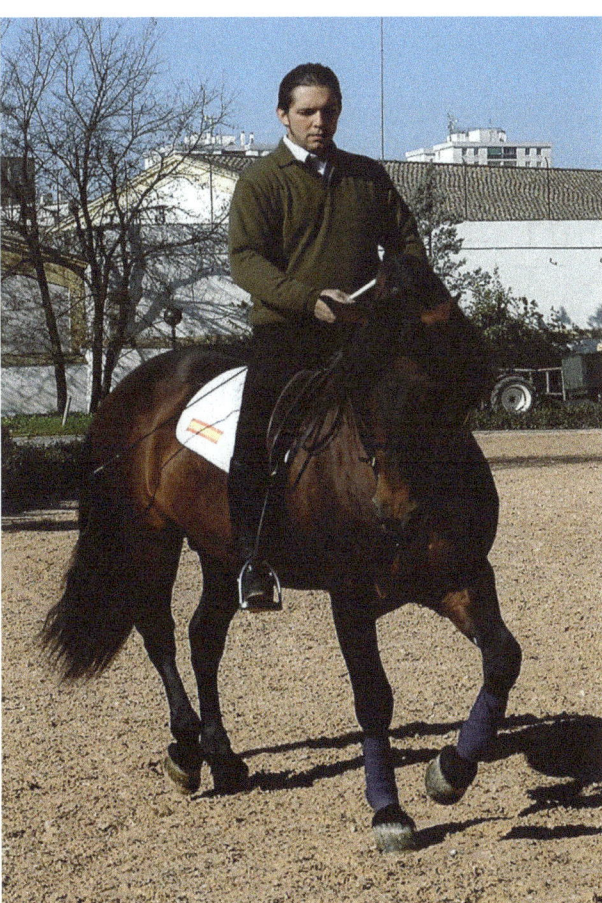

Fig.5.10. The appearance of "bending in the ribs" arises from the upwards curve and rotation in the thoracolumbar area. A genuine bending of the thoracic spinal column is limited due to anatomical and biomechanical factors.

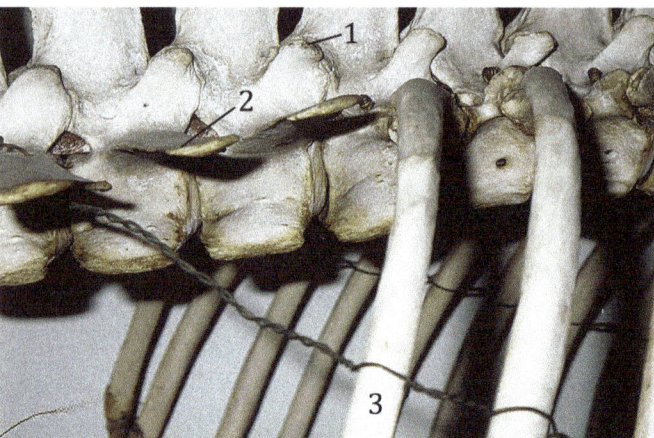

Fig. 5.11. Lumbar spine and thoracolumbar intersection

1. *Proc. mammillaris of L1*
2. *Proc. transversus of L2*
3. *18th rib*

one lumbar vertebra less than warmbloods, that have a more rectangular shape. The lumbar vertebrae have spinal and transverse processes where important muscles for spinal movement are attached. They are linked to each other with multiple joints and due to their construction, where they have no ventral support, they are very prone to becoming blocked. (Fig. 5.11)

On the one hand, this is associated with the fact that the very mobile thoracolumbar intersection is at the same time the bearing surface for the last third of the saddle, and together with the centrifugal and shearing forces that the rider brings, they create disadvantageous lever on the back of the horse. One also finds the lumbar wave, composed of the M. longissimus dorsi

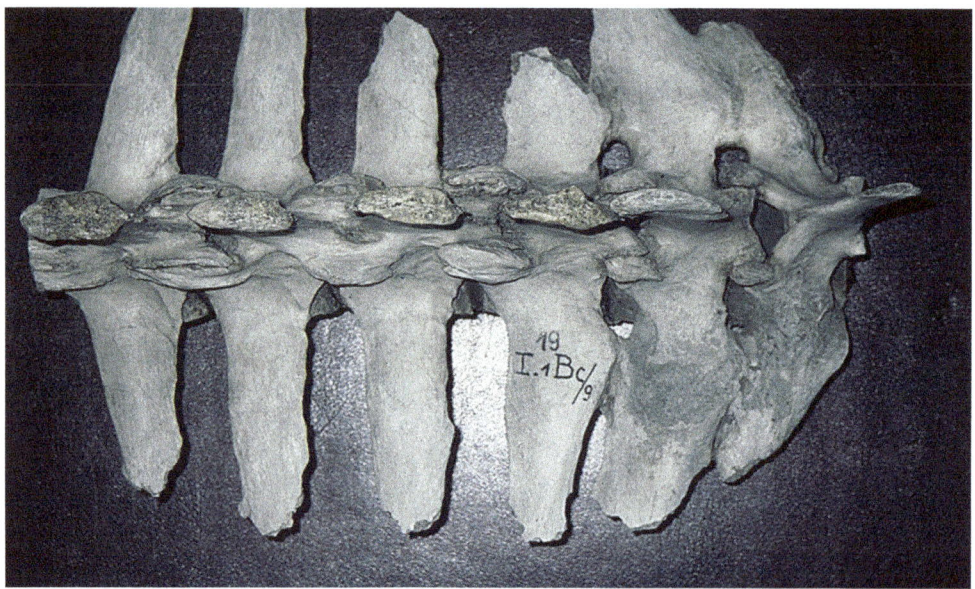

Fig.5.12. Ankylosis of the transverse processes in the lumbar area (here from L4-L6). Early and intense burdening of still growing Thoroughbreds can lead to fusion of the transverse processes, limiting sideways movement

in this area. When the ileo-sacral joint is blocked, this part will induce intense tension and thereby provoke osteopathic lesions.

Both the thoracic and the lumbar spinal columns are capable of flexion and extension in which the range of motion in the upwards arching is considerably more than the lowering in this section of the spine.

An anatomical peculiarity worth mentioning in the horse is the intertransversarii muscles when too-strong demands are made on these muscles, too early ankylosis[3] can occur, as is often seen in racehorses. This fusion of the spinal cord will limit lumbar flexion. (fig.5.12)

> *In practice: Whether a horse can be a weight carrier or not depends on the caliber and arch of the ribs and on the length of the back. The greater the distance between the mid-line and the arch of the ribs, the wider the bearing surface of the saddle, making the distribution of weight better on the back. Short, wide backs are more stable, for they are not so springy and due to their compact structure, they do not show fatigue as fast. However, one should not be deceived by this, but continue with consistent building-up of muscles in order to ensure longevity. Short, compact horses bounce less and these horses instead, show a tendency for bony problems such as periostitis, kissing spines etc In the event of fatigue, their spines will carry the weight of the rider. Long backs will swing more and are more comfortable, but are also more susceptible to muscular disease, as the longer back muscles will acidify easier and the appearance of fatigue will show more clearly. Pressure points in the saddle area, resistance when being saddled, contact and collection difficulties are some of the consequences of non-systematic training methods on a long back.*

The main muscles of the back, the M. longissimus dorsi and the M. iliocostalisare also very important muscles as they primarily assume the function of stabilizing the spine (fig.5.13) The M. ileocostalis additionally has the ability to cause lateral flexion through unilateral contraction. Contraction of the M. longissimus dorsi will induce extension of the back bones whereby the distance between the vertebrae becomes smaller. When a horse has been incorrectly ridden, this position can advance kissing spines. Normally both longissimi dorsi muscles work rhythmically and equally. They relax in the protraction phase and contract in the retraction phase. This enables harmonious tensing and relaxing. The M. latissimus dorsi as well as the thoracic part of the M. trapezius are also responsible for a flowing course of movement in the area of the saddle. A depression behind the shoulder is a sign of an inactive trapezius muscle, in most cases this is owing to a too narrow

---

3   A stiffness of a joint due to abnormal adhesion and rigidity of the bones of the joint, which may be the result of injury or disease.

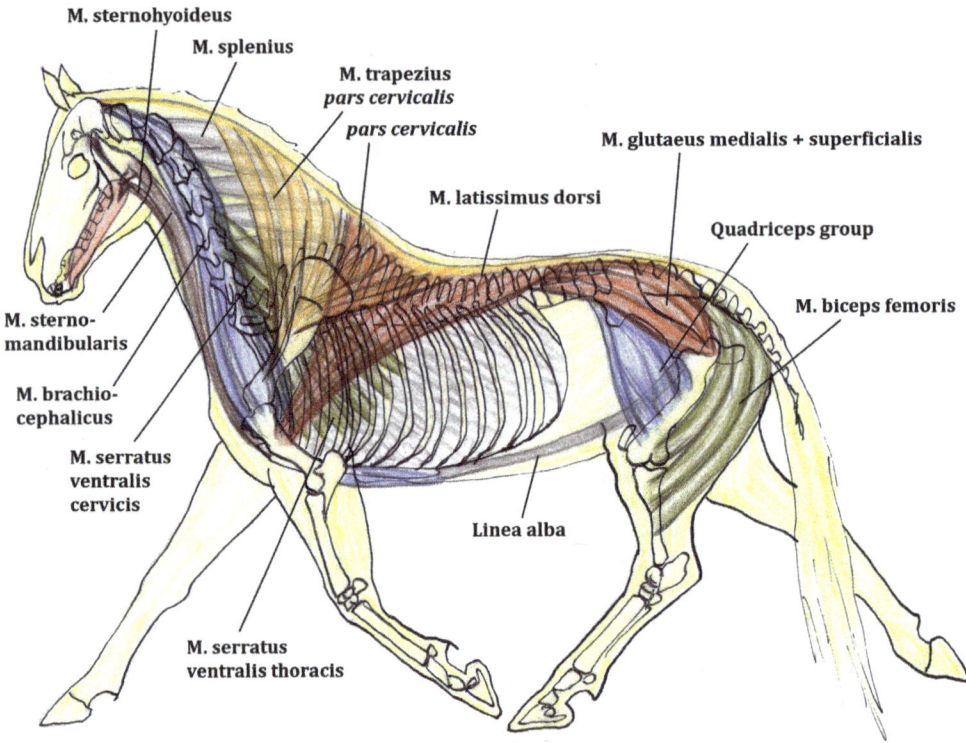

Fig.5.13. Diagram of muscle groups that are important for the rider.

saddle leaving this area tense and painful to pressure.

The trapezius originates in the fascia of the withers, and inserts on the caudal part of the scapula and partakes in retraction. Tension and pain in this area manifests itself through lifting of the head, whereby the M. brachiocephalicus, that participates in extension of the front leg, also tenses. Tension in these two muscles causes shortened strides and the horses develop a relieving posture with trigger points in the trapezius muscle, that in turn will curtail the action of the foreleg. When the caudal branch of the M. latissimus dorsi at the back end of the saddle is irritated, the tension in the muscle will hollow the back, the croup will appear horizontal and the extension the foreleg is once again limited. It is therefore recommended to give one's best attention to the fit of the saddle and even pressure distribution. (See Chapter 7.1)

Even though the back muscles have always been given great importance, one should not forget the function of the antagonistic abdominal and psoas muscles. The obliquus externus and internus abdominis muscles, combined with the M. iliocostalis take part in bending when contracted unilaterally. When the rider applies his leg aid on one side, the horse's upper leg fascia will contract as a reflex and provoke lifting of the leg. The psoas

The Science and Art of Riding in Lightness

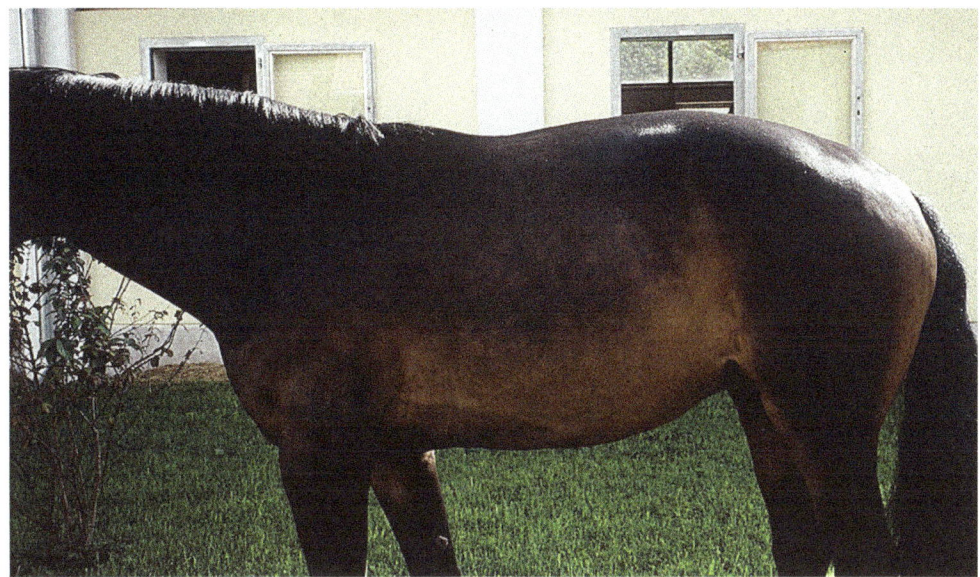

Fig.5.14. Typical image of a roach back

muscle plays a significant part in the lowering of the croup. Strong demands are made on these muscle groups, especially in the collected gaits.

Roach back, hollow back:

When the spinous processes of the lumbar vertebrae are too long, a roach back can be the result (fig.5.14) that is not esthetically pleasing and it can pose a problem in finding a fitting saddle.

From a functional point of view, this deficiency is less significant than the hollow back, for a lifting of the back is possible; however, this is not a desirable back shape. This shape of back is a problem when it is accompanied by a short, weak neck, for this combination will seriously affect the horse's balance and equilibrium under the rider. These horses can be used without any problems in carriage driving, although a certain element of aesthetic pleasing should not be disregarded.

Kissing spine syndrome:

When the vertebral bodies are not used correctly, tension in the area of the back muscles can cause the so-called kissing spine syndrome. This can be verified with x-rays as a narrowing of the distances between the spinous processes. (See Chapter 19.2.2)

In many cases it comes to the same thing when the back muscles are used incorrectly and lead to asymmetry and shortening of the muscles, where the permanent pressure can cause periostal deformation on the involved vertebrae. (fig.5.15). Kissing spine syndrome can be rehabilitated by specific

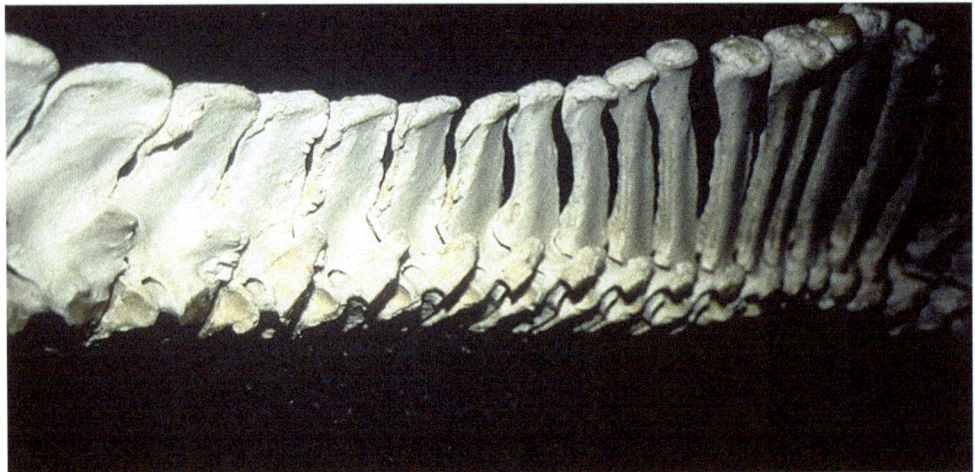

Fig.5.15. Kissing spine syndrome. The periostal deposits on the spinous processes can be clearly seen. In jumpers the thoracic vertebrae are strongly compressed in the landing phase, whereby kissing spines can develop due to reactions of the periosteum.

changes in the training of many sports horses and is not really an issue in the purpose of sports. When a horse in work uses his back and rounds it, it will automatically open the distance between the spinous processes, the muscles will be stretched and the abdominal muscles will become stronger, thus ensuring the best long term success.

In the extreme cases, where the spinous processes are so closed together, it is almost impossible for the horse to round his back. This can be seen in hollow backed horses or horses that are croup high, especially those that have the conformational problem of very straight hind legs as well. These horses are very difficult to collect and often get a high elevation of the head, but the back does not realistically work. In their endeavor to collect themselves, they appear to be divided in two, with a comparatively immovable and inelastic topline, whereby they can neither develop extra stride length nor regular cadence. They appear wooden. This is especially seen in the baroque breeds, where one is rarely tempted by the high neck attachment to ride these horses in a deep position, and there is a much bigger tendency towards this shape of back. Even the horses that lend themselves to being "easy to collect," must be trained according to the training scale in the classical way, so they can shine in the lessons of the high school.

Diseases of the back muscles

I cannot discuss all pathological details of diseases of the back muscles in this book. However, one cannot forget the relationship of the muscle physiology with the training, that a muscle can only work efficiently when it has the ability to relax completely in order to then fully contract again. This simple mechanism is necessary to assist the building up of muscle, ensuring that the muscle can be sufficiently supplied with nutrients and oxygen. In the same way, it is possible to remove waste products; for example lactate, from the muscle. A horse must be inwardly relaxed to accomplish this activity, for a horse that is permanently in psychological stress cannot easily accomplish this biological feat when his muscles are always tense. Toxic products are not metabolized sufficiently, vessels become smaller and can only supply limited amounts of oxygen, waste products irritate delicate motor ends, producing pain and an abnormal hardening of the muscle (myogelosis). Myositis and tying up are the results of improper and especially irregular training.

Energy in the form of ATP[4] must be available for the muscles on a daily basis by means of a tailored ration to mark the needs of the horse in the same way as regular daily training. ATP is the purest form of energy, the start of the biochemical process of metabolism with the help of oxygen to supply the muscles with sufficient fuel to work. When the muscle comes into an energy deficit as a result of over-training and lack of oxygen, the body will release energy on short notice through fat burning and thus achieve high performance energetic metabolism. Unfortunately this kind of energy release brings more toxic waste with it, that provokes muscle soreness and myogelosis. In order to generate muscle growth, (5-6) high quality repetitions of an exercise is sufficient for enough stimulus but not to tire the muscle. The constant interplay between contraction and relaxation in the training is furthermore essential to develop healthy and powerful muscles. Any part of the body that is kept in one position for a long time, will cause pain and resistances will be the result.

Young horses in particular, who start to throw their heads after a few minutes of going on the bit, do not do this out of dislike, but it is a sign of muscle pain due to the consistent position they adopt in a still untrained body. Immediate stretching after short successful repetitions advocates motivation and avoids hyper-acidity and stiffness on the next day of training. For this reason it is advisable to finish every training unit with calm forward and down trot work, even with well-ridden horses. The remains of the metabolic products that were accumulated during training will then be eliminated.

Thoracic muscles
M. iliocostalis
I: Tuberositas m. iliocostalis of the 18 ribs, and Procc. transvesii of the last neck vertebra.

---

[4] Adenosine triphosphate, coenzyme used as an energy carrier in the cells of all known organisms; the process in which energy is moved throughout the cell.

F: Sideways bending of the lumbar and thoracic spinal cord, expiration

M. longissimus dorsi
I: Transverse processes of the thoracic and lumbar vertebrae and ribs
C: Lies between M. iliocostalis and M. spinalis and is the longest muscle in the horse's body, presents the location for the saddle.
F: Extends the spinal cord (Lordosis)
M. spinalis
I: Spinous processes of the thoracic vertebrae
F: Extends the thoracic and lumbar spinal cord
Mm. multifidi
O: Transverse processes of the thoracic and lumbar vertebrae
I: Spinous processes of the same thoracic and lumbar vertebrae
F: immobilization of the joints, sideways bending and rotation of the intervertebral joint spaces, proprioception

M. psoas major
O: ventrally on the transverse processes of the lumbar vertebrae and the 17th and 18th rib
I: Minor trochanter of the femur
F: Flexion of the lumbosacral joint, sacroiliac joint and the lumbar vertebrae, unilateral contraction can cause rotation of the lumbar area, bends the hip joint and turns the femur to the outside

M. psoas minor
O: Ventrally on the vertebrae of T16-T15
I: Psoas minor tuberosities of the ilium
F: Flexion of the sacroiliac joint and the lumbosacral joint

M. quadratus lumborum
O: iliac crest
I: Ventrally on the transverse processes of the lumbar vertebrae
F: Sideways flexion of the lumbar spinal cord

M. Obliquus externus abdominis
O: Outer surface of the 6-18 ribs
I: Linea alba, inguinal ligament
F: Flexion of the thoracolumbar spinal cord with bilateral contraction, turning and sideways bending with unilateral contraction

M. obliquus internus abdominis

O: Tuber coxae, inguinal ligament
I: Medially on the distal section of the last rib
F: similar to the M. obliquus externus abdominis

M. rectus abdominis
O: Costal cartilage, sternum
I: Cranial border of the pubic bone via the ventral pubic ligament
F: Flexion of the thoacic, lumbar and croup area when bilateral contraction; turns sideways, bends when unilateral contraction
M. transversus abdominis
O: Transverse process of lumbar vertebrae and the cartilage of the ribs
I: Linea alba
F: combined with M. obliquus externus, internus and M. rectus abdominis, makes an important antagonist for the back muscles and serves as a "ventral brace"

M. Thoracic serratus vetntralis
O: 1-9 ribs
I. Inside of the shoulder blade
F: combined with the M. serratus ventralis cervicis the most important carrier of the torso, takes part in inspiration

M. internal and external intercostals
O: intercostal chambers
I: ribs
F: in- and expire

The forelimbs

The forelimbs are column shaped and are connected to the torso merely by muscle attachment. (Serratus muscles) This kind of construction is for support and absorbing burdens.

As mentioned before, the head and neck, because of their high dead weight, will shift the center of gravity to the front and this is an ideal type of construction for the horse as flight animal, as this kind of suspension will act as a shock absorber for the impulsion generated by the hindquarters. This is significant in the landing phase after a jump, where there is substantial traction force on the serratus muscle, and it is therefore very important to warm the muscle up properly before the upcoming activity in order to avoid muscle injury. The serratus muscles are divided into a cervical and a thoracic part, which means that tension can cause flexion problems in the neck to one side. The serratus muscles attach medially to the border of the shoulder and join the 8 true ribs in a fan-shape.

Since the center of gravity lies more towards the front as a result of anatomical conditions, the forehand carries about 55% of the weight, which symbolizes that a 500kg warm-blood will have an applied load of 137.5kg per front leg. This surplus load can become several tons when the horse lands after a jump. This suggests that every horse has only a limited amount of jumps in his legs.

During sudden bursts of canter, the thrust from the hindquarters will travel forward, and the back will first arch up, then drop down in the stance phase, putting all the forward movement on the now supporting front legs. This is when the serratus muscles and support ligaments serve as suspension and shock absorbers.

The tendons, being the end-points of the muscles, are in the same way supplied with a shock absorbing safety mechanism, that allows a 4% over stretch without tearing the tendon. This arrangement is very important for a flight animal such as the horse, seeing that sudden sprints provoke changing moments of burden in the joints. This is when an elastic yielding is possible.

Even though the diameter of a muscle can often be 60 times that of a tendon, a muscle is never able to tear a tendon just by its own strength, seeing that the tear strength for tendon fiber is around 7-8 kg/square mm.

As a result, tendon fibers will only tear at 4-11 times the load of resting, whereby that produces a pull of around 950-2000 kg.

Based on biomechanical laws, the superficial digital flexor and the suspensory ligament are taxed more in the stance phase and the deep digital flexor is taxed more in the break over phase.

The lacertus fibrosus and the check ligament of the deep digital flexor offer the forelimbs a sinewy bracing possibility of resting while standing without any specific muscle power. Furthermore, check ligaments serve as security constructions to protect tendons from over stretching. This is also the reason why horses can continue to move in extreme cases of loading, even with damage already done to the tendon fibers, for these security constructions will momentarily restrict the lowering of the fetlock. It it were not for them, there would be many more spontaneous tears in the loading peaks with much higher pain and horses would be more or less immobilized, thereby surely costing a flight animal his life. Therefore, it is very important to prevent tendon injuries, as this is indispensable for keeping the horse healthy for a long time.

The angle of the shoulder is decisive in determining the length of stride and should be inclined at 90-100 degrees. More important than the angle of the shoulder, is the maximum angle of opening of the elbow. The more open, the easier it is for the horse to stride out, making bigger steps possible.

The steeper the shoulder and the shorter the forearm, the shorter the length of stride, whereas a correspondingly longer upper arm and metacarpal bone give rise to higher knee action. In the area of the shoulder joint, one finds the bursa of the bicep tendon that serves as a sliding bearing for the tendon of the biceps. Inflammation in this area because of mechanical trauma, falls etc can influence the stride length, causing the horses to have an asymmetrical gait.

The shoulder blade is composed of a bony and a dorsal cartilaginous part and has a conspicuously palpable spine that divides the scapula into two parts. The neck of the scapula forms an important transfer point for the N. subscapularis at the cranial side, whereby lesions of this by virtue of blow injuries can cause muscle atrophy in the area of supraspinatous and infraspinatous muscles. A conspicuous emergence of the scapular spine with partially impaired movement is a definite clinical parameter for this disease pattern.

The shoulder cartilage as the most caudal element of the scapula and the angle of the shoulder blade are of significant importance to the choice of the correct width of the saddle, seeing that the shoulder blade moves several centimeters caudally with every forward movement of the front legs. Improperly fitting saddles with trees that are too narrow can result in pressure points and ossification of the cartilaginous parts. Asymmetry because of ossification is always a problem in the choice of a saddle and can almost not be compensated for, given that the saddle will always be inclined to be lopsided due to the misalignment of the scapular borders. This will in turn cause diagonal instability and create irritation of the supraspinous ligament in the lumbar area.

The ideal angle between the humerus and the elbow is 130-140 degrees. Located caudally between the border of the shoulder blade and the humerus, are the important triceps muscles that flex the shoulder joint and stretch the elbow joint. In the case of faulty loading, one can locate trigger points in the area of the caput longum and caput laterale in the medial third. The M. brachii distend cranially from the tuberculum supraglenoidale to the tuberositas radii, and then join the M. extensor carpi radialis via the lacertus fibrosus. The M. biceps brachii extend the shoulder, flex the elbow and influence the action of the foreleg through the lacertus fibrosus, since the M. extensor carpi radialis inserts on the cranio-proximal edge of the third metacarpal bone. The elbow, as a hinge joint, has a primarily stabilizing function. The olecrani bursa can, in the event of an irritation, look very imposing as a capped elbow. But when it does not form a fistula or chafe on the girth, it is only a blemish. When it calcifies at the tendon attachment on the tuber olecrani, it can impede the movement of the horse.

The angle from the elbow to the carpal joint is approximately 180 degrees and the fetlock forms an angle of 45-50 degrees to the pastern and hoof joint at the end.

At a full gallop, the fetlock and the second and fourth metacarpal bones can actually touch the ground, which often result in micro fissures of the metacarpal bones and chronic degeneration of the sesamoid bones. Due to these intense moments of loading, the tendons, especially the suspensory ligament, is of the utmost importance, as this takes on an intermediate position as the M. interosseus medius between the muscle and the tendon. Through the two suspensory ligament branches that is redirected cranially on the sliding bearing behind the sesamoid bones to the combined extensor tendon, it is capable of supporting the fetlock joint.

The caudal lateral border of the carpal tunnel is formed by the Os carpi that is connected to the medial parts of the carpus with the Retinaculum flexorum.

In cases of osteopathic lesions of the carpal joint, there will be an increased pull on the Retinaculum flexorum, thereby making the diameter of the carpal tunnel smaller and greatly affecting the mobility of the structures lying inside it. Less blood circulation of these structures on the inside with resulting pain and disturbed functioning of tissue are the consequences of this disease. Both the tendon and the tendon sheath can be affected by this. As a reflex, the corresponding muscles can shorten, thus limiting the range of movement of the horse. Horses with recurring tendon problems should be thoroughly examined in this area, as regeneration can only make process when the damaged area is sufficiently supplied with blood and oxygen.

The movement of the carpal joints are limited to flexion and extension and a roughly 30 degree possibility of ab- and adduction, giving this joint an extensive range of motion.

Spanish and gaited horses often have what one calls "camponeo" (Spanish: bell player gait) that can be subdivided into high and low camponeo.

The high componeo, due to its excessive mobility in the carpal joint, produces a swinging, swaying movement in the cannon bones when the horse flexes his front legs. This movement was very popular at one time in Spanish horses, as this grandiose gesticulation was a spectacle for the eyes. Through this extravagant movement, however, the susceptibility to abrasive wear and tear was too high and the length of stride is very restricted. In breeding today, much more merit is given to the correctness and straightness of the movement.

The low campaneo is to be looked upon as a minor fault and is often seen in horses with a wide chest. The campaneo movement is seen a below the fetlock joint.

The fetlock joint is made up of the third carpal bone and the first phalanx and is, in essence, a hinge joint and therefore only has a limited possibility for sideways movement. In the same way, the characteristics are similar in the pastern and coffin joint, but the coffin joint; being protected by the hoof, is only indirectly subjected to a test of mobility.

The hoof bone has two cartilaginous extensions to the side, that are, together with the digital cushions, of utmost importance for the pumping mechanism of the hoof.

The navicular bone is a flat, wedge-shaped bone that forms part of the navicular system that is composed of the Bursa podotrochlearis, impar ligament and the deep digital flexor. The navicular serves as a diverting pulley for the deep digital flexor and is exposed to great biomechanical forces during jumping and extended trot, and is therefore, time and again, a cause for lameness. The difference of pressure executed by each step taken will provoke varying moments of loading on the podotrochlea, causing alteration on the Margo distalis in terms of recovery.

The horse stands on the tip of the third toe that has adapted itself outstandingly to the flight inhabitant of the plains. Only the second and fourth metacarpal bones and the chestnuts point to the historical developmental from the dog-sized eohippus that moved on five toes.

By the same token, the ulna of the horse has shortened to form the elbow protuberance and this hinge joint has an intrinsic stabilizing function. When the elbow is too close to the ribcage, the range of movement will be insufficient. A flat elbow can generate an inelegant, waddling gait and cause instability in the joint. Due to the anatomy, the radius of the movement in the elbow joint is limited to extension and flexion and therefore has no relevant movement to either side. The wider the opening angle of the elbow joint, the freer and more effortless the horse can lengthen his stride.

Abduction of the front legs in the lateral gaits or mobilization for the most part come from the shoulder joint, that likewise can be flexed and extended. The triceps as well as the trapezius muscles and the M. latissimus dorsi are given great biomechanical importance in these movements. The pectoral muscles must be capable of maximum stretching in order to make it possible for the front leg to step forward and sideways. Due the proactive action of the M. brachiocephalicus on the forehand, it is essential that the horse is not positioned too much in the direction of the movement as that would inhibit the forward-sideways motion sequence. If the horse has too much position, the restricting tension in the above mentioned muscle can cause limited deployment and puts strain on the contra-lateral shoulder that should move freely outward (half-pass, shoulder-in), the result is that the horse looses balance. What's more, when the horse's head is pulled too far to the inside, it has a negative influence on the inside hind leg, since it cannot lower the haunches through more bend in the hips but instead wants to push to the outside. The inside hind leg will therefore not be encouraged to step further under the body and the straight forward impulsion will be slowed down.

The shoulder muscles.

M. trapezius
O: The Pars cervicalis originates on C2 and the nuchal ligament along the withers. The Pars thoracica originates between the withers and T10
I: Both insert on the shoulder blade
C: Most superficial muscle, atrophy can occur when the saddle is too narrow
F: Forward movement and adduction of the front legs

M. rhomboide
O: Pars cervicalis: C2 and funiculus nuchae up to the withers. Pars thoracica: spinous processes of the withers up to T8
I: scapular cartilage
C: lies under the M. trapezius, important is the interplay when the neck muscles are relaxed.
F: takes the front leg back, lifts and fixates the front leg and also lifts the neck.

M. deltoid
O: scapular spine
I: deltoid tuberosity of the humerus
C: meets the M. brachiocephalicus and together they insert on the humerus
F: Move the front legs forward

M. supraspinatus
O: Pars supraspinatus scapulae and the cranial cartilage of the shoulder blade
I: The front of the humerus directly beneath the shoulder joint.
F: extension of the shoulder joint, stabilizes the joint, moves the leg forward

M. infraspinatus
O: Pars infraspinatus and the caudal cartilage of the shoulder blade
I: front of the humerus under the shoulder joint, next to the tendon of the M. supraspinatus
F: :flexion and stabilization of the shoulder joint

M. latissimus dorsi
O: Thoracic and lumbar vertebrae
I: caudally on the humerus
C: lies under the pars thoracicus of the M. trapezius, good to palpate
F: Flexes shoulder joint, takes font leg back

M: triceps brachii
O: scapula (caput longum) humerus (caput laterale and caput mediale)
I: tuber olecrani

C: easy to palpate, often tense with local trigger points
F: extends the elbow joint (caput laterale and mediale), flexes the shoulder joint (caput longum)

Pectoralis muscles
O: sternum, 1-9 ribs
I: inside of the humerus
C: important trunk supporter, existing of 4 different portions (M. pect. transversus, M. pect. descendens, M. pect. profundus, M. subclavius)
F: adduction of front leg (crossing in half-pass) Fixing the shoulder, move legs forward and back.

Leg muscles

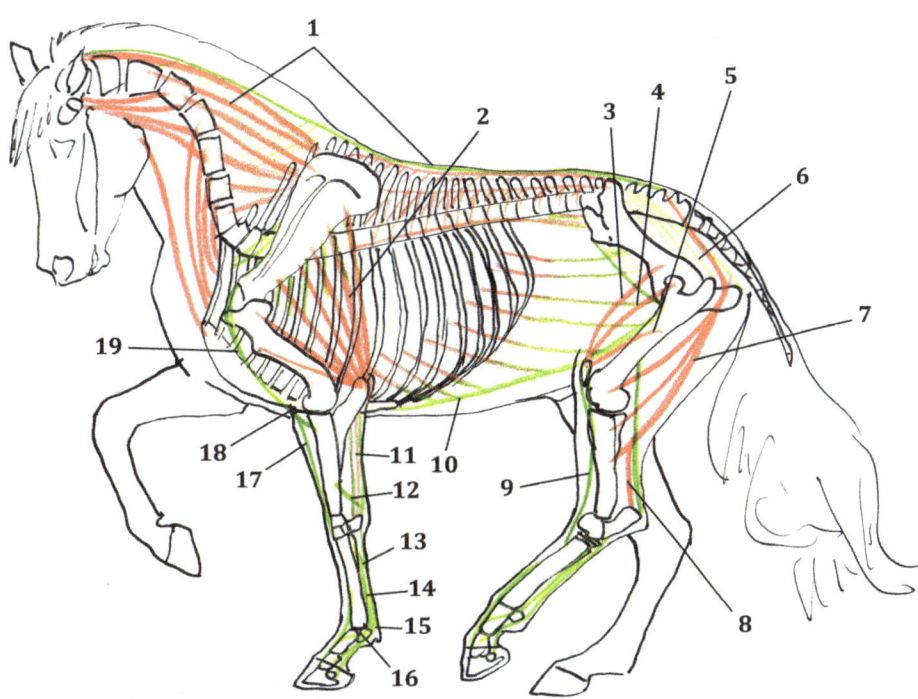

1. Nuchal Ligament
2. M. triceps brachii
3. M. rectus femoris
4. M. quadriceps femoris
5. M. vastus lateralis
6. Ligamentum sacrotuberale latum
7. M. biceps femoris
8. M. gastrocnemius + M. flexor digitorum superficialis
9. M. fibularis tertius
10. Linea alba
11. M. flexor digitorum superficialis
12. Ligamentum accessorium
13. Check ligament
14. M. interosseus medius
15. M. flexor digitorum profundus
16. Support leg of the M. interosseus medius
17. M. extensor carpi radialis
18. Lacertus fibrosus
19. M. biceps brachii

Fig 5.16 Important muscles and tendons of the front and hind legs

Extensors
O: all originate on the outside and front of the leg in close proximity to the elbow joint
I: Third metacarpal, P1, P2, P3
C: all the muscles have their muscle belly above the carpal joint and continue as tendons down the distal third (M. carpi radialis, M. ext. digit. communis, M. ext carpi ulnaris, M. ext. digit. lateralis)
F: Extends the above joints, including the carpal joint.

Flexors
O: Caudally and medially on the leg in close proximity to the elbow joint
I: Third metacarpal, P1, P2, P3
C: they also continue in the distal thirds as tendons (M. flex. digit profundus, M. flex. carpi ulnaris, M. flex superficialis, M. flex. pollicis longus)
F: flexes the above joints, including the carpal joint

The hind limbs

The sacrum is only fused at the age of five years and is shaped in the form of a cross. It is for this reason that it was called the holy bone in ancient times, the "Os sacrum." The Os sacrum has three articular surfaces on the cranial border, where it joins directly with the last lumbar vertebra as well as the articular surfaces of the transverse processes of the last lumbar vertebra. Horses that are strained too soon, as is often the case with racehorses, can develop ankylosis in the transverse processes as well as in the sacrum due to extreme physiological overload in the lumbo-sacral junction. Reduction in flexion of this area is the logical implication, making the tilting of the hips in bending the haunches almost an impossibility. The slightly slanting articular surface [iliac wings] of the Os sacrum connects the iliac wings and together create a real synovial joint, namely the Articulatio sacroiliaca (fig.5.17)

The *sacroiliac joint* is a very important structure as far as the

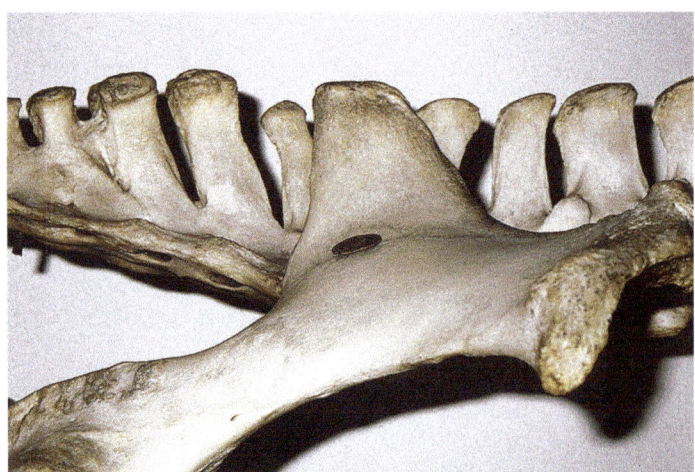

Fig. 5.17 Sacro iliac joint

biomechanics and collection of the hindquarters are concerned. It is the only synovial connection with the hind legs and therefore, transmits the developing thrust directly onto the spine. The high mobility in the sense of flexion and extension allows the horse to tilt the pelvis with the help of the psoas muscles and, in this way, creates the impression that the horse becomes "shorter" and able to bring his hind legs further under toward his center of gravity. The very small cross section of bearing area proportionate to the hindquarters, together with high mobility of the sacro-iliac joint creates much stress on the joint area extremely liable to break-down in terms of osteopathic lesions in the horse. Due to the enormous pressure and torque strength, falls and sharp turns or trauma to the hip bone etc can induce rotation on the relatively solid pelvis. In turn, this gives rise to functional misalignment of the tuber sacralia (fig.5.18a) and mobility restriction that can be mostly reversed with osteopathic procedures. Signs of this can include shortened length of stride and difficulty with collection on one side. Normally the tuber sacralia are fairly symmetrical with a noticeable impression between the two bones. Physiological asymmetry of the functional soundness is the result of the changeable tendenous structures of the joint. Physiological discrepancy can be up to one centimeter, without the horse suffering a blockage in the joint.

Atrophy of the corresponding gluteal muscles and adductors is not uncommon. (fig.5.18b) The foramina sacralia, together with the last two lumbar nervous emmersion points, form the outlet portals of the nervous structures that further down, unite to form the sciatic nerve. This nerve cord, as thick as a finger, supplies the hindquarters and is easily irritated because of the Ligamenta sacrotuberalia lata. Blockages in the ileo-sacral joint provoke mechanical irritations especially in the area of the gluteals and show up as lumbar syndrome with sciatic neuritis that naturally influences the way of going of the hindquarters. When the croup is fixed in extension, with the lumbar area barely utilized, the result will be shortened strides, rhythm disturbances and pain when turning. Collection or jump-off as well as increase in speed with the racehorse will explicitly be impaired or made impossible.

The haunches

Definition: *The haunches constitute the entirety of the big joints of the hindquarters: the hip-, knee- and hock joints. Bending of the haunches in the rider's language describes the closing of the hind leg joint angles. (Fig.5.19)*

The increased bending of the hocks result in a lowering of the hindquarters and the horse seems to be "sitting down." This closing of the joint

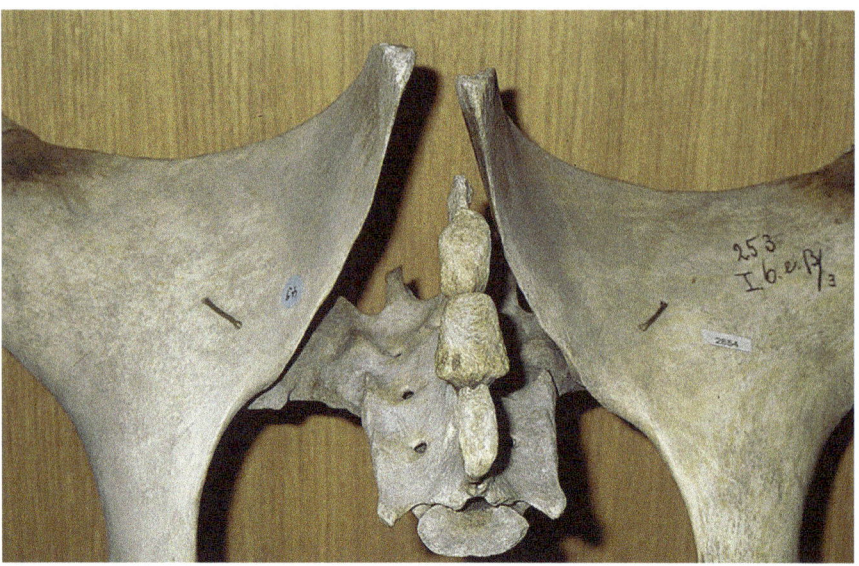

Fig:5.18
Blockage of the sacro iliac joint   a. Depiction of asymmetry in a model

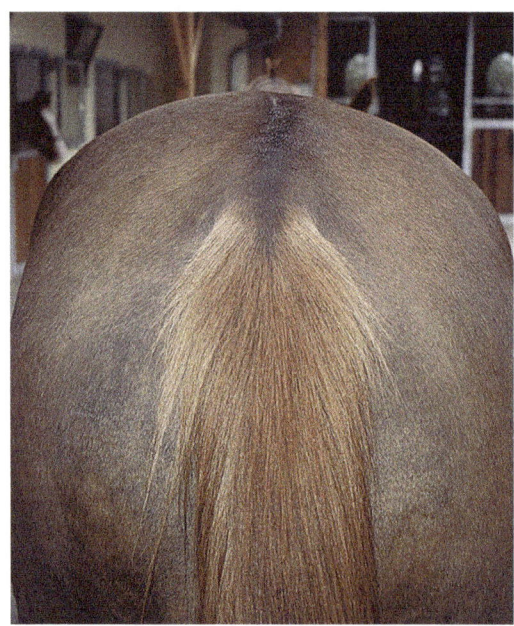

b. Atrophy of the right M. gluteus medius as a result of a blockade in the sacro iliac joint

angles calls for years of constructive muscle build-up in order to withstand such strenuous demands. This makes it clear that this characteristic of collection is not attainable through any shortcut. The horse should, in doing so, use bouncy strides or jumps, whereby the term bent haunches describes a particular elasticity and power for carrying weight. The angle of hindquarters is innately qualified to absorb the burden and thus relieve the forehand by moving the center of gravity to the rear, thereby making the action of the forehand freer and effortless and the elevation higher. The gluteal muscles, the M. fasciae latae, psoas major and minor muscles and the M. biceps, are significantly engaged in this biomechanical process. The quadriceps, with the co-operation of some smaller groups of muscles, guide the hind legs under the body and function as antagonists to the semi-membranosus and semi-tendinosus muscles.

Flexion of the hind legs makes finding the hip joint easier. The angle between the pelvis and the femur should be between 90 and 100 degrees so that the horse can sit down easier with the hindquarters. The Ligamentum accessorium connects the femur to the acetabulum and limits sideways kicking of the hind legs. As a matter of fact, horses can actually kick sideways through a simultaneous rotation of the lifted leg in the lumbar area.

The best biomechanical angle of the stifle in a sporting horse is 90-100 degrees, and 130-140 degrees in the hock. This will ensure optimal functioning. Steeper gradients will interfere with the ability for collection and jumping capability.

The head of the femur is deeply embedded in the acetabulum and is joined to the acetabulum with an intra-articular tendon. The hip joint is

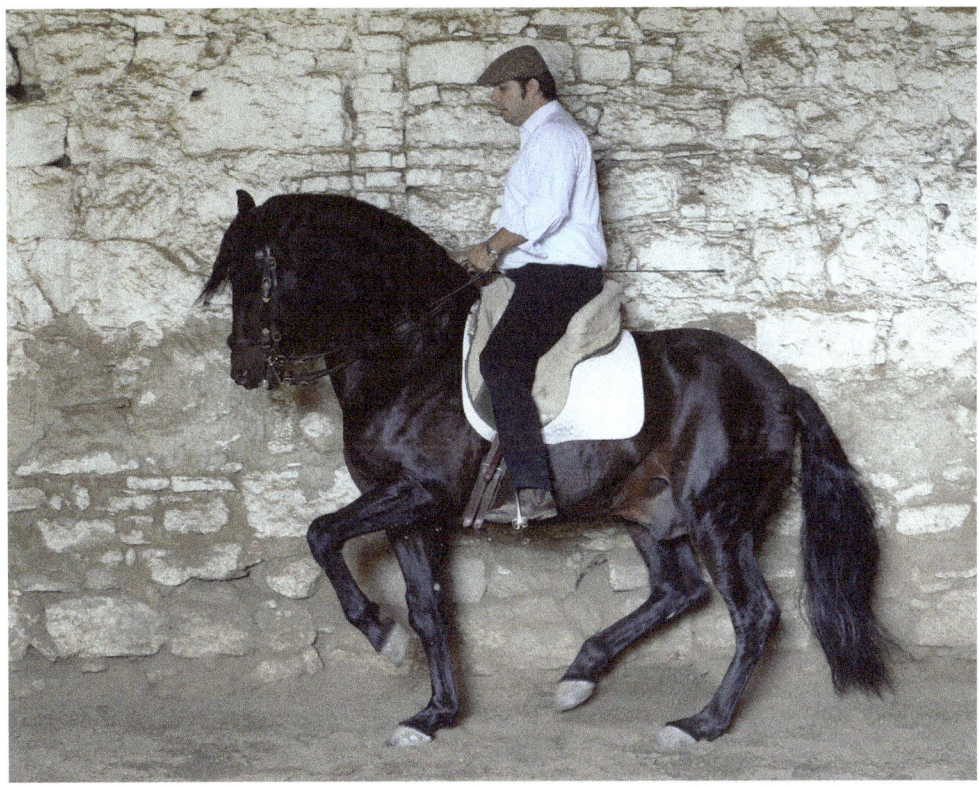

Fig.5.19. A good rassembler in the Piaffe. The forehand is perpendicular and the haunches are bent very well, so that the left fetlock almost touches the ground. The loins are well rounded and the tail hangs in a relaxed way.

capable of flexion and extension and possesses an enormous adduction possibility with a somewhat smaller abduction potential.

The stifle joint is made up of the femoro-patellar joint and the femoro-tibial joint. The medial ridge of the femur is more developed and offers the horse the possibility, through the reciprocal apparatus to hitch the patella into the groove without muscular power, but through simple over-stretching of the knee joint. The mechanism just described can only be sustained when the hoof-toe axis lies between 50-55 degrees. When this axis is broken back, there will be a position deviation in the third metacarpal as well, for this should be in a vertical position in order for this mechanism to function. When this happens, the position must be held with active muscle input and the horse will have light tension in the gluteal and hamstring muscles, which then means that they will start their daily training with acidic muscles. This mechanism was of vital importance for the flight animal that lived on the plains, for it meant that it could rest without lying down. In addition it is also conducive to the horse's well-being.

Apart from the collateral ligaments in the femoro-tibial joint, there are also the cruciate ligaments. This construction is capable of enduring great moments of load. The patella is kept in position by three tendons, in which the medial collateral ligament often provokes movement dysfunction, for it can easily be overstretched; for example, through falls, dislodging etc Injuries to the tendons will show up especially in the extended gaits as a result of instability of the stifle joint, causing breakdown in the rhythm and an unwillingness to step under the body more (trot racers) around the corners for the overtaking maneuver.

The tibiotarsal joint as the biggest joint is important for the flexion of the joint. Horses that show a lot of action in the tibiotarsal joint, but very little bending of the haunches and little activity in back, are so-called "leg movers." These horses, due to the lack of gymnastic training of the back and hindquarters muscles and therefore failing strength to carry weight will show a faster wear and tear of these parts, seeing that the thrust should come from the hocks and almost exclusively be absorbed by them as well. The shock absorbing action of the elastic muscles no longer have any effect. In many cases this exaggerated action of the hocks can be seen in the three year old action horses, who have been trained in the shortest possible time without sufficient building up of the muscles, emulating the highest attainable neck position with a taut back, pretending to have achieved a high level of training that they could not possibly have. Refer to the detailed description of the training scale in Chapter 10.

The distal tarsometatarsal joints (so-called bone spavin joints) and intertarsal joints are of lesser importance for the movement possibilities of the hock joint, but the pathological processes like arthrosis and arthritis have made a name for themselves.

The calcaneus should be pointed out as it serves as a pulley system for the Achilles tendon with its bursa (which is the capped hock in pathology) Interesting from the biomechanical point of view is the fact that the stifle and hock only move in combination with each other. That means: with every flexion of the stifle, the hock must also flex and the same applies for extension. Anatomical substrata of this construction is the M. fibularis tertius, that originates on the lateral ridge and forks to insert craniolaterally to the tarsus, and the M. flexor digitorum superficialis. The latter originates caudal and somewhat proximal from the lateral ridge, fuses with the M. gastrocnemius as the Achilles tendon distally and inserts on the calcaneus. In the event of an accidental tear of the M. fibularis tertius, the stifle and hock can flex separately from each other. This injury can be treated with physiotherapeutic procedures; for example laser, magnetic field therapy, and lonthoporese. The horses can often return to sports after subsequent rehabilitation.

The angle of the fetlock of the back foot (50-55 degrees) is steeper than the front foot which means the pushing force is improved. The rest of the joints in the hind foot are similar to that of the front foot.

Hind leg muscles (See also Fig. 5.16.)

Mm. glutei (M. glutaeus medius, superficialis, profundus, accesorius)
O: Tuber coxae, wings of the ilium, ilium and M. longissimus dorsi
I: lateral on the femur
F: Extension and inward rotation of the hips, abduction of the hind legs

M. biceps femoris
O: Os sacrum and seat bone
I: Patella, tibia and calcaneus
F: Extension of the hip joint, flexion of the stifle in the stance phase

M. tensor fasciae latae
O: Hip bone
I: Stifle joint
F. Flexion of the hip joint, extension of the stifle, moves hind legs forward

M: quadriceps femoris (Mm. vastus lateralis, medialis, intermedius and M. rectus femoris)
O: Femur and ilium
I: patella and just under the stifle joint on the lower leg

F: Extension of the stifle joint, main flexor of the hips

M. semimembranosus, M. semitendinosus
O: Os sacrum, Ca1, Ca2 and seatbone
I: Patella, tibia and calcaneus
F: Extension of the hip joint (M. semi-membranosus), extension of the stifle in the break-over phase, flexion of the stifle in the stance phase (M. semi-tendinosus), antagonists to M. quadriceps femoris

Adductors (M. sartorius, M. gracilis, M. pectineus, mm. adductor magnus and brevis)
O: Os pubis
I: femur and tibia
F: Adduction of the hip joint, antagonists to the gluteal muscles, M. sartorius functions as flexor and outwards rotator for the hips, M. adductor functions as extender and inwards rotator and M. pectineus fixes the hip joint.

Extensors (M. extensor digitorum longus, M. ext. digit. lateralis)
O: cranially on the femur, tibia and fibula
I: Tarsal joint, fetlock, pastern and hoof joint
F: Flexes the hock and extends the toe

Flexor (Mm. flexor digitorum superficialis and profundus, M. gastrocnemius)
O: Femur, tibia and fibula
I: hock, fetlock, pastern and hoof joint
F: Extends the hock and flexes the toe

Ligamentum sarotuberale latum

Another significant ligament that runs between the sacrum and the seat bone is the Lig. sacrotuberale latum. This ligament plays an important role in blockages in the pelvic area as it becomes taut through rotation of the pelvic girdle and can then aggravate the sciatic nerve. In this way a mechanically induced neuritis of the nerve can be provoked.

Check ligament

The check ligament is often the cause of lameness in the front legs. The radial check ligament joins the radius with the M. flexor digitorum profundus and also inhibits a too deep lowering of the legs higher up. It inserts on the radius, originates from the superficial flexor tendon and inhibits extreme lowering of the fetlock joint, thereby avoiding damage to this joint under heavy loading.

The *M. interosseus medius*, also known as the suspensory ligament is somewhere between a ligament and a tendon, given that it inserts caudally on the proximal third of the metacarpal bone and has no muscular origin. It runs distally along the back of the metacarpal bone and then supports the sesamoid bones with one part and with the other branch ends at the extensor tendon. This ligament has a considerable function as a support for the fetlock and prevents hyper-flexion of the fetlock.

5.2. The "good" rider—The correct aids

Time and again the demand for anatomical constitution, gait quality and mental aptitude of what the sport-horse should and must have is brought forward. However, the status of the rider as provider and trainer is questioned to a lesser extent.

By virtue of this responsibility when faced with another living being, the question should be asked as to what characterizes a "good" rider. Is it the ability to sit long enough on a bucking horse without falling? Is it the rider who owns a badge from some equestrian federation? Or is it the rider who participates in competitions? Is the fact that the rider is a member of an Olympic team enough evidence that he is a good rider? Or is it the rider that empathetically struggled for years on a ruined horse and can finally ride it without any difficulty that should be classified as a good rider?

The opinion of the author is that all riders who have compassion, empathy and respect for the horse, who are able to motivate, train and control the horse with logical and methodical training methods, without doing any physical or psychological damage to the horse, can be considered as such. In similar form, Brigadier Kurt Albrecht said:

"The real disciple of the art of riding does not crave the approval of others, it is more the feeling of being one with his horse. When this harmony is absent, at best, one will have perfect technique, but never perfect art."

From this, one can deduce that a certain amount of humility and capacity for self-criticism to all intents and purposes is necessary so that one does not fixate on erroneous paths with his horse on this long road of training. *Every resistance has a reason and has to be questioned and reflected upon, so that one can save the horse from unnecessary suffering and aggravation.* Self-discipline and self-control are two important virtues a rider should have. Uncontrolled fits of rage towards the horse do not help anybody and often damage the mutual trust forever. Podhajsky used to say:

"One should not foolishly ask something foolish from a horse."

This is still valid today.

However, in order for the rider to get along with the horse and deal with him using fine aids, a flexible, independent seat is the basic technical background that is needed. If a rider is not capable of using his hands independently from the rest of his seat, there will always be a failing of soft communication between horse and rider. The soft giving hand is fundamentally waiting for the incoming impulsion from the hindquarters and may never move backwards in its action. A hand that works backwards will always disturb the forward impulsion, causing tensions in the back and neck of the horse.

An unrelenting and inelastic hand will have contact difficulties and rhythm disturbances as an outcome.

The finely tuned interplay between the driving legs and the waiting hand co-ordinates an almost invisible communication to the horse through the well-balanced seat, making it seem like it is guided by the mere thoughts of the rider. In this ideal image that one should aspire to, the relationship between man and horse creates a momentary work of art, where the journey is the reward.

The great master, de Pluvinel already stated that time and a methodical approach is necessary in order not to damage the horse physically or mentally:

"The charm of a young horse is like the fragrance of a flower—once it is elapsed, it can never return." [The Maneige Royal, Xenophon Press 2010]

5.2.1. The aids

Definition: *An aid is the way the rider can communicate with the horse.*

The rider, sitting on the "navigation bridge," the horse's back, can communicate in four main ways: voice, reins, legs and weight aids. In this list there is no emphasis given with regard to the potency or effectiveness of the single aids. The interplay of the single aids, when they are finely adjusted, will produce discreet, almost invisible influencing of the horse.

It is for this reason that a well-balanced, independent seat is a basic prerequisite for every riding discipline. (Fig:5.20) Even the rider that "only" rides out in the country will be able to cope better with dangerous situations when he has a well-balanced seat, seeing that he can influence the horse better and move with the horse in a more elastic way, re-establishing any momentary loss of control in no time. An incorrect position in the saddle can lead to contact difficulties, due to one-sided overloading. An unbalanced seat results in problems straightening and later on, collecting the horse. The head of the rider, weighing between 5-6 kg, can greatly influence the forehand of the horse when the rider has his head more forward. When one ponders how little application of force a well-balanced rider, who has brought his center of gravity into alignment with that of the horse, applies in order to ride high

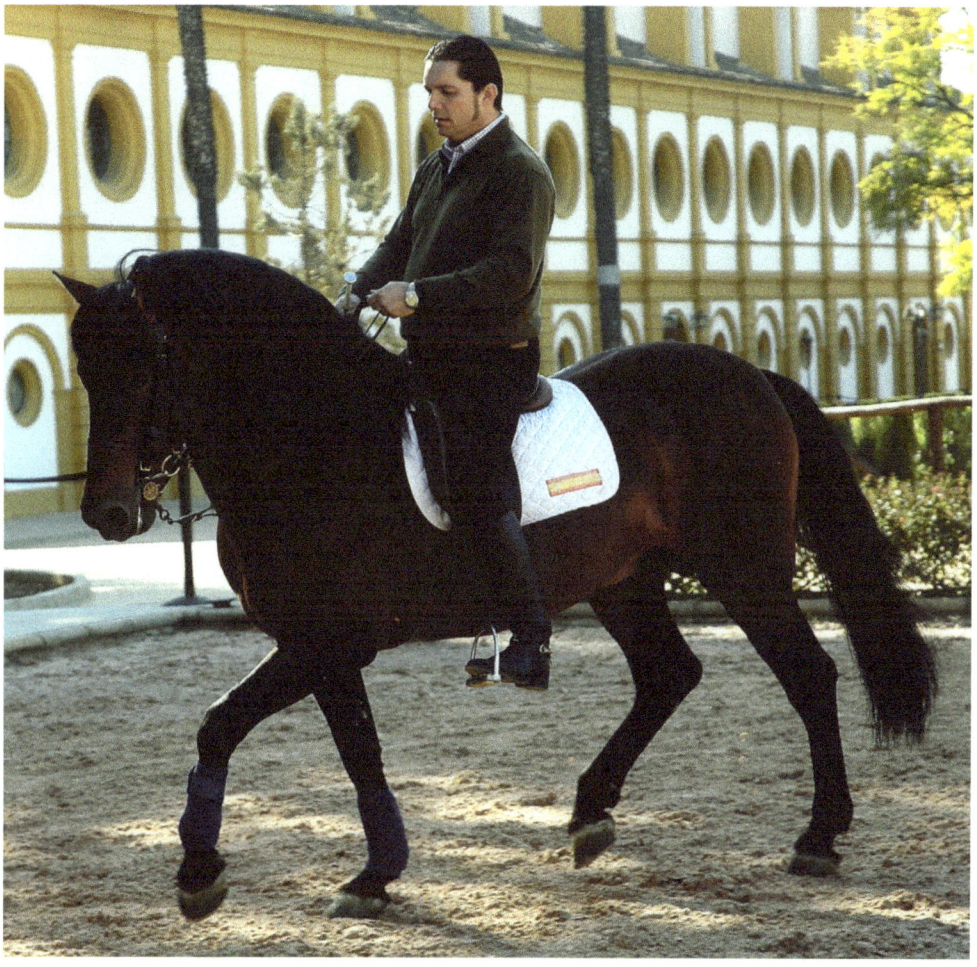

Fig: 5.20 A well-balanced seat with an independent hand are essential for delivering correct aids. The rider's body axis from the shoulder over the elbow down to the heels must be in vertical alignment in a straight and continuous line.

school lessons with seemingly playful ease, it becomes clear how an unsettled seat and incorrect position can greatly influence the balance to its detriment.

The coordination of the dosage can transform every aid from reassuring to penal. It is for this reason that one should always take care to achieve the maximum reaction with a minimum input.

> **Note:** *Only the rider who can control himself, might be able to control his horse!*

Voice

The voice of the rider is definitely the most important way of influencing the horse; not least because this is the first contact the horse has when he first meets man. The young horse gets cultivated by the voice on the lunge, the voice aids refined and by the time the young horse is ridden, he can understand the introduction of the next gait or return to the previous gait. When the voice is used in a deep and quiet tone, it can have a very calming influence. Whistling also has a calming effect on most horses. Animated and harsh words can demand more lively steps from a horse; and can, in the case of an imminent punishment, alarm the horse. Rhythmic clicking of the tongue can support the horse to find a rhythm when working on the lunge or in-hand and even under saddle. Even though the action can be very strong, one should also try to use the voice aids as economically as possible, so the horse does not get used to it and become dull, necessitating the consequent impulsion to be much stronger in order to obtain the same impression.

Rein Aids

Definition: *Rein aids are defined in the first place as the information that is transmitted on the horse's mouth from the hand of the rider. The rein aids should always be applied slightly after the leg aids. When the hand and leg aids take place simultaneously on the horse, the horse will halt, and in this case, the half-halt will then be interpreted as a complete halt.*

Baucher coined the phrase: "leg without hand and hand without leg," but this is often falsely interpreted, as it comprises the fine and sophisticated interplay between giving the leg aid and the waiting hand. The impulsion generated from the legs must either be left, or in the form of half-halts, be more actively one sided on the corresponding, mostly outside hind leg of the horse. In this way the flexion of the leg can be influenced just before it happens, the flexion activity will be slightly slower and therefore prolonged. The haunches become more flexed, leaving the impression that the horse sits down more, lowering more in the hind and lifting more in the front. (Fig: 5.6) Through this adjustment of the hind legs one can partially explain collection.

The half-halt can be executed in one or both directions with upward checks in the direction of the corner of the mouth. (Fig. 5.21a) The half-halt should never be working backward and acting on the tongue, for the effect of a relaxed lower jaw cannot be achieved in this manner. Significant for the understanding of this mode of action of half-halt on both reins, is the simultaneous soft influence on both sides of the corners of the mouth, whereby the relaxation of the lower jaw is achieved on the one hand and elevation of the head and neck on the other hand, producing displacement of the center of gravity towards the hind-end.

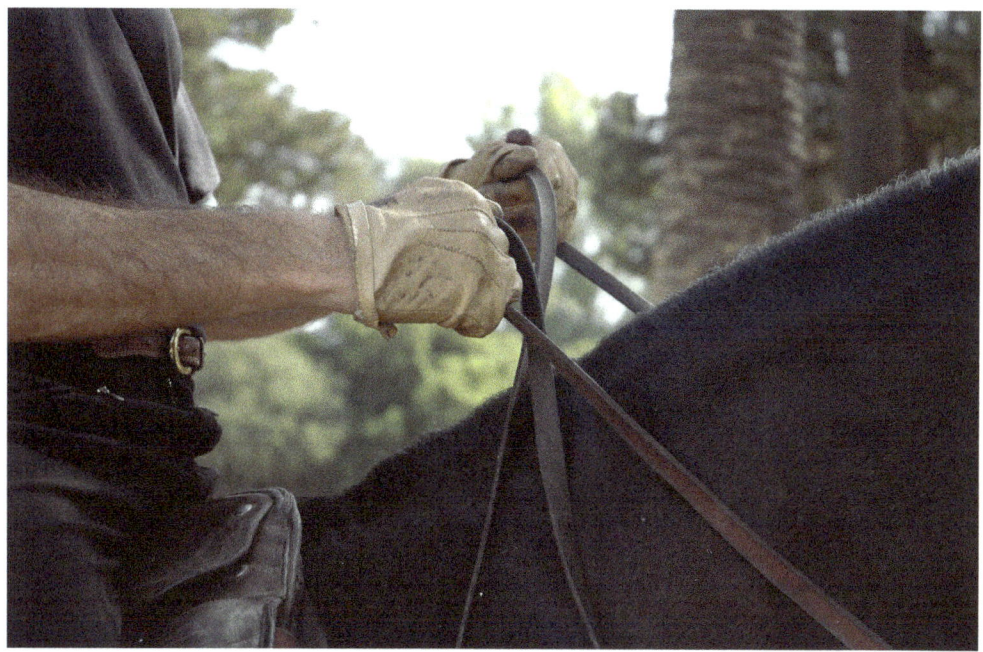

Fig: 5.21a. Half halt with both reins

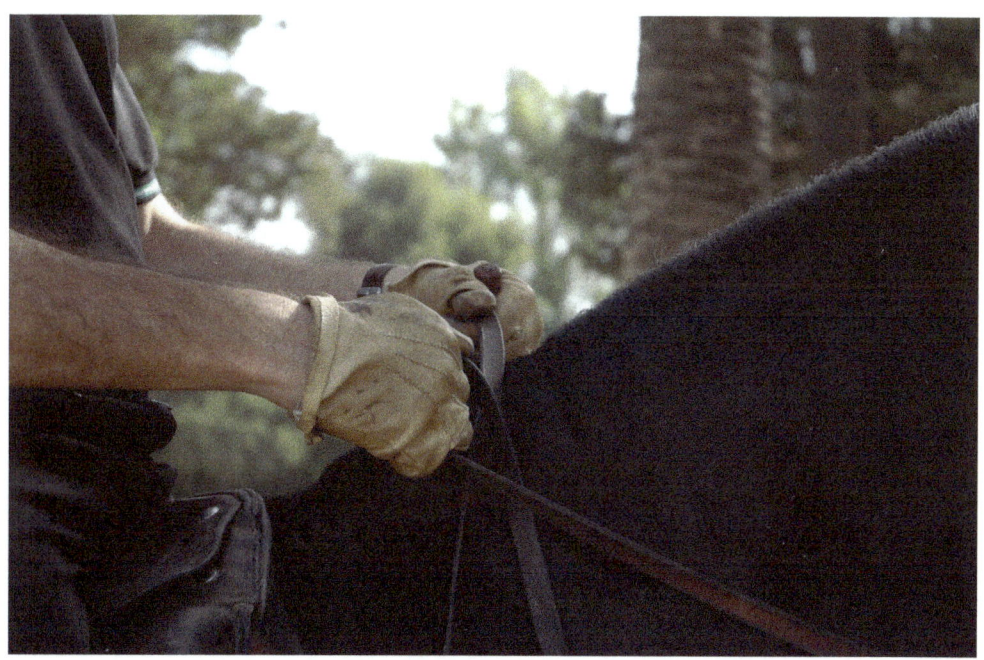

*b. Lowering of the hand after the half halt (*descente de main*)*

The horses seem shorter and take the forward impulsion generated from the legs as a reason to flex the haunches more through the lowering of the croup, thus taking on more weight. What is important, is the finely adjusted interplay between hand and leg, where the hand may never work backwards in a pulling action. The half-halt with both reins should provoke a displacement of the center of gravity to the hind, whereby the horizontal balance change into a vertical balance that is shifted backwards.

Definition: *The horizontal balance is the rectangular posture of the horse where the weight is evenly distributed between all four legs, but having said this, it is anatomically in this sense not really achievable as most of the weight rests on the forehand by nature. Nevertheless, the horse appears to be rectangular in form with his head and neck only moderately elevated.*

As a result, one has an optimal utilization of the neck as a balancing pole in everyday training, together with good back activity that follows, without overloading the haunches. By elevating the head and neck, one tends to move the center of gravity more to the back-end and the horse appears to be shorter, and thus setting up the so-called vertical balance.

Definition: *Vertical balance is the result of systematic gymnastic exercise of the horse, where the increased bend in the haunches results in a shorter base of support for the legs. The horse becomes more stable in his balance and therefore more agile.*

Horses that become heavy on one hand, can be corrected by using a one-sided half-halt on the side that is heavy. The result is a lifting of the shoulder on that side and an indirect impact by the rein on the diagonally opposite hind leg.

When the horse goes too deep in the front, this can be corrected by bilateral [both sides] action of the half-halt in interplay with the leg aids to help to return the lost balance. In spite of the uplifting action of the bilateral half-halt, one should not forget that leaning on the bit is the result of a hind leg that is not active enough.

Essential for the use of the half-halt is the pulsing vibration of the rein. After setting up the desired effect (yielding in the poll, becoming lighter, elevation, etc), the horse must immediately be rewarded with a release of the rein, the so-called "*descente de main*." (lowering of the hand: fig.5.21.b)

The French school, known for its particular lightness (*Legerité*) differentiates basically between five various rein aids, besides the half-halt and the complete halt.

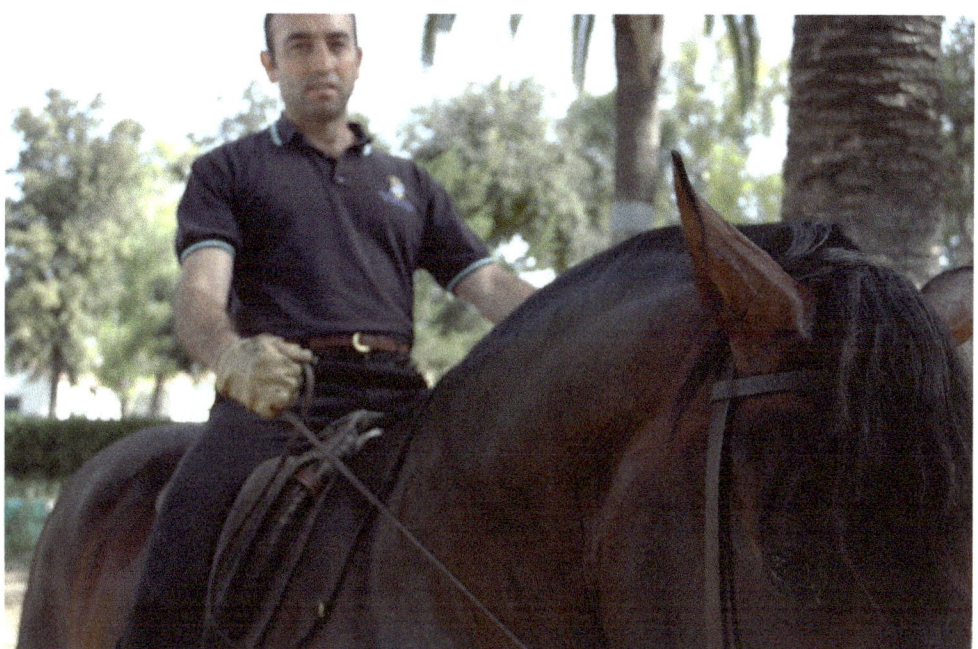

Fig:5.22: Opening rein aids

The opening rein: With the opening rein the rider opens his hand position in a wide berth to the inside and thus moves the inside rein away from the neck of the horse. (Fig. 5.22) The leg aids stay active equilaterally, the inside leg causes bend and the outside remains supporting. This will cause the horse to follow a circular line with an inside bend, as the inside shoulder leads the way and is free to step far forward since it is not loaded. This interaction is also brilliantly suited to recover momentary loss of contact, when the horse was frightened and tightened his neck for example.

The opposing effect: This is a one-sided rein action on the mouth of the horse together with ipsilateral sideways stimulating leg aids (fig:5.23). This will cause the croup to move to the outside, whilst the inside shoulder is more loaded. In this case the inside shoulder serves as the pivot point and the horse is positioned against the movement. This action is used in the turn on the forehand in order to obtain more control and flexibility of the neck.

The indirect effect: With the indirect effect, the reins are used in the direction [of travel] over the mane (fig:5.24), whereby the outside pushing leg aid causes the horse to step over with the outside shoulder and thus move with the forehand around the hindquarters.

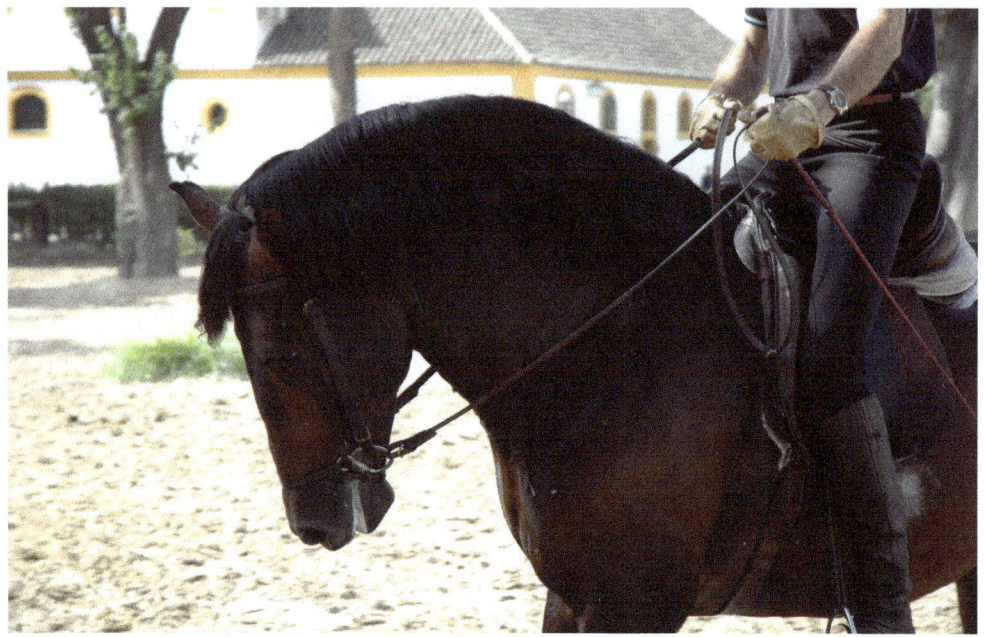

Fig:5.23. opposing effect

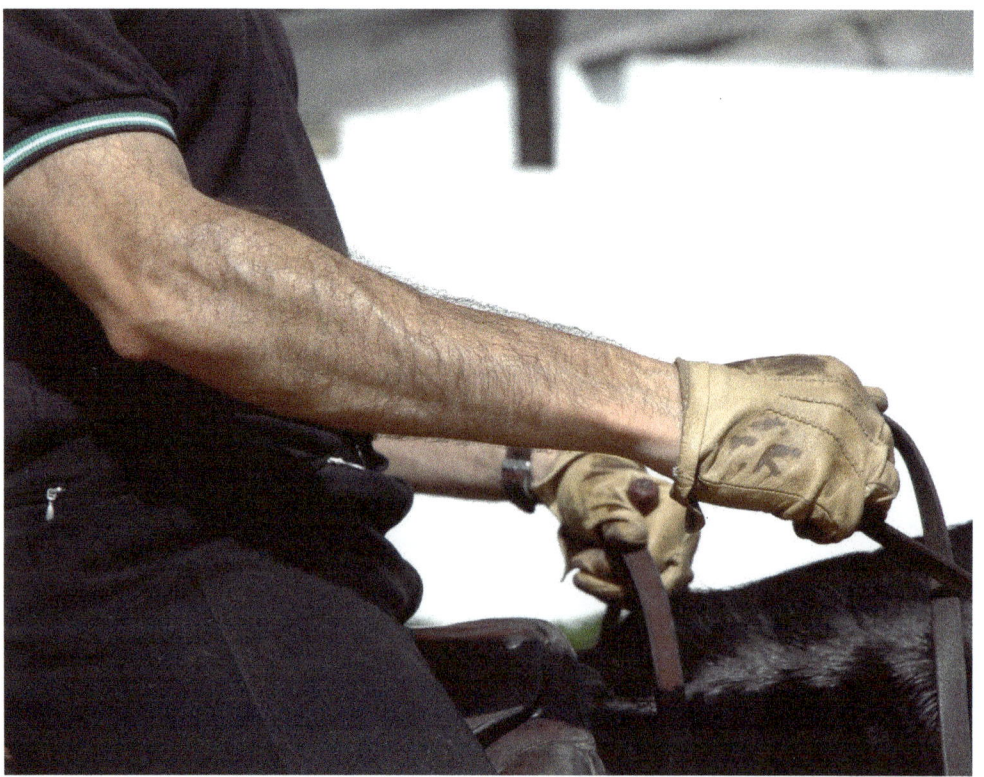

Fig:5.24: Indirect effect

Fig. 5.25 Leg Aids

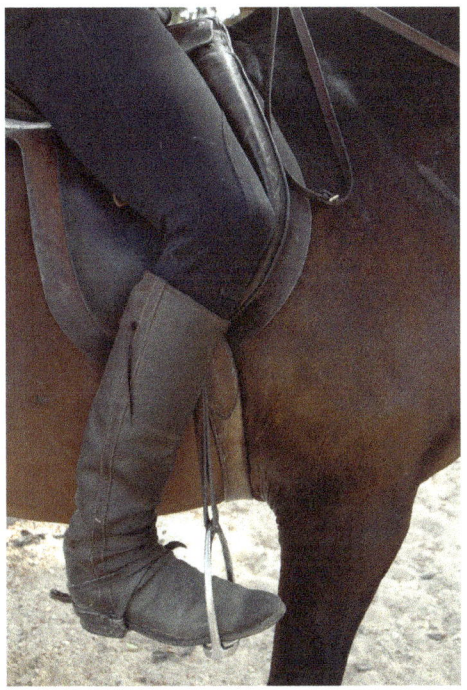
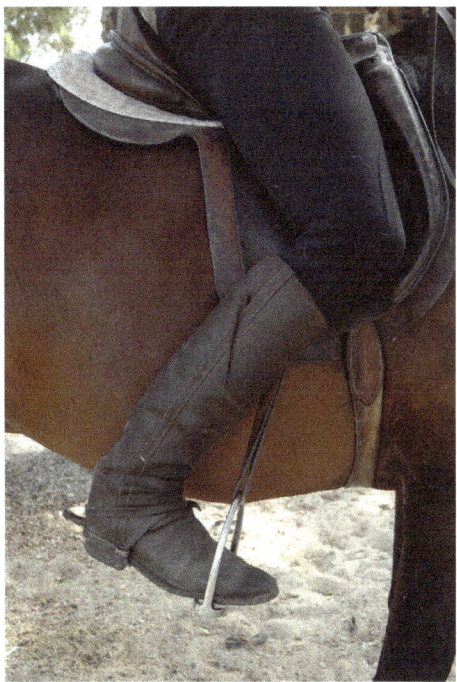

a. Forward driving leg   b. Lateral driving leg

The indirect opposing effect Similar to the indirect rein aids, the inside rein is directed towards the mane and the outside leg creates pressure. Through this effect, the horse will shift his croup to the inside while the shoulder will move to the outside in response to the indirect rein aid. A release of the inside shoulder and an enhanced bend in the spinal column will be fostered. Using this aid, one can develop a turn on the forehand in renvers [haunches-out] from this position, this considerably improves the suppleness of the horse.

The indirect opposing effect to the back: The difference to the indirect opposing effect is that the inside rein does not get directed towards the mane; instead, it opens towards the direction of the rider's abdomen. At the same time the inside leg pushes, triggering a lateral movement which frees the outside shoulder through the activity of the inside hind leg. This is excellent introducing lateral aids to the young horse, and later for developing half-pass.

Leg Aids

The leg aids are fundamental for maintaining forward movement as well as lateral movement. Without driving power from behind, the hand cannot receive anything, and riding can just as well be knocked on the head.

One differentiates between forward and lateral driving leg aids as well as the supporting leg aids.

The **forward driving aids** will encourage the desire to move forward through rhythmic application or tension of the calf muscles (fig:5.25a). The impulse of the legs will cause a reflex contraction of the fascia on the abdomen and a slight lifting of the corresponding hind leg will result. When this reflex is thus conditioned through the training process, one can appropriately employ the response of the corresponding hind leg. Nevertheless, the forward driving leg should also be active in the halt and in transitions so as to not provoke a dwindling transition. The horse must be driven with the forward leg aids to step under his center of gravity in such a way that the sustaining and waiting hand of the rider should feel the impression that the horse wants to lift himself off the forehand through the springiness of the transitions. This has nothing in common with abrupt halts provoked by the hand, because a springy transition is only possible when the back of the horse is elastic and supple.

The **sideways driving aids** must always be employed in combination with the forward driving leg aids; a backwards tendency should be avoided at all costs. This will only teach a horse that he can withdraw [suck back] himself from the aids of the rider and become uncontrollable in the process.

Furthermore, this contradicts the classical sentence of Steinbrecht, that says "ride your horse forward and straighten him." In the lateral gait, the sideways driving leg should act rhythmically in time when the leg lifts off the ground, in order to allow for a longer swing phase and thus guarantee the crossing over. This will stretch the outside muscles of the hindquarters as the hind leg must step more under the center of gravity with the help of the sideways driving leg aid.

The **supporting leg** [or guarding leg] acts in a restricting way on the outside of the horse; for example, on a circle or in a lateral movement, in order for the horse to maintain the degree of bend or position (fig: 5.25b). The supporting leg aid must always be active in conjunction with the outside rein that defines the bend or position. Otherwise the horse will stagger in a curve to the middle of the arena and control will be lost over the inside hind leg as a result.

At this point it is good to refer once again to the alternating interaction between the impulse from the leg and the waiting hand of the rider, since a simultaneous action of the two aids will produce a halt. The waiting hand regulates and shapes the forward impulsion from the hindquarters in such a way that it becomes possible for the rider to sculpt the pattern of the muscle. The hand must never work backwards and in such that it blocks the hind leg on that side. Tension in the neck and lumbar areas could be pre-programed in this way, but are avoidable.

In concluding the leg aids, mention must be made of the action of the spurs. Spurs simply serve as refinement of the leg aids and must never be seen as a means to maintain forward movement alone. Continuous and/or excessive use of the spurs will only dull the horse. Horses that are "dead" to the legs are introduced to fine aids with great difficulty, for they have learned to suffer the hardship of the pain from the rider with a passive consistency.

The moment when the forward impulsion cannot be maintained anymore should also signify the end of the art of riding. It is for this reason that the young horse especially should be carefully introduced to the spurs as they will often kick out as an impulse due to a ticklish reaction and therefore interpret the lesson in the wrong way. It is therefore advisable to habituate the young horse first to the voice and girth aids. Once the horse is secure in what is expected of him, one can carefully introduce the use of the spurs.

The rider's weight aid

The subject has already been broached as to how sensitive and delicate a horse reacts to changes in balance. This is especially conspicuous when a young horse is started and because he has not found his balance under the rider, the horse moves unsteadily under every gesture the rider makes. In the same way the untouched mouth of the young horse is still fine, sensitive and active.

In practice: *This basic willingness to respond should be kept at all costs, for the horse trained to become a dressage horse should react with the maximum lightness to minimal influence from the rider. These conditions are present in most young horses and must not be ruined by unsystematic training combined with a high measure of pressure to perform.*

In this combination we are once again reminded of the words of the great French riding master, de Pluvinel, that have lost none of their validity in the intervening years: By virtue of the balanced and independent seat, the three-point seat (two seat bones and the pubic bone), it is possible for the rider to influence his weight distribution by rotating about the axis of his own body, sit deeper through relaxation of the buttock muscles, and by rising from the saddle.

The dressage seat (or the basic seat) should be the starting position of every influence over the horse, whereupon elegance goes hand in-hand with functionality and effectiveness. The line from the shoulder through the elbow to the heels must be a consistent and continuous one, as this is the only possibility the rider has to have his own center of gravity in accord with that of the horse. (Fig: 5.20)

Once this basic balance has been found, it is very easy to more or less to disturb the balance with little changes, and in this way change the direction of the movement and even produce high school movements. It is fundamental to always align the shoulders of the rider with that of the horse, for already by the turning of the body axis one can initiate a change of direction. If for example, one requires a half-pass, the inside seat bone must be weighted along with increased weight on the inside stirrup. By means of this inside weight on the seat bone it is possible for the horse to relax the outside M. longissimus in order for it to stretch and thus cause a bend with the extra help of the inside bending leg of the rider.

By the same token the situation is the same when riding lateral gaits, where the rider should always sit in the direction of the movement and therefore allow the horse to step into the desired bend.

The only exception in this context is portrayed by the shoulder-in, where the rider sits on the inside seat bone to stretch the outside long back muscle, but due to the inside position of the horse, the rider actually sits "against" the direction of the movement. In this specific case it is necessary, in order to achieve a lowering of the inside hip, whereby the inside hind leg is animated to take more load through more adduction. Furthermore, this increased loading capacity will induce more freedom of the outside shoulder, develops collection and improves the freedom of the shoulder considerably. This can be achieved as long as this bend is achieved through the inside leg aid and not by pulling the head to the side with the hand.

The more collected horse can work on a smaller the base of support and the horse becomes easier to direct and to turn. A majestic, powerful movement is generated, and the horse appears to be liberated in the front.

> **Note:** *The measure of collection is not necessarily slowness, but rather the increased will to go, based on the expectant hand that reduces the dimension of the gait. (Nuno Oliveira)*

PART II: TRAINING AND PREVENTING PROBLEMS

6. The Schooling of the Horse

6.1. The question of the specific riding technique: French, Spanish or German after all?

It has become the fashion today to adapt the riding style of the country of origin of any breed of horse, then implementing it in your own country. In many countries, the different riding styles emerged organically from working with livestock and from the inherent absolute obedience required of the horse to ensure the safety of the rider. The resulting riding styles were very efficient, as the original use was proof enough of its existence. The usually brusque methods used to obtain absolute obedience in dangerous situations, often causes a loss of delicacy in communication between horse and rider, as this kind of riding is practical and bound to the specific original purpose.

Classical dressage training has the purpose of making the horse obedient, agile and comfortable for the rider, while keeping it healthy for as long as possible through systematic training. This very modern view was already taken by the founder of the systematic training of horses, François Robichon de la Guérinière [*École de Cavalerie,* Xenophon Press 1992], who up to present day, remains the pioneer of the classical art of riding.

France can, in this context, then be described as the cradle of the classical art of riding, as all important works on riding, starting with de Pluvinel, and Guérinière up to Baucher have their origins in this country. The French art of riding is based on the concept of "*Legerité,*" or lightness, and the slogan "Balance before movement." The practical implementation would be that the horse must be free from all muscular tension even before it begins moving in order to achieve maximum lightness and the finest contact with the hand of the rider.

According to Baucher, all tension in the body is reflected by an inactive, hard mouth with an inflexible poll and lower jaw. Therefore, he sought to rectify the problems in the body of the horse through systematic mobilization and stretching exercises. His flexion exercises at a standstill and, later on, during movement are the precursors to the modern mobilization techniques of today. A horse that is always light in the hand and reacts willingly to the leg of the rider is the specified goal of the French system. Baucher wanted a collected horse that could be easily steered, turned and controlled in order to execute his art in maximum *Legerité* [lightness].

On the other hand, German (or F.N.) riding seeks a continuous contact and a constantly collectible horse as essential. Nonetheless, both the German riding system and the Spanish Riding School in Vienna see the school of the French master F. R. de la Guérinière as "classical," thus rendering the question of a riding nationality relative.

Commercial competition riding most certainly plays a substantial role in the horse business today and is most certainly a driving factor in the further development of the sport and breeding. It is on this account that "classical riding," which is seen as an art form, is often placed at the opposite end of the spectrum.

> **Definition:** *In the first place the definition of classical must be addressed. According to the dictionary of Meyers it is explained as harmonious, complete, self-contained.*

Interestingly enough, this dictionary does not refer to riding per sé, but one recognizes significant characteristics of riding in this.

It is generally known that art lies in the eye of the beholder, therefore, no one should judge what should be rated as such. Riding as sport and riding as an art are no exceptions to this; as it always lies with the rider what performance and interpretation is to be undertaken.

This does not mean that how the horse is kept, and prevention of physical and psychological damage while training, should be forgotten. The guiding principle "he who moves slowly in the art of riding will arrive quicker to the goal" should be adhered to.

With this in mind, systematic training should also be of assistance to the horse. Artistic elements, that are common in certain styles of riding, are not excluded from systematic training and vice versa. Accordingly, one cannot speak of a better system when said system is continuously developed, improving the horse and not allowing him to suffer physical and psychological damage. Combining the two, (at first glance different) beliefs, could possibly be of great benefit to the health of the horse, which should always be put first in the partnership between horse and rider. The art in training lies in finding the individual way for each horse—in finding a way to improve his faults and bring out his strengths without wearing him out during the training. This also applies when a horse does not seem to fit into a conventional system. The important part is that the horse shows us how trainable he is. A clever and sensitive trainer can model a horse according to his specific capabilities. It is also a great art to know when to stop and praise the horse, for this is the only way to establish a trusting relationship between the horse and his rider.

The art of riding is an ever changing process, based on the natural ability of the horse, and one should not constrict this dynamic process with inflexible and rigid rules. The art of riding does not permit false teachings that are harmful to the horse to be administered freely.

The great rider and former chief rider of the Spanish Riding School in Vienna, Arthur Kottas-Heldenberg, once clearly showed the two ways and defined it as follows: "There are only two ways of riding—the right way and the wrong way."

The correct, often unpleasant, lengthy and rocky way, however, sets the foundation for meaningful cooperation with the horse, to make it more beautiful and pleasing to the rider. The wrong way entices with short term translucent success. That which has an unstable foundation is harmful to the horse.

6.2. Riding disciplines and their specific problems

The characteristic patterns of movement of the horses participating in the respective branches will be critically analyzed in this Chapter. The pre- and post-competition care that arises as a result will require different preparation and treatment of trigger points that are specific for each discipline. The growing requirement and specialization of a vet and physical therapist in this field is daunting. It is evermore difficult to meet all demands. A short description of the different branches will improve the general understanding of the "occupational" problem areas.

6.2.1. Dressage

Note: *The dressage horse is known as the body builder of horses. Dressage horses must float through the arena in a rhythmic, cadenced and light-footed manner, while the movement should be powerful and collected at the same time.*

Because of the composition of a dressage test, the horse must be able to perform slow, consistent, powerful movements for a longer period of time (up to 8 minutes). Dressage horses do not reach the anaerobic phase of metabolism as often as a racehorse, but this kind of burden is a mental strain as well as a physical one. Mental tension before competition can put unnecessary stress on these sensitive specialists and makes economical movement really difficult. In this discipline it is therefore extremely important to keep the horses' temperament as balanced as possible and not scare them from performing well. Achieving and keeping both the mental and physical suppleness is the key for the dressage horse as the results will make themselves known in the test scores.

The carrying ability of the hindquarters should be even more trained, as well as the neck and poll areas, for these seem to be the most vulnerable in this discipline. The back, as the connecting link between the front and the hindquarters, must swing in an elastic way allowing the rider's aids through. Depending on the degree of collection, the back must be able to round. Lengthening of the gaits requires an elastic and shock-absorbing forehand, where the range of movement seems to be effortless and the muscles can absorb the tremendous thrust from the hind legs.

When this is not the case, the shoulder muscles become tense and the tendons and joints are overtaxed, making tendinitis and navicular disease possible. The fetlock and the splint bones are also highly stressed in the trot extensions.

The long back muscle is exposed to severe stress when the rider sits on a horse that has not been sufficiently prepared. The horse will suffer especially in more collected work and in the extensions, causing unevenness and problems with being ridden. The contraction of the M. longissimus dorsi will fix the vertebrae and make it difficult for the rider to sit. Subsequently the horse has to take the full impact on his skeleton. These horses look like they are divided, and it is very difficult to get them round again. The area of the flanks over the kidneys must be powerful and flexible for this is the connection where the power of the hindquarters gets thrust on the vertebrae. When this area is tense, unevenness and problems with collection become obvious. The horse goes against the hands of the rider and the movement of the croup looks horizontal.

It is clear that a dressage horse has various parts of his body heavily burdened in the collection and extension exercises. Other than the correct warm-up, the following can be offered as rehabilitation and prevention:

1. Relaxing of the neck and poll. Massage and stretching of the shoulder and back muscles. Stretching of the hind legs, especially forward to lengthen the hamstrings. Lifting the back by stimulating the reflex point on the stomach.

2. Magnetic blankets and boots can be used successfully in the warm-up phase and post competition to aid in the transport of waste material.

3. Acupuncture can be used as trigger point therapy to correct the energy balance, as can laser therapy when a specialist in acupuncture is not available.

4. Regular lungeing twice a week with a suitable aid (for example a modified Pessoa system) or cavaletti training can bring variety and gymnastic advantages to dressage work. Going for a hack as mental equilibrium can also work wonders.

5. Thermography can be used as prevention, as changes in heat patterns, for example in the tendons, can be seen weeks before the actual clinical lameness manifests itself. Lameness can therefore be drastically reduced by early intervention of changing the training plan or cooling the tendons.

> **In practice:** *Errors occurring frequently: Hard and inflexible rider's hands, insufficiently independent seat, horse becoming dulled through permanent leg aids, no interplay between tension and relaxation, lack of carrying ability, wanting to achieve something too fast, lack of suppleness, too little variety.*

6.2.2. Jumping

> **Note:** *In contrast with the dressage horse, the jumper has several tons of weight on the hind legs (take-off) and then several tons on the forehand (landing) for a short period of time. The physiology of jumping causes compression of the spinous processes in the withers and enormous tension on the serratus muscles and the tendons.*

The energy of the jumper is normally sufficient as the duration of the course is normally short enough, even with all the short sprints and turns, and the horse seldom reaches the anaerobic phase. A bigger problem is the sudden turn, pull and stop pressure on the body of the horse. Tears in muscles and tendons can be the result of sudden changes of direction on the fully loaded legs, especially when the horses have not been warmed up properly.

Trigger points in the shoulder areas are not rare and can be the reason for unwillingness to jump. The head and neck is more or less free in most of the jumpers, but enormous pressure can be exerted on the mouth and poll in sharp turns and half-halts before each jump in the jump-off. Development of the lower neck can often be a problem in jumpers, where the use of running reins are commonly an attempt to correct this predicament. Trying to force the head down in this matter causes greater pull against the rider's hand and even more powerful development of the lower neck muscles, thereby never achieving the corrective effect. The forward and down stretch is especially valuable for jumpers, as the back should bascule in a rounded way over the jump.

The muscles in the hindquarters, that must push off strongly before a jump, are extremely susceptible to tears and also to calcification. This area should therefore be warmed up carefully.

The hocks and knee joints are just as vulnerable as the sacra-iliac joint to injuries.

The back muscles are prone to tension especially in the Latissimus and trapezius areas. The degree depends on the gymnastic effect of dressage movements used and the pounding of the total weight of the rider right behind the shoulder blades when the horse lands after a jump.

1. T.E.N.S. treatment of the back and hamstrings as well as stretching of the neck and shoulder area is advantageous. Targeted use of a soft laser on localized trigger points, and acupressure mobilization techniques can be very

helpful in releasing tension.

2. Manually rounding the back and magnetic blankets and boots also have a positive effect on the performance of the jumper.

3. Regular gymnastic dressage training encourages elasticity and can be improved even further with lungeing and free jumping. The use of training aids, however, should be thoroughly thought-out and should not be used according to current trends.

> **In practice:** *Errors occurring frequently: Too strong hand influence, too little systematic dressage training, jumping big jumps too often (wear), lack of suppleness and ease, use of strong bits and training aids, too much pressure from the rider causing mental stress.*

6.2.3. Doma Vaquera and Western Reining

The disciplines of Doma Vaquera and reining unites riding with working livestock.

Doma Vaquera, the Spanish forerunner of reining is distinguished through working purely at the walk and canter, in which the horses not only have to perform lateral work and fast turns (pirouettes and *media vueltas*) but also stop from a full canter (Fig. 6.1 and 6.2). Further difficulty in this discipline are flying changes, up to changes of leg every stride. Flowing transitions and fast reactions are required, which inevitably causes strong loading on the back and hindquarters of the horse as well as on the tendons of the front legs. In contrast to the sliding stop in western riding, the Vaquera horse must come to an abrupt halt without sliding too far.

The area of the long back muscles are extremely prone to tension, as the horses seldom get worked through the back and kissing spine syndrome can be, as with the jumper, the painful result of inadequate preparation of the horse's body. Abrupt turns take their toll on the neck and poll, as the vaquera horses, in contrast to the western horses, have to work with their heads in relative elevation. This results in tension in the poll and temporal-mandibular joint. Extreme stepping under the body with the hindquarters has the consequence that the horses have sacroiliac problems, which may be helped with osteopathic treatments. The saddle can also cause problems in the caudal region of the supraspinous ligament, especially when the horses actually work with livestock; for example when the *garrocha*[5] is used to trip a bull at a full gallop. The sudden jerk when the bull falls causes punctual loading at the back edge of the saddle and hematomas and infection can result. The construction of the vaquera saddle has the horse positioned in the front and

---

5 A long rod with tip of metal used to direct animals in the field.

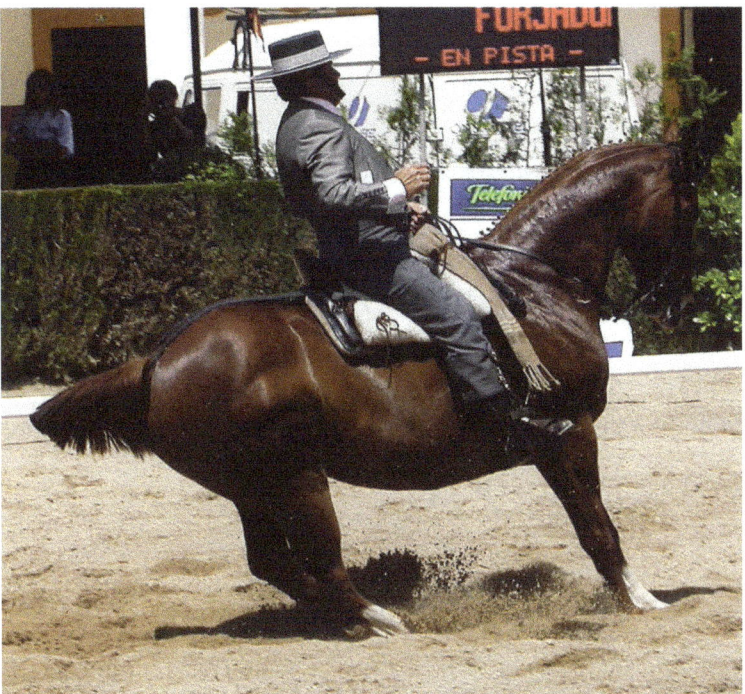

Fig 6.1. The *parada raya*, the abrupt stop from a full gallop, is probably amongst one of the most difficult exercises in the Doma Vaquera. The extreme tipping of the pelvis puts more pressure on the sacro-iliac joint, while the canter has to be intercepted by the front legs, which in turn causes severe loading of the tendons. This photo show a correctly executed *parada raya*.

the back with iron bars, with straw bundles in between that function as the tree. Enormous pressure points in the area of the trapezius muscle can arise as a result of a saddle that is too narrow.

Traditionally, the vaquero had to ride straight for hours and only had to perform a few turns with short sprints without really bending. The classical vaquero saddle was also built for this purpose (Fig. 7.7). The wide bearing surface made problem-free, uniform weight distribution possible during the long working hours. In the competition sport nowadays, the horses have to show more bend as well as collection and the traditional saddle does not allow for this due to its length and construction. The saddle will shift diagonally when the horse has to bend and the horse is unable to move behind the shoulders and at the caudal arch of the ribs.

In the discipline of reining, the spin and the sliding stop are key exercises. The horses move with a relatively low head carriage in a slow walk or canter.

In the spin, the horses turn very fast around the hindquarters, but not in the canter rhythm as is the case in classical dressage, where the loins and hamstrings have to be severely stretched.

In the sliding stop the horse has to stop from a full gallop with extremely seated hindquarters and the utmost arching of the loins, while still continuing to walk with the forelegs, which is what causes the impression of "sliding."

This exercise requires extremely strong and resilient hamstrings and loin muscles. Tearing and calcification in the semi-membranosus and semi-tendinosus muscles are frequent with excessive training. The sacroiliac area is also heavily strained by this extreme arching.

Less experienced horses also suffer in their front limbs such as the shoulder girdle and the trapezius muscle areas. This can quickly lead to overloading of the check ligaments of the deep digital flexor tendons. It is often forgotten that western horses are already broken in at a very young age, 1.5 to 2 years, and the overloading of the training, combined with the still growing skeleton, can have devastating effects. Wear and tear of the joints, ligaments and tendons are therefore no exception in these horses.

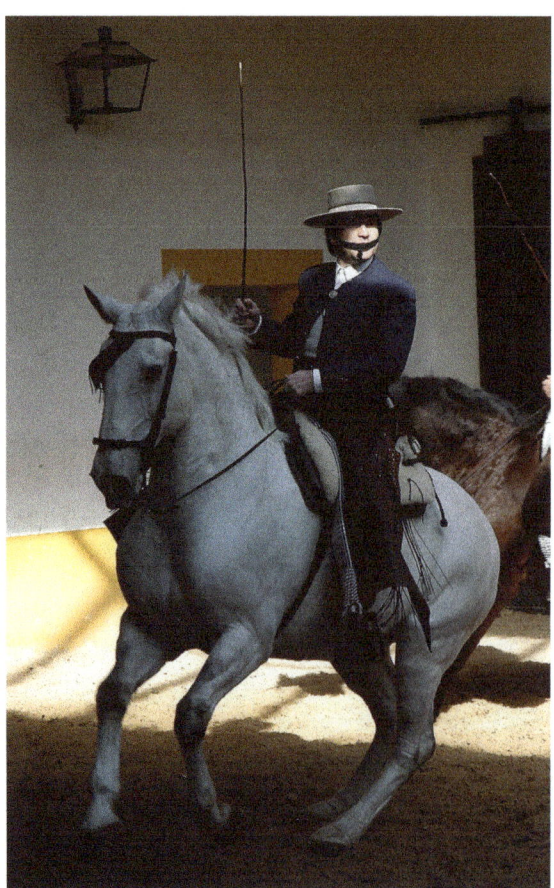

Fig. 6.2
The "vaquera turn on the haunches" is demonstrated by the Spanish rider, Angel Cid. It is a fast turn on the haunches in two or three movements and is used for fighting bulls in the field to change direction rapidly. The classical canter pirouette is a short canter turn around the haunches in 6-8 strides with a very cadenced up and down movement of the hindquarters done much slower.

Another special discipline in western riding is cutting, where the horse has to perform turns, acceleration and sliding stops at lightning speed in order to separate a calf from the herd. These super-fast turning maneuvers, mainly initiated by the horse himself—not within the normal range of movement for the spinal column—will subject it to early wear and tear. Ankylosis of the transverse processes of the lumbar vertebrae, arthritis of the joints between the vertebrae are all signs of athletic overload.

The shoulder muscles should be relaxed and ready to cushion the impact, so in order to avoid tears in the muscles it is important for the horse to be warmed up properly.

Barrel racing—as the fastest discipline in western riding—asks for a lot of speed with a lot of fast turning and the front legs are subjected to major turn and drag forces. The tight turns around the barrels calls for a very high capacity to bend. Due to the laws of biomechanics, these dramatic turns can only be achieved through rapid maneuvers and changes of direction. The results of these actions are mainly joint inflammation and damaged tendons, as well as bracing of the neck and back muscles.

1. TENS-treatment, massage and magnetic field therapy of the affected body parts can be extremely helpful in this sport. Trigger point and acupuncture treatments can contribute to the elasticity and mobility shortly before a competition.

2. Systematic gymnastic exercises should nevertheless be a part of the physical and psychological preparation of these "extreme" athletes.

In practice: *Prevention of frequent errors: Doma Vaquera: asking too much elevation of the head, being "on the bit" too early, lack of working the horse through the back, the working trot is often omitted as a working gait in the fully trained horse, abrupt turns and stops without sufficient preparation, inadequate warm-up before the daily work, irregular training, sharp bits to solve a problem with bending. Western: through misunderstanding of collection, only slow way of going without impulsion with head in a low position and no overstepping. Over-bending the neck in order to achieve longitudinal bending through the body. Strong, often exaggerated use of the hand with big movements and hand held high. Absent inside leg aids make bending the horse more difficult.*

6.2.4. Eventing

Note: *In this sport, the horses need to faultlessly compete in three different disciplines: dressage, jumping and cross-country.*

Training eventers are certainly the most intensive and most time consuming (several hours per day) of all riding disciplines, in order to not only gain in muscle power but also in stamina. Due to the chronology of eventing, the horses are always at risk of developing anaerobic metabolism. They produce too much lactic acid in the bloodstream, which makes supplementing with electrolytes and water absolutely essential.

The horse should be fine on the first day of dressage. The degree of collection is not extremely high, not even in the top classes, as the horses probably do not have as much possibility to bend their haunches due to the extreme endurance capacity that is needed.

The cross country course on the second day requires tremendous athletic performance, with up to 50 kg of weight loss per horse per competition, as they only gallop with frequent rhythm changes, and have numerous obstacles to clear. The obstacles on these courses are fixed and this requires both jumping ability and courage. The proprioception of the horse is significantly tested by different kinds of terrain, jumping up and down, jumping into water etc Apart from the endurance required, the horse also needs courage and a good eye to judge the distances correctly.

In the big competitions, there is also a race course, and the distance must be completed at a full gallop. This requires incredible extension of the horse's position, and tests the full capacity of the horse's heart and lung volume. In this phase the accumulation of lactic acid can become a problem as the demands on the organism are relatively long in relationship to the energy reserve. These distances often take around 15 minutes to complete, stressing the heart and lungs to maximum capacity, and the energy reserves for short sprints is just not sufficient. Careful preparation, which includes interval training and regular controlling of the pulse and breathing, to reach the perfect performance, is indispensable.

On the third day the horses must jump a circuit which draws on the last reserves of the horse. Once again the decisive factor lies not in the height or difficulty of the course, but that the horse completes it successfully and in an orderly tempo.

1. On the basis of the major requirements from the body of the horse, TENS, massage and mobilization techniques should be performed regularly. Cooling of the legs with ice (cool bags) is recommended after each time they have been strained. I recommend regular thermo-graphic monitoring, as a difference in the heat pattern can be seen before a clinical lameness shows up. Going easy on the horse and cooling can alleviate this difference in temperature.

2. Magnetic field therapy and acupuncture can also help performance and keep the horse fit and elastic for longer.

> **In practice:** *Common errors: Too little or not enough gymnastic exercises, over-training with too much endurance training, a high percentage of thoroughbred blood in the horses can make them more difficult to handle, especially in the cross-country phase.*

6.2.5. Leisure riding horse

Interestingly enough, to date no-one has thought too much about the special needs of the so called leisure riding horse, even though these horses are exposed to considerable and especially irregular stresses. Most of these horses spend the entire week in the paddock with their stable companions and on the weekends have to put up with long rides out for several hours without sufficient preparation through regular training.

Severe cases of tying up, azoturia, tendon and joint inflammation may result from this. In many cases the situation can be aggravated by unsuitable bridles and ill-fitting saddles, and back problems make the horse even more reluctant to be ridden.

Leisure riding horses often have gymnastics required of them, but due to the ignorance of the rider it is not correctly performed and the correct muscle growth and flexibility is never reached. (Fig. 6.3)

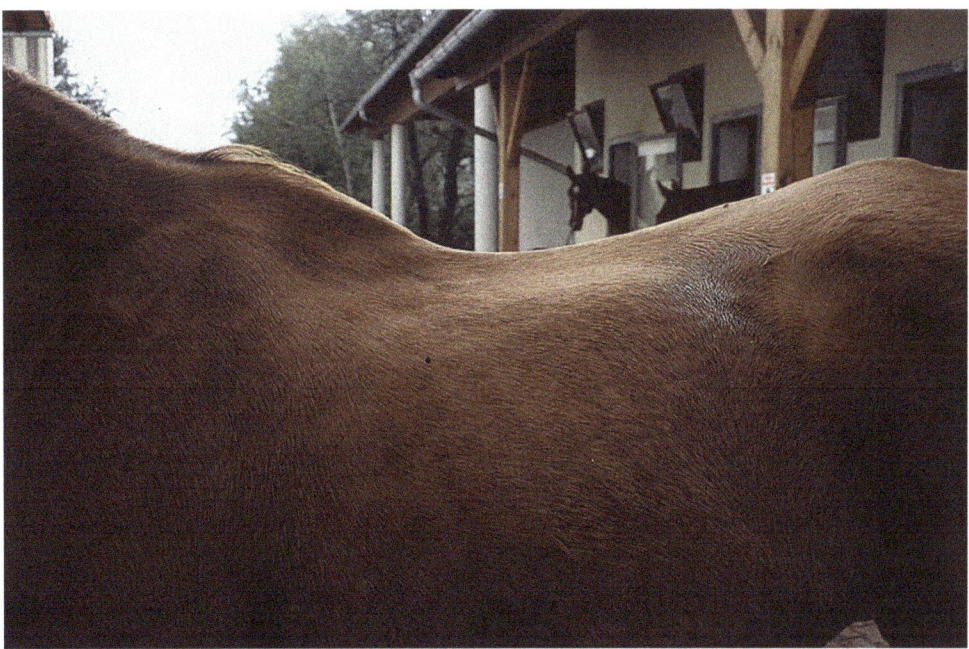

Fig.6.3. This extremely high degree of muscle atrophy is often seen in leisure riding horses due to insufficient and irregular training. Note the protruding spinal processes behind the loin area, also known as hunters bump, which is the result of enormous muscle atrophy in the area.

Due to frequent irregular training, the muscles cannot develop adequately, and choosing a correct fitting saddle becomes almost impossible. If the saddle is chosen to fit the angle of the shoulder blade, the lacking muscles can provoke pressure points from the saddle. When a slightly smaller saddle is chosen to avoid pressure points, the muscles lying directly underneath are prevented from developing, making any increase in muscle very difficult.

Pressure behind the cartilage of the shoulder blades causes a lot of tension, making the length of stride shorter especially in the front legs. Trigger points in the neck and shoulder area are the consequences.

Nevertheless, the owners of these leisure horses should be credited that they do a lot with work from the ground in the form of "horsemanship" and these "horse whisperers" are often preoccupied with the emotional side of the horse and find peace of mind with their leisure friend.

Regular massage and acupuncture can definitely be helpful for these horses, nevertheless one should not only look at the correctness of how the horse is kept (in the paddock), but also be concerned with planning regular training sessions with correct equipment in order to avoid too many problems with the body of the horse.

In practice: *Frequent problems: Irregular and unsystematic training, lacking gymnastics and suppleness, ill-fitting tack, bad seat of the rider disturbing the horse's balance.*

6.2.6. Racehorses

Note: *Race horses are started very young while still growing. Apart from limitations of temperamental make-up, these horses have significant discrepancies between stress levels and underdeveloped physical capacity to cope.*

Even though horses that mature earlier are used in both branches (flat racing and trotting), it must be remembered that horses that are broken in at 1-1.5 years, are both physically and mentally still "kids." The growth plates of a horse only close at 5 years of age, and overloading the system, as can happen in racing, can result in serious damage to the bones (including stress fractures). Splints and "bucked shins," the inflammation of the periosteum on the cannon bones, are often signs of overloading the system and lead to lameness.

The skeleton adapts naturally to the strong demands made. Oftentimes, training-related tying up, acidosis and lameness occur due to the discrepancy between the stress and the body's capacity to cope with it in the still-growing horse. As racehorses are not expected to be flexible in the classical sense, the focus is more on endurance, stamina and speed, and muscular tension results in many problem zones. The horses are frequently not capable of delivering their best performances due to the various muscular problems (tying up, azoturia, myositis). Increase in the muscle enzyme can be tested in a laboratory. A single race can lead to the destruction of several square centimeters of muscle tissue. This is replaced by inelastic scar tissue. Flexibility is lost.

Flat racing

The main gait for racing is the gallop, and there is a definite difference between stayers, sprinters and steeple chasers

Stayers must be able to gallop longer distances, which places particular demands on the cardiovascular system and on muscle metabolism. Lactic acid can easily form in the muscles. The horses doing well are mostly bigger, rectangular shapes with deep chests and good respiratory capabilities.

Sprinters must be capable of reaching maximum speeds in short distances, without the need for too much catching up. The most suitable for this are short, compact horses with muscular and well-developed hindquarters that can accelerate quickly. Traction torque in the hindquarters of these horses causes muscle tears.

Steeple chasers are the so-called obstacle horses, that should have staying qualities in addition to jumping ability. For this purpose, bigger riding horses with long legs are used to make it easier to overcome the obstacles. The fences are not high, but they are built with brush that is semi-fixed, requiring good balance from the jockeys. The extra stress from jumping comes when the horse's back is burdened on the landing phase. The forelegs are inherently under tremendous stress and the muscular tension in the back is often so dramatic that the horses flinch their lower backs severely with the lightest palpation. These horses are never made to do any gymnastic exercises, and have therefore rarely learned to carry the weight of the rider correctly, so they endeavor to carry the weight by tensing the M. longissimus dorsi and bracing their necks against it in an attempt to absorb the shock in their axial skeleton. The muscles do therefore not function with an elastic connection between the forehand and the hindquarters.

What they have in common is that they are broken-in between 1 and 1.5 years of age. The very lightweight jockey sits on the weak, underdeveloped back muscles that have not been prepared for work in any way.

The racing seat has punctual pressure on the trapezius region, since the racing saddle should be as small as possible to be the least weight to be carried.

The instability of the saddle offers the jockey no possibility to sit properly on the horse, which means the reins function as a balancing mechanism. Most racehorses are used to running fast the more they get pulled in the mouth. This reaction arises from the reflex of the young horse; namely, to try and flee from the pain felt on the bars of the mouth when they are first mounted.

Depending on the type of use, there are different kinds of training intervals, to stimulate either fast twitch or slow twitch muscle fibers. The development of the cardiovascular capacity takes priority. In the classical school, it takes the third spot after successful adaptation and strength training.

On their way to the finish line, steeple chasers must clear various obstacles, which created additional stress and torque loading on the shoulders with respect to the joints and muscles. Because of the unstable standing seat of the jockey, the rider uses the reins to balance himself, often making the jump itself uncomfortable for the horse, who cannot round himself in a bascule but must jump hollow, without using his back properly, as can be seen in the old prints of yesteryear. The spinous processes of the thoracic and lumbar vertebrae are in this way severely compressed, and bony changes are visible already in young horses on x-rays.

Due to the high speed, the loin vertebrae are especially vulnerable and the sacroiliac joint is also strongly stressed. One can often find fractures and ankylosis on the transverse processes in the lower back. (fig.5.12)

The fetlock joints of the forelegs will often go into hyper-extension, which may result in the splint bones coming into contact with the ground, causing fractures and bucked shins.

Trotters

Trotters almost reach the same speed in trot as flat racers achieve in gallop, 45 km/h being the norm. In the sport of trot racing, the horses must move exclusively in trot. In order to reach these unbelievable speeds, the horses must trot with their hind legs apart to step past the front legs so as not to step on the tendons of the front legs. Of course this puts extra strain on the much more flexed sacroiliac joint.

The use of the so-called over-check, which forces the horses into an unnatural head carriage where they can remain in the trot with more shoulder freedom, has the disadvantage that the thoracic vertebrae gets pushed down, favoring the development of kissing spine. Tension in the muscles and irregularities in the walk and trot are common problems in trotters, who are rarely allowed to move forward freely in a forward and down posture (fig.6.4.).

Lungeing of the trotter is, as is with the racehorse, only running on a circle without any gymnastic effect. It is therefore not possible for the horses to achieve an effective, biomechanically sensible gymnastic therapy for the

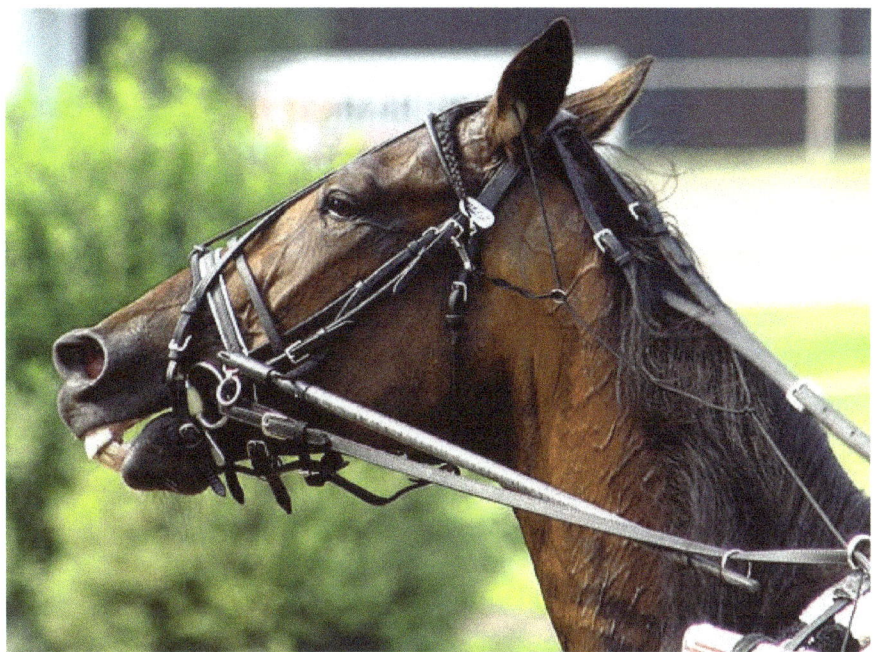

Fig.6.4. The artificial head carriage provoked by the overcheck does not allow the trotter to develop correct back muscles. The back becomes increasingly stiff and lordosis is the consequence, making rhythmic swinging of the back impossible. Muscular tension is the result of this faulty skeletal loading.

back muscles, as they have not learned how to use their backs correctly in their training.

The hard and intensive training and relatively hard surfaces are also not very good for the joints. Wear and tear is noticed much quicker. Problems with lactic acid in the form of tying up and azoturia often happen due to the unnaturally high head carriage and incorrect stresses on the body, frequently resulting in bad performance and horses that can no longer be used.

1. Regular thermo-graphic checks on the legs are just as important as the use of acupuncture. Mobilization techniques and TENS treatments should be used for localized trigger points.

2. Laser therapy can be successfully used on overloaded joints. Magnetic blankets can help in the reduction of lactic acid when used after a race.

3. In the race-free intervals, the horses should be allowed to stretch down in order to compensate for the incorrect head carriage in race training.

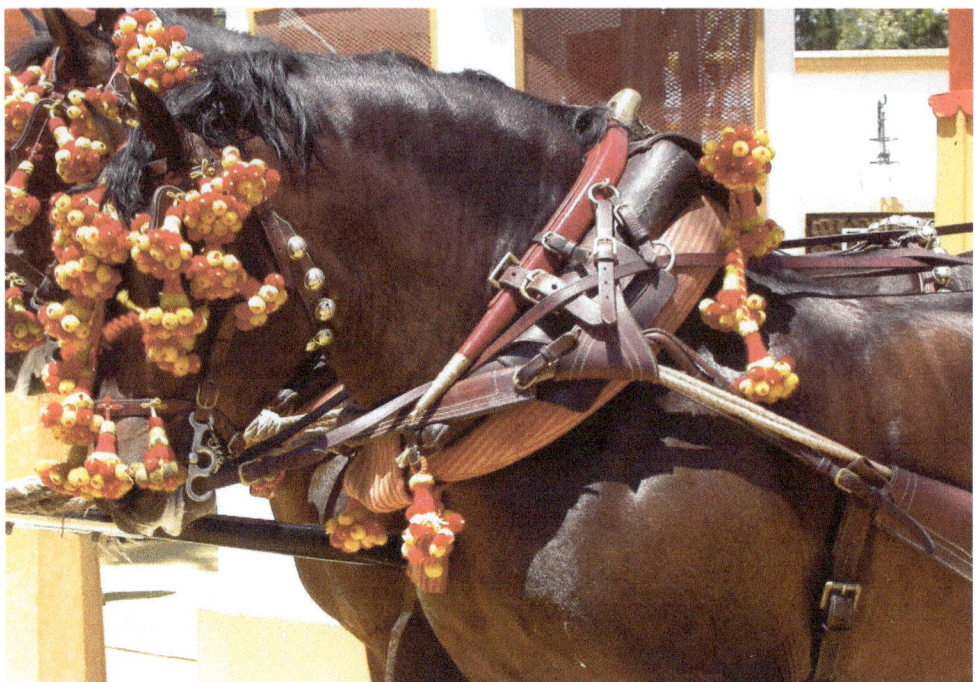

Fig.6.5. When a collar is used, the horse can employ his whole body weight to pull and to brake, provided it fits properly. This photo shows a beautiful traditional Spanish pair with collars.

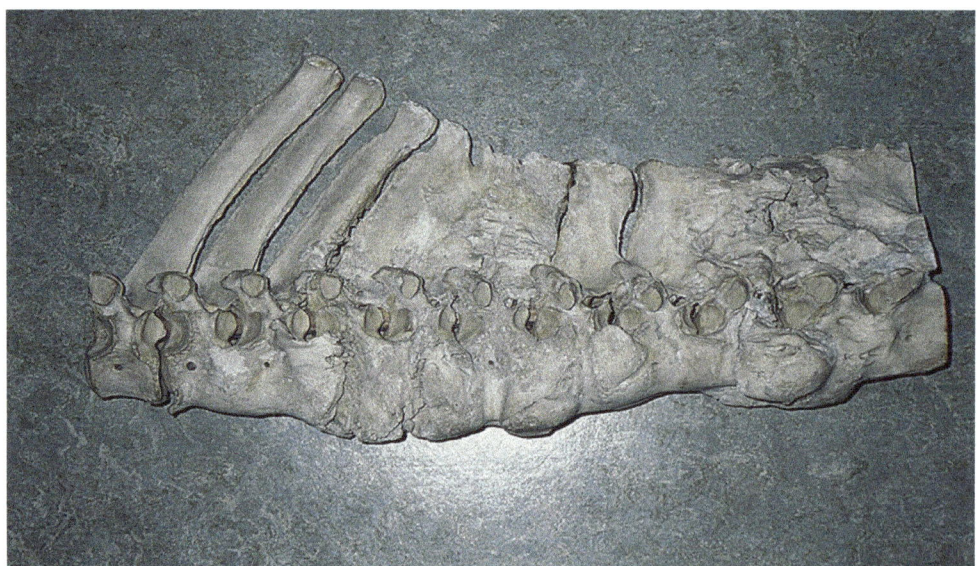

Fig.6.6. Horses that have had to pull heavy loads, may develop skeletal changes in the thoracic vertebrae due to the strong compression during the braking phase. This photo shows total fusion and ankylosis of the thoracic vertebrae, making the spinal cord completely stiff with no movement possible.

6.2.7. Carriage horses

Even though carriage horses have no rider on their backs, there can be significant stresses on their bodies especially in the marathon and cross country disciplines. In hilly terrain the horse must be capable of using his body to accelerate or to brake, where both thrust and tractive forces must be overcome. (Fig. 6.5. and 6.6.)

Carriage horses, like dressage horses must be strong and must have good bodies. This is achieved through proper training, including turns, transitions, pulling, braking and stopping on a slight slope. Lungeing and double lungeing also have valuable gymnastic advantages for these horses. Carriage horses should be checked regularly for lesions in the hindquarters and in the shoulder areas. Massage and mobilization techniques can be of great help.

Gaited horses

In this Chapter, the problems of gaited horses will be discussed. Due to the many different gaits, lameness examinations are almost impossible to do, as the horses often do not have a normal trot pattern. It is extremely difficult to assess the pureness of any gait.

Icelandic ponies also have a tremendous tolerance for pain, making diagnostic usefulness very doubtful when it comes to sensitivity to pressure. A small reaction from these little horses is often significant when compared to that of another horse, as they do not "communicate" on a voluntary basis. Furthermore, the saddles of gaited horses should be looked at under a magnifying glass, as the opinion of relevant professional circles is that a saddle that lies further back and pushes on the kidney area makes a horse more "collectible" by making the shoulder more free to improve the mechanics of the gait. The high head carriage—above the rein hold position—in the rack is viewed as beneficial for "collection." There is no biomechanical examination that can validate this. Many of these horses have extreme tension in the muscles of the back. The high occurrence of kissing spines that occurs in the Icelandic pony population can be proven by x-rays. This condition may have resulted from incorrect gymnastic training.

The footfall of the rack, which has no moment of suspension, makes a comfortable, vibration-free and easy on the inter-vertebral disc movement possible for the rider, which is why it makes assessment of tension and lameness very difficult.

In professional circles the irregular rack is considered "pacing" and the purity of the rack suffers because of it. Unfortunately these horses mostly refuse to trot properly, which makes gait analysis useless.

More important in this context is the long-term practical experience and palpatory skills to interpret and rectify lesions and changes in the body of the horse, as one cannot expect too much reaction from these good-natured animals.

Important areas to examine are the loins, neck vertebrae and the sacroiliac joint. Most Icelandic ponies are only broken in at the age of five years, which in itself is worthy of praise, but one can often find changes in the skeleton as defined in kissing spines, which might be traced back to the too high head carriage for the rack (fig. 5.15.)

The panel saddles used in the sport are often not in accordance with the curve of the horse's topline and the too long panels press into the area of the last lumbar vertebrae, causing tremendous pressure damage. The horses do not want to trot, refuse to come on the bit and can eventually not even be ridden in the rack. These are all signs that something is amiss.

Regular thermography in winter is more difficult because of the thick coat, but in general it is a good diagnostic tool. Massage and mobilization therapy can improve both the life and the performance of the competition horse.

These rules apply to most other gaited horses, like the Paso Fino, Paso Peruano etc, whereby the Pasos, with their Spanish heritage, have a much higher sensitivity and the test results are much more satisfying. Controlling the fit of the saddle is once again very important, as many of these saddles come from the country of origin and they may be beautifully made and decorated, but don't necessarily fit the horses and that, of course, can cause tension and irregularities in the movements.

6.3. The green horse, the young horse, the school horse

The H. Dv. 12, The German Cavalry Manual on the Training of Horse & Rider [Xenophon Press 2014] clearly differentiates between the green and the young horse, where the importance of the various equestrian requirements in the still developing horses emerges.

Definition: *The green horse is 3.5 to 5 years old, and moves free on the lunge and under the rider, both in the school and outside in the country, in order to find its balance. The young horse is 5 to 6 years old and is worked more seriously in the school (fig.6.7) with the greatest importance given to the first four phases in the training scale. Straightness will end this phase of training.*

It is only after this phase that a horse is specialized according to its strengths, in dressage or jumping. This will guarantee that a horse has good

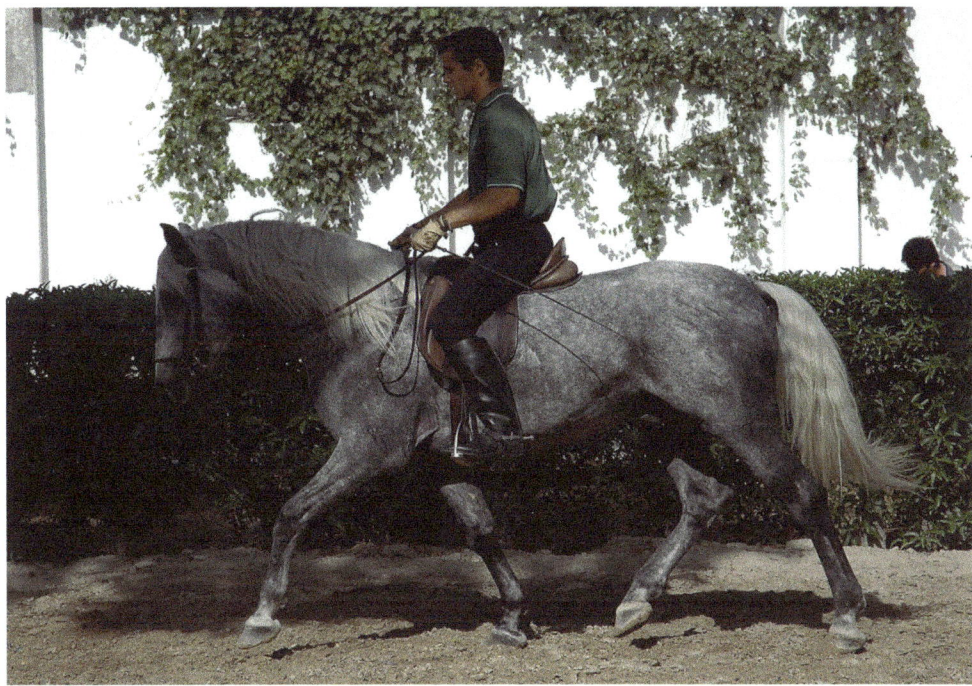

Fig.6.7. The photo shows a green horse in natural contact with the bit, moving with good rhythm in a trot with sufficient impulsion.

basic training, while at the same time having the opportunity to reach physical and psychological maturity without too much athletic stress. The three phases of adaptation, building strength and endurance is also optimally utilized in the first years of lungeing and rides in the country.

It is noteworthy that in *The H. Dv. 12, The German Cavalry Manual on the Training of Horse & Rider* [Xenophon Press 2014] the horses were taken in for training at a relatively late age and that they had been given time for their development in order to be ready for the work in the cavalry. When one considers that the average age for a cavalry horse was between 15 and 17 years and that the sport horses now have an average age of only 9 years, the time factor given promoted the longevity of the horse.

A concept that has disappeared into oblivion, namely the school horse, that is very well-trained in all the classical lessons, where riders can learn the necessary sensitivity needed for obtaining the lessons under the watchful eye of a good trainer. The value of a school horse in the traditional sense is priceless. Theoretical knowledge can never be felt in any way other than on a correctly trained and ridden horse. This is why the saying "riding can only be learned through riding" has lost none of its truth to this day.

7. Equipment for the Horse

7.1. The saddle fitting

There are basically four different types of saddles, based on the way they are constructed: the English saddle, the military or full shifting panel saddle, the working saddles which include western and vaquera saddles among others, and the treeless saddles.

7.1.1. The English saddle

The English saddle has either a wooden, synthetic or metal spring tree and is appropriate for use in any riding discipline, mainly because of the light and portable design. The point of the tree is situated in the front of the saddle and determines the width of the tree, which should be customized for each individual horse according to his anatomy. This part of the tree also gives stability to the saddle and the rounded top component forms the pommel of the saddle. The rest of the tree continues toward the back in a somewhat curved manner and ends in the cantle. The length of the seat is decisive. The narrower the two parts in the middle of the seat, the smaller the bearing surface on the horse's back, making the weight distribution unfavorable, but has a positive influence on the comfort of the seat for the rider. The stirrup bars with the safety catch are found in the front part where the twist and the seat intersection is, and a further pressure point can develop in this area on the trapezius muscle if the saddle is not properly fitted. The length of the flap and the use of knee and thigh rolls depends on the discipline for which the saddle is made. The billets are attached for use with a long or short girth, and these can also cause various pressure points on the horse's back.

The bearing surfaces on the back of the horse are called the panels and the clearance between the two is known as the gullet. This gullet should have a continuous width of at least three fingers right up to the back of the saddle, so as not to interfere with the movement of the spinal column. (fig.7.1.)

The relative lightweight construction and little possibility of pressure distribution cause the saddle to effect the back of the horse in a very precise way, which makes it beneficial for dressage and other disciplines where the emphasis is not extensive hours in the saddle. However, when these saddles are not correctly fitted, they can damage the back of the horse. (Fig. 7.2)

The criteria discussed above for the correct fit of a saddle apply to all kinds of saddles, as these are guidelines for the anatomy of the horse.

A correctly fitting saddle is especially important with rehabilitation patients and will have a significant influence on the continuing healing

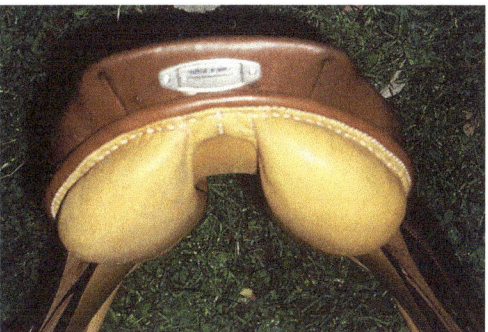

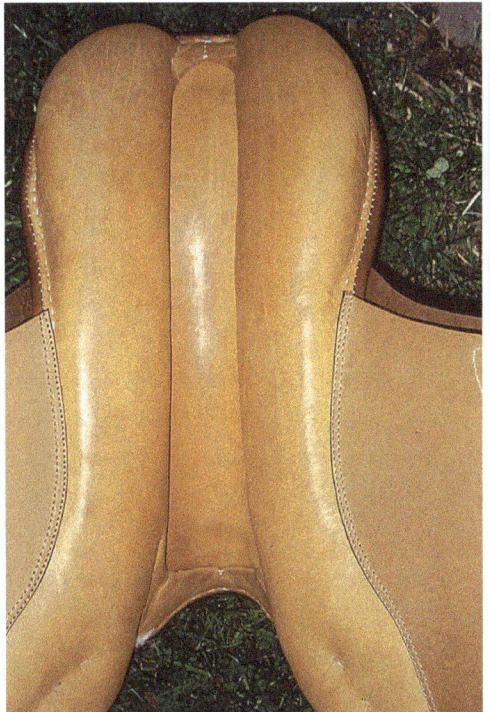

Fig. 7.1. A sufficient gullet of at least three fingers wide to accommodate the movement of the spinal column.

Fig. 7.2. Asymmetric panels. There should be at least three fingers width between the two panels, so as not to interfere with the movement of the spinal column. One should always look for symmetry of the panels, and not only in used saddles. In the above example there is a distinct asymmetry, where the more used side will cause more punctual pressure points and the rider will sit crooked on the horse.

process. Irrespective of the riding discipline, every saddle should do justice to the anatomical requirements of the horse, as a physiologically efficient pattern of movement under a rider will not be possible otherwise.

As anatomical references we have the cartilage of the shoulder blade that, through the angle of the shoulder blade, forms an anatomically unchanging factor (with the exception of the cartilage that can ossify when the pommel is too narrow), the swing in the back of the horse as well as the lateral deviation during movement of the spinous processes of the thoracic and lumbar vertebrae.

A variable factor is the muscles. Here the M. trapezius, M. latissimus dorsi, M. longissimus dorsi and M. iliocostalis need to be mentioned. The deep depression behind the shoulder blade is often falsely interpreted as a distinct saddle position. Truth be said, this is more a question of atrophy of the M. trapezius and M. longissimus dorsi due to a too narrow saddle that cannot allow muscular development due to the constant pressure. Any regular contraction of the above muscles will be made impossible due to the compression of the muscles. Little blood and nutrients can be transported under the saddle during movement. It is for this reason that the muscle cannot build, but rather atrophies, and the activity of the back and the action of the forehand can be seriously affected. The horses show problems with contact and diminishing gaits.

In cases such as these, the horses should be lunged and worked in-hand for months in order to build up the muscles. In this state of atrophy, no saddle can promote the muscle building around the withers without pressure points. "More padding" will have fatal results on the development of muscles in this area.

It is especially important to take this into consideration with young horses, as a saddle can quickly become too narrow when the horses grow. It is therefore not logical to use the most expensive "made to fit" saddle for a young horse from the beginning. As a rule of thumb, the green horse to Grand Prix horse will change 4-5 saddle sizes.

Young horses, depending on their type, will have a pointed oval shaped back and through progressive training and growth will obtain a more rounded form.

The cartilage of the shoulder blade will move 3-5cm backwards with every step of the foreleg extending of each front leg. The shoulder will often bump against the point of the tree, which proves the saddle is too narrow. Within 10-15 minutes this area will become numb and muscle destruction will progress. One can often see small "sacks" of fluid a hand's width under the edge of the scapula. This is a collection of tissue fluid that descends with the

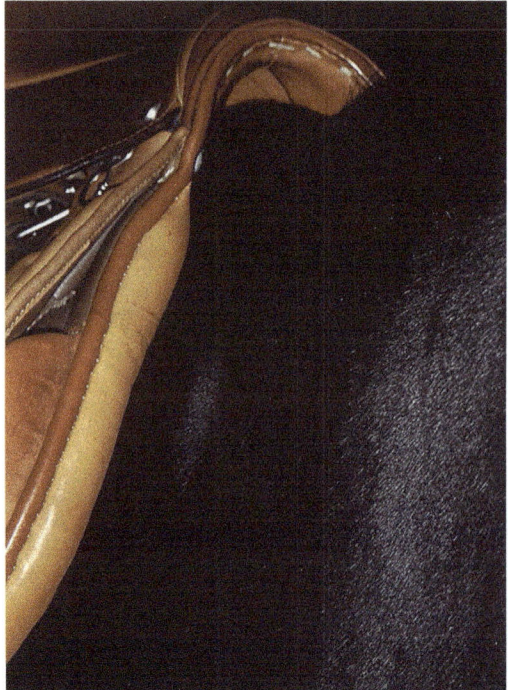

Fig.7.3: The width of the saddle is correct when the point of the tree is parallel to the angle of the shoulder blade and a clearance of two fingers is possible in between the withers and the saddle when the rider sits in the saddle.

help of gravity as a result of muscle damage.

Painful areas behind the shoulder blade induce a contraction of the M. trapezius, thus blocking the activity of the forearm and reducing the range of movement. A reflex reaction of the horse, triggered by the pain, will accompany this, contracting the neck extensors. The M. brachiocephalicus is pushed out and tensed up. This, in turn, will restrict the extension of the shoulders even more, making the gait tight and second-rate.

If this pressure acts too long on the cartilaginous edge of the shoulder blade, it can lead to ossification and permanent deformation and asymmetry, where every saddle will be brought to a twisted position, and fitting a saddle on a horse with this problem can be really difficult.

Apart from the uncontrolled and permanent stimulation on the heart-circulation acupuncture points, this pressure area is the most frequent catalyst for "poor performance syndrome." Especially in the race horse industry, the small saddle creates maximum pressure on this area. This will have an adverse effect on the actual race.

It is for this reason that the point of the tree should always be parallel to the angle of the shoulder blade in order not to impair the mobility of the shoulder.

In the ideal situation the point of the tree should be cut back slightly to allow more space for the anatomy of the shoulder.

A clearance of two to three fingers between the pommel and the withers of the horse should be accounted for, depending on the weight of the rider. (Fig. 7.3 and 7.4a) If this clearance is too big, it is a sign of a too narrow fit and the center of balance will be transferred to the back and kidney area (fig.7.4b). In this case, the saddle should be one number wider. A wedge-shaped padding or extra flocking of the saddle should, under no circumstances, be tried as a compensation, for this saddle is quite simply too narrow for the horse.

The curve in the horse's back is regularly a neglected variable for the ever more fashionable baroque horses. Andalusians, Friesians and Lippizaner often have a higher croup. Due to the square form of these horses, the saddle should have a different curve so as to not press on the kidneys and only touch the back in the front and caudally in the typical bridging phenomenon. (fig.7.4c and 7.5) Resistances are pre-programmed and working round is not possible. These horses have contact problems and are unable to track up. They can have rhythm disturbances and even excessive shying and rearing.

7.1.2. Full shifting panel saddle

The full shifting panel saddle, that was originally designed for the cavalry has a wide gullet as opposed to the English saddle with laterally

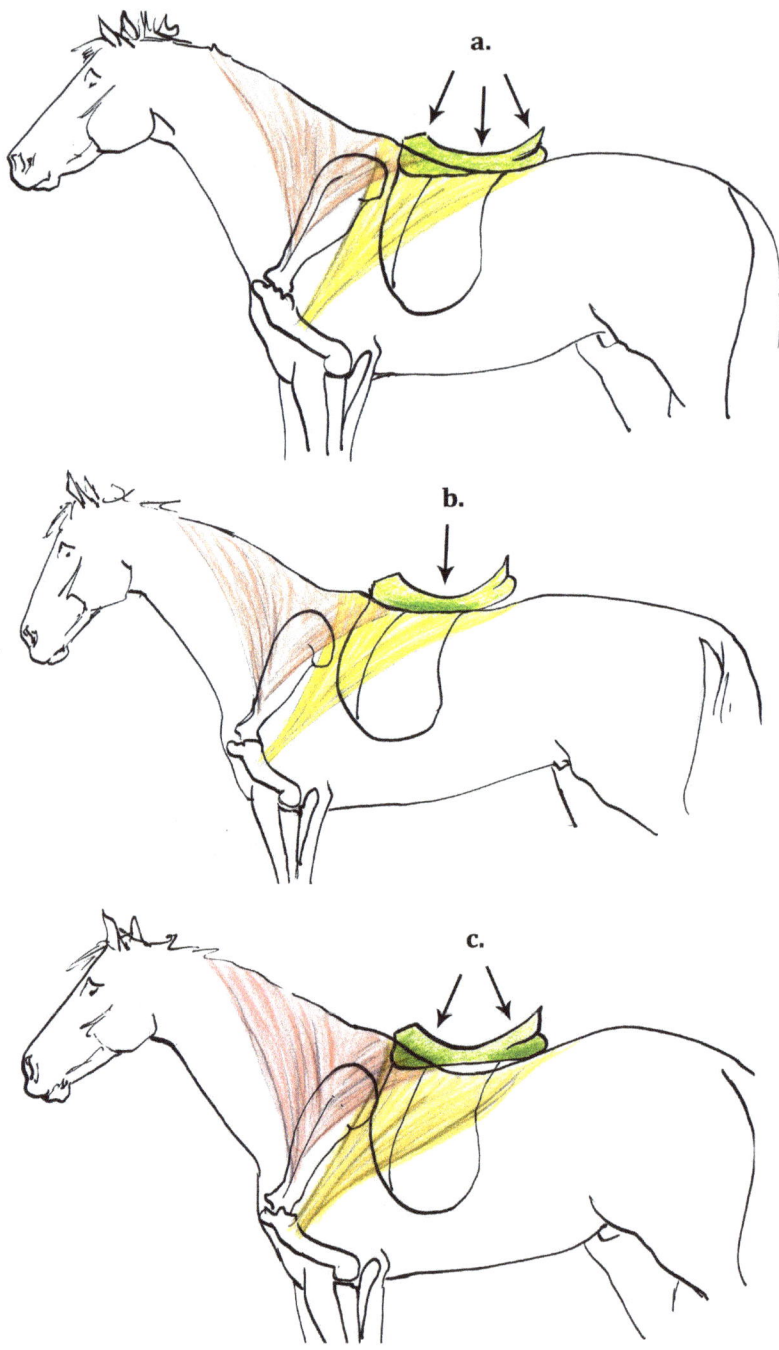

Fig: 7.4(a) A well fitted saddle (b) too narrow fit will cause the pommel of the saddle to rise too high and the center of balance is moved to the back (c) with an extremely curved back and too straight saddle, the saddle does not lie snug on the back of the horse (pink=M. trapezius, yellow=M. latissimus dorsi)

The Science and Art of Riding in Lightness

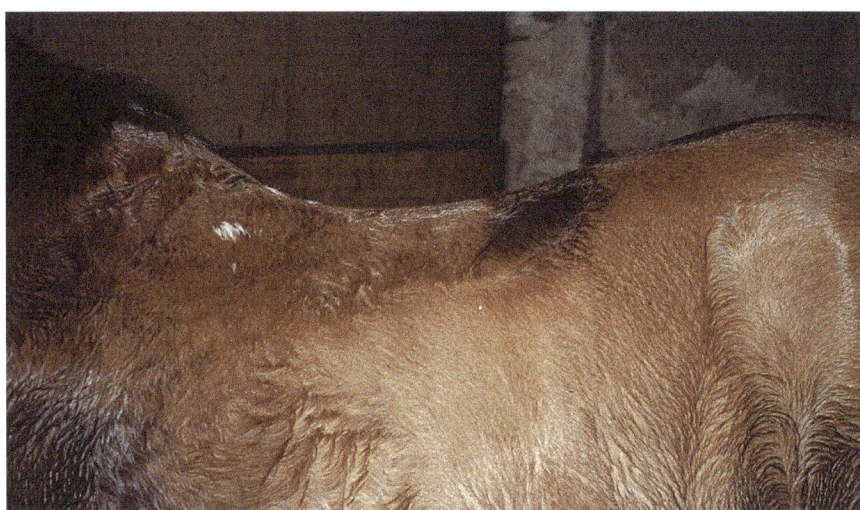

Fig. 7.5. Horses with hollow-shaped backs should be carefully considered so that the saddle ought to follow the curve of their backs. This was not the case here; strong pressure was put on the kidney area (sweat mark) which will also manifest in problems being ridden.

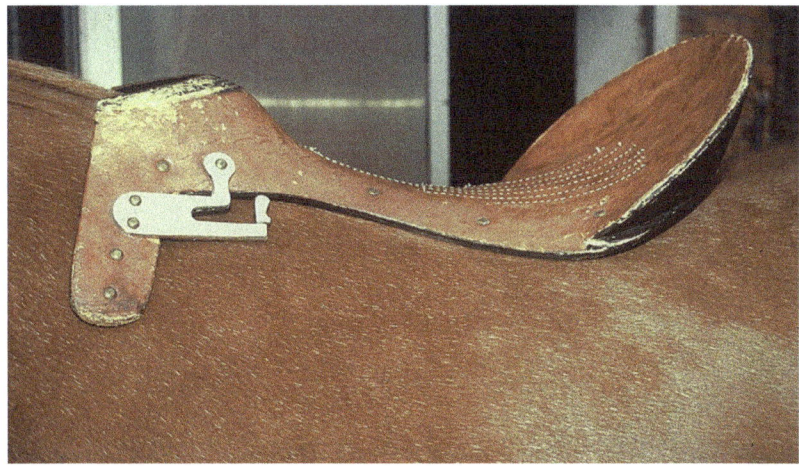

Fig:7.6. Wooden tree. The tree parallels the skeleton of the saddle. The point of the tree lies just behind the shoulder blade and must be at the same angle as the shoulder blade. The stirrup bars lie in the level of the trapezius muscle and must not compress the muscle. The tree must be adapted to the topline of the horse, without any concentrated load in any one place.

moving, well padded panels that allows for a fit on most horses. In this way, weight loss on long hikes can be counterbalanced, which would not have been possible with the unchangeable, rigid English saddle and would have been the cause of many pressure areas. Although it is an uncomfortable saddle for the rider, it's construction where it lies high on the horse's back allows for a good circulation of air which would prevent the horse's back from overheating on long hikes. Through the construction of metal and leather, it was easily possible to change defective parts of the saddle or fasten any additional baggage to it. The greased woolen blanket, folded 6 times according to the military service regulations, not only had the function to protect the saddle from the horse's sweat, but also served to reduce pressure and friction and impede muscle-wasting together with the flexible panels during the long rides.

The American military saddle was the McClellan saddle. This was open through the seat which made the flow of air under the rider possible.

7.1.3. Western saddles

Western saddles, depending on the way they are built, can spread the weight evenly on the horse's back when they are correctly fitted. This type of saddle does not have pads that can be re-flocked, so it is essential that the tree be an accurate fit to the horse's back. The rider sits directly on the tree and very few changes can be made to the finished saddle.

These prefabricated wood, rawhide, or fiberglass trees must not only conform in the skirt, but also in the twist of the saddle. (Fig. 7.6) Fiberglass trees can always be changed in their width afterwards with the appropriate workmanship, something that was not possible with traditionally manufactured saddles. The fork, which determines the width of the saddle, must be wide enough to give the shoulder clearance. When this is not the case the shoulder blade cartilage can ossify, making the horse asymmetrical which cannot be rectified at a later stage.

The different widths come in full-quarter, semi-quarter and Arabian sizes, where the first one should fit on a well-developed Quarter Horse. Western horses normally have very short backs, and though the greater bearing surface and length of the saddle, it is often saddled too far forward over the shoulders which puts too much load on the shoulder. The length of the saddle must be adapted to the length of the horse's back. This makes it more difficult to fit a western saddle than an English saddle, but it is of the utmost importance.

A further complication is the minimum distance of 2 fingers at the back border of the saddle between the spinal column and the skirt, since too little space can lead to abrasions and spinal column irritation. When the skirts are too long, the inside hip bones can be chafed when the horse is asked to bend. It is for this reason that the length of the saddle is so important.

The shape of the saddle depends on the western discipline, for example, the cutting discipline demands a longer horn and reining or roping employs a shorter horn. The different methods of girthing, known as ridging, corresponds to that of the English saddle, and can deal with the distribution of pressure on the back of the horse. The stirrup attachment takes place through the fender that can be adjusted at the bottom instead of the top as is the case with English leathers.

7.1.4. Iberian saddles

Spanish and Portuguese saddles are called Iberian saddles. The Spanish saddle has two varieties: the Vaquero and the Española saddle.

The most important criteria of the Spanish and Portuguese school saddle is the wooden tree, the deep seat and the elevated galeria in the front and the back of the saddle which gives the rider a very firm hold in the saddle. The particularly high galeria of the Portuguese saddle makes it impossible to do rising trot. The Spanish Española has lower galerias and is flatter and straighter in the seat. The rider should have a well-balanced seat if he intends to use this saddle. A more convenient alternative, that is something between the Española and the Portuguese saddle, is the Spanish "foal" saddle or Potrera, that combines the high galerias with more freedom of movement and in which the rider can rise the trot.

All of these saddles have horse hair padding. Breaking-in the saddle without a numnah [saddleblanket] to achieve a perfect fit on the horse's back takes a rather long time. Many Iberian saddles are too narrow in the last third of the gullet and presses on the lumbar vertebrae. Therefore, one should always pay attention that there is adequate space between the panels. To give the saddle more stability, always use a breastplate and a crupper.

The construction of the Spanish Vaquero saddle takes on an exceptional position in this context, (fig.7.7) in that the front and back portions have metal rails in whereas the tree of the saddle is traditionally handcrafted with straw bundles. The panels of horse hair are very thick and the idea is that it should adapt to the back with the help of the sweat from the horse. The girthing is with a surcingle that ties the saddle tightly in the middle on the horse's back. The thick sheepskin numnah causes the rider to have more distance from the horse, but the seat has a high degree of comfort.

Unfortunately, with this considerably long and heavy saddle (20kg), it is often forgotten that even a relatively "back friendly" saddle should equally do justice to the minimum anatomical requirements in order for the horse to move under it without discomfort.

The arch at the back is often too narrow and due to the construction, it is also not expandable. This will lead to loss of movement in the lumbar area with considerable loss of bend as horses will suffer from bruising when the saddle does not fit. The same can happen when the fork in the front is too narrow, as most of these saddles are modeled on Arabian crosses that have much less substance than the more sturdy Andalusian type.

Vaquero saddles should therefore never be bought off the rack, but should always be individually produced for every particular horse.

All Vaquero saddles are traditionally ridden with an integrated crupper that should prevent the saddle from slipping forward. The stirrups are mounted in a special attachment with a mandrel, where the stirrup leathers get looped twice through the box-stirrups to guard against the leather breaking which could be fatal in work with fighting bulls. The horse hair panels are also very thick and sometimes need to be broken-in to adapt optimally to the topline of the horse, and it is for this reason that this saddle often is ridden without a numnah. The cotton towel to protect clothing from sweat of the horse, called a *manta estribera* is traditionally affixed to the pommel, finishes this saddle. Modern variations of the Vaquera and Portuguese saddles can have additionally fitted galerias at the front and together with the elevated shell-shaped cantle at the back, that has an Arabian origin, and offers a secure seat in the bull-fight or in the training of young horses.

The spine of the horse has a more or less lateral movement, depending on the horse, and one must make allowances for the sideways protrusion of the spinous processes. This makes a gullet width of three-fingers-width essential,

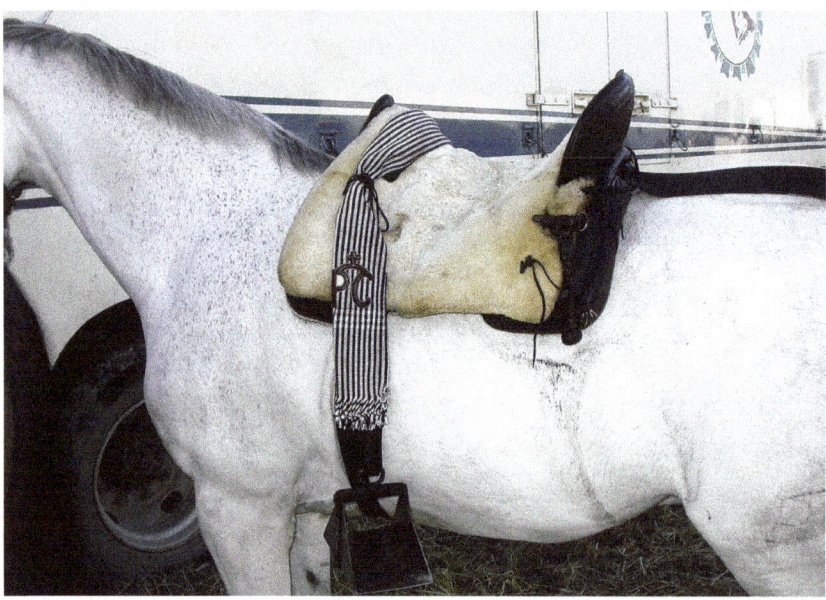

Fig.7.7. Vaquero saddle. The length of the saddle will lessen the lateral bending of the vertebral column considerably. But when a Vaquero saddle is properly fitted it will spread the weight of the rider over a broad surface which makes it a good choice for long rides. These saddles are always ridden with a crupper.

so that this important biomechanical component is never obstructed. All bending and sideways movements become impossible, especially at the back of the saddle, if the gullet is too narrow. The spinous processes become positively blocked and the structures that lie on top (for example, the supraspinous ligament) become irritated and inflamed. Problems with bending, bridle lameness, rhythm disturbances and deficient willingness to collect are some of the results of a gullet that is too narrow.

In summary, one must use the following criteria for fitting a saddle:

1. The size of the tree must be wide enough to allow movement
2. The bearing surface next to the spinal column must be even and soft
3. The gullet [anywhere along its entire length] must never come into contact with the movable part of the spine.
4. The pads must be evenly soft and may not be flocked too tightly, for this will cause a concentrated, selective load that can massively influence the motion sequence of the horse's back. By the same token one should make sure that the pads are not asymmetrical or crooked, for this will lead to further inappropriate stress on the backbone of the horse, and bring the rider out of the horse's center of gravity.
5. As a matter of principle, one should use as little padding as possible, but as much as necessary in order to establish the most favorable fit for the horse's back. 10cm thick panels are a real handicap especially with the Spanish saddles, even though the saddles have the benefit of a larger bearing surface for weight distribution across the costal arch.

7.1.5. Icelandic pony saddles

In this context, the Icelandic pony saddle is somewhat questionable, as it is neither an English saddle nor a full shifting panel saddle in the real sense. This hybrid incorporates all the disadvantages of both models in the most unsuitable manner.

The narrow contact surface of the English saddle is made worse through the inflexible *trachtenähnliche*[6] extensions to the back and will often press mercilessly on the kidney area due to this extreme straight form. These saddles are often too long and due to lacking curvature in the tree, they tend to form a bridge. In many cases the center of gravity is too far back and this leads to overloading or a physiologically incorrect loading of the lumbar vertebrae; the horses try to escape the desired gait of amble for example by going into pacing.

---

6   The panels which are made differently than modern English saddles; these panels are stiffer and longer, extending back further, similar to those used on western saddles.

To aggravate matters even further, the saddle is often put on further back than necessary and used with a back to front riser pad in order to improve the "willingness to collect" in the gaited movements. If one has studied the training scale, one will recognize the typical method of riding Icelandic ponies is vastly different from the classical way.

7.1.6. Panels, elastic trees, broken trees

It is obvious that the tree of a saddle should not be broken and this can be tested with ease when the saddle is put on one knee and the pommel is pulled towards the person doing the test. (Fig. 7.8) When the seat casts folds, it is almost a sure thing that the tree is broken and that the saddle should be withdrawn from circulation. Broken trees can seriously damage the back of the horse, especially in the middle, for the saddle no longer has an even bearing surface and buckles more under the weight of the rider, pressing on the vertebral column.

Something similar happens to saddles with flexible trees or treeless saddles. As a result of lacking structural requirements, the leather bodywork presses relentlessly on the withers (in treeless saddles) or on the breast and lumbar vertebrae in sagging or too elastic saddles.

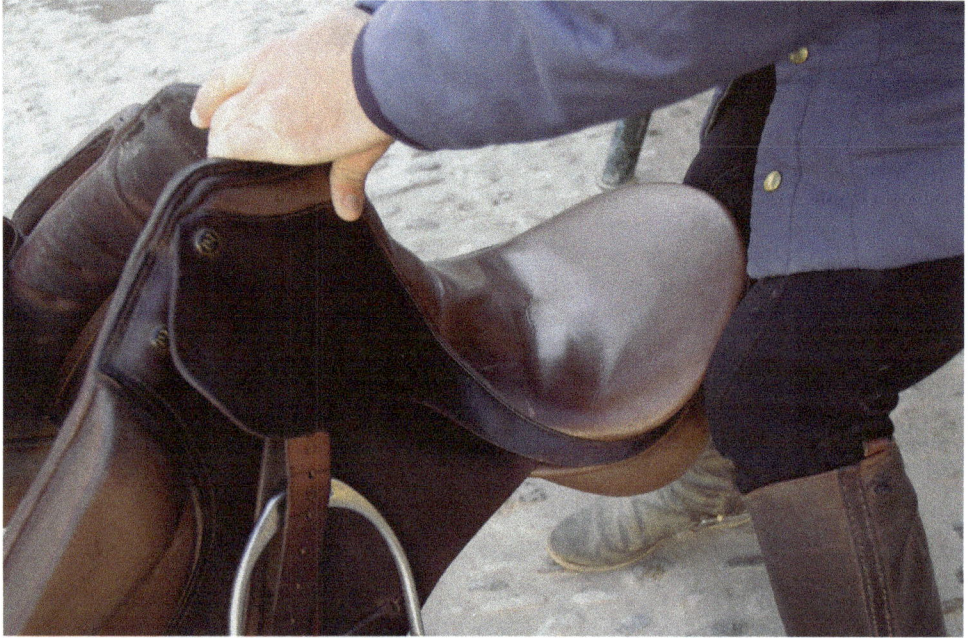

Fig. 7.8. Broken tree. A simple test as shown in this picture to check for wrinkle formation on the seat. These saddles must immediately be taken out of circulation, as they are a definite source of injury to the back of the horse.

In order to test if a saddle is damaged by a fall, simply put your hands on the head plate and try to change the width by pushing this together or pulling it apart. Under normal circumstances nothing should move or change.

The demand that a saddle should move with the horse's back is warranted and good, but only to a justifiable extent in that the saddle complies with the criteria above. A tree that "adapts itself" cannot function, for either it is too unstable due to the deformation tendency and thus causes pressure points or does not adapt adequately and then pinches because of that.

The idea to change the head plate over a period of training, is basically welcome, but these changes are only useful when the other parts, for example the pads, can also be exchanged. It is for this reason that the do-it-yourself manufactured saddles with which one can personally change the head plate is inadequate for our intended purpose.

All types of designs where there is a lack of steadiness and that cannot assure a proper fit on the horse's back, are not useful in the classical art of riding due to the lack of stability. Quite the opposite—these saddles can even cause pressure points and undesirable overloading due to the missing freedom at the withers and missing gullet. "Bareback pads" that are so loved by ponies and children are perfect for children that are being led on ponies, but from a biomechanical point of view, these are not really saddles to be recommended.

The elastic trees are similarly difficult, as they should adapt to the horse's back by reason of their particular flexibility. However, when one considers that the tree of the saddle should offer stability, this endeavor is almost nonsensical. Only through stability is it possible to ensure an even distribution of pressure. A saddle that is flexible in the dorsoventral, or always readjusting to the curve of the horse's back, can have the same devastating consequences as a broken tree —namely localized pressure on the spinal column of the horse. (Fig. 7.8) Proper use of the back is thereby not enabled and all efforts to get the horse to round his back become almost impossible.

Trees that have longitudinal flexibility are, due to their construction, are also less back friendly; when they are fitted well behind the shoulders, the longitudinal yielding makes it press more on the longissimus part. This will cause a vice-like action in the area where most of rider's weight is. The horses show a tendency to drop their backs due to this localized pressure.

Due to the above reasons, it is always a good idea to critically challenge "new ideas" and painstakingly test them for their usefulness.

Once these criteria are complied with, the last question concerns the center of gravity, and according to the type of saddle, it is sometimes a bit to the front (dressage) and sometimes more to the back (jumping) but should never reach the flanks (kidney area).

Saddles can function in a more severe or mild way, depending on their construction. A more severe saddle forces the rider into a predetermined position due to a very high cantle and extremely padded knee rolls (many dressage saddles) and this makes the influence of the lower back of the rider very extreme. Such saddles should be used only in a very limited way when breaking young horses, since the predetermined position of the rider would put too much pressure on the back of the young horse as compared to saddles with a flatter seat.

The straighter the seat and the fewer the knee rolls, the better and more balanced the rider's seat should be. This will also give the rider the possibility to feel the horse more directly and to interact with him more masterfully.

The stirrup bar attachment should also not be ignored. Its location will significantly influence the correct seat of the rider as it will often cause a chair seat or a fork seat when it is not suitable. As a rule of thumb, the linear measure length between the rider's center of gravity and the stirrup bar should be obtained from the measure between the distance from the ball of the foot and the ankle (normally between 15-18cm).

This is also the area where superior traction and pressure forces coming from the rider will momentarily be located only on the trapezius muscle area [of the horse], as is the case in the light seat, rising trot and jumping. This region should be examined very carefully when fitting a saddle, to be sure that no extra pressure is added through bad panels.

The billets or the attachment of the girth is likewise significant, as this will also form part of the foundation for even distribution of pressure on the horse's back. When the saddle is girthed up too tight [unevenly] on one side, it can slip to one side and be pulled out of balance.

Fore-girth straps are leather straps that are affixed additionally on the tree that securely tie down the point of the tree and constrict the freedom of the shoulder, for this reason they are not to be advised. By the same token the much loved fore-girth, popular in some dressage stables, that claim to stop the sliding forward of the saddle, is, if anything, a hindrance to the motor function of the shoulder. It limits the continuation of forward movement from the M. trapezius and M. longissimus dorsi to the neck. The fore-girth is made of a metal arch with bilateral pads that were intended to prevent the saddle from slipping forward and is attached to the saddle just in front of the shoulders with the help of a leather girth.

V-girthing in the front and back panel areas can also restrict the rounding of the horse's back, especially when the girth is pulled really tight.

The most viable are still the three billets that are attached to the middle of the tree, where the first and the last ones are used, this assures an even spread of pressure on the horse's back. The use of a long or a short girth is a matter of taste, where the short girth is favored in the sport of dressage owing to the closer contact on the of the horse's belly, seeing that the buckles are not interfering under the flap and the rider's legs.

7.1.7. Influence of the saddle on the Shu-points of the horse

The Shu-points are described as the points of the bladder meridian that will notify the examiner of the energetic state of the meridians in the body. They are found bilaterally, a hand's width from the spine and therefore also in the saddle area of the horse.(Fig. 7.9)

As anatomic reference points, the rami superficiale and rami ventrales of the spinal nerves should be mentioned, as they are located just under the surface of the skin. A lower resistance in the skin can be measured, and histologically, a collection of blood and lymph vessels can also be found there.

Due to the visceral-cutaneous reflex, disruptions of the organs can manifest via the vegetative nervous system as segments that are tender to

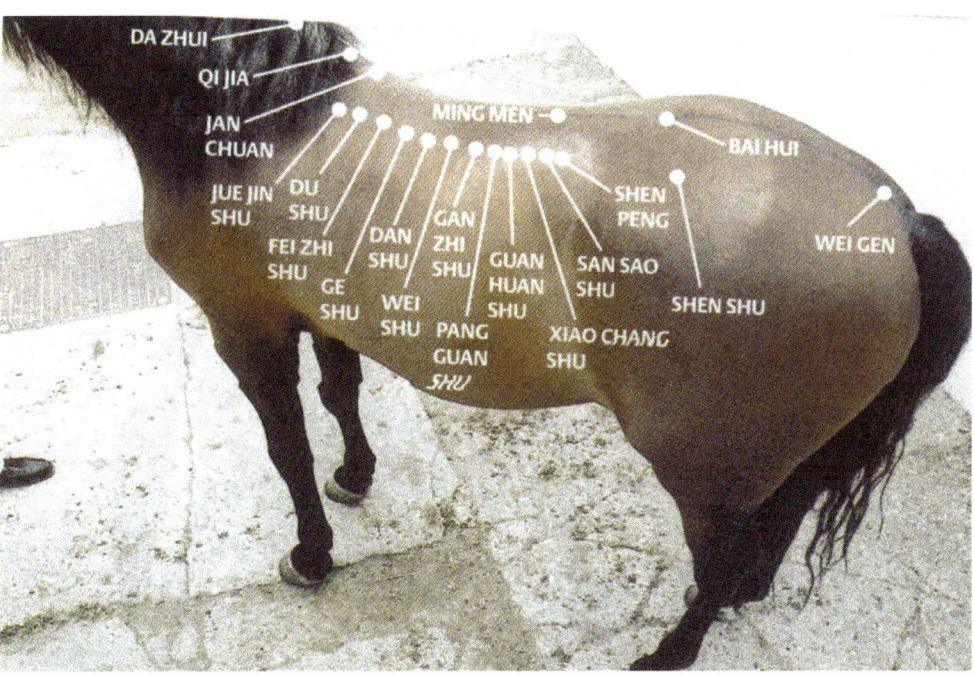

Fig. 7.9 "There are very important acupuncture point (shu-points) from the bladder meridian in the saddle area that would be negatively influenced by a badly fitting saddle. Therefore, adverse stimulation of these points can negatively impact the functioning of the entire energetic system of the horse." (from Traditional Chinese Acupuncture (TCA) of the horse, *by Robert Stodulka, Sonntag publishing 2003)*

pressure on the skin. This influence can also be vice versa and the acupuncturist can therefore have an impact on the organs with the aid of the corresponding acupuncture points.

It is not crucial whether the acupuncture is done by needles, laser or acupressure, since results can be obtained with all of these modes of treatment. In this context the irritated points of the bladder meridian can be understood when a badly fitting saddle is used.

The points Bl 13, Bl 14 and Bl 15 are found behind the shoulder blade and are points for the lungs, pericardium and heart. The logical consequence of a too narrow saddle would be a pectoral pain caused by constriction, and is usually interpreted as "girthy." Horses that cough every now and then when being ridden, may also show sensitive Bl 13 points.

Horses that suffer from "Poor performance syndrome" can display severe reactions when palpated on these points, since the entire weight of the rider is distributed in this area, especially when the rider canters in the light seat; naturally, this would be exacerbated by an ill-fitting saddle.

Horses with heart defects often have a pinched mouth which can, when clinically examined, very quickly lead to an established diagnosis.

When the panels of the saddle are too curved, and the contact is concentrated in the middle, this can, apart from the see-saw effect, lead to an impediment of the diaphragm, where Bl 17 gets stimulated and free breathing is prevented. The horses will also seem to be split in half, the back is hollowed and cannot be rounded, for the pressure causes a contraction of the M. Longissimus dorsi.

Bl 18 and Bl 19 are assigned to the function of the liver and the gallbladder respectively, according to TCM, and have various functional outcomes on the muscular system; for example tension, myositis, and tying up syndrome. Saddles that push down on the flanks, will irritate the kidney area increasingly, and the desired activity in the back will be severely hindered. Thus the horse will tense up. When the loins are not free to move, there will be an accumulation of lactic acid, the result being aching muscles and psychological irritability, which will inevitably lead to insubordination. The caudal parts of the M. Latissimus dorsi can similarly be irritated by the stimulation of Bl 18 and Bl 19. That will, in turn, lead to a reduction of the extension of the forelimb, because the muscles are in a reactive contraction all of the time.

When the tree of a saddle is broken, or the gullet is too wide, the result can be pressure points on the underlying capillaries, which will inevitably turn into obvious saddle pressure points.

The billet and girth construction are also important in this context, for they can block the yin meridian in an energetic manner when the girth is pulled too tight. The affected meridians include the conception vessel, the stomach, the spleen, the liver and the gallbladder meridians, all of which will influence the activity of the hindquarters.

All in all, the energetic components of the system should not be forgotten and regular routine examinations by a TCM practitioner should be a part of the horse's well-being.

7.2. The Appropriately-Fitting Bridle

7.2.1. Basics of fitting a bridle

Along the same lines as choosing a well-fitting saddle, it is absolutely necessary to select equipment for the sensitive head area where an immense number of nerve endings and blood vessels are located.

In the commercialized horse world there are often very expensive branded leather goods available, that unfortunately do not always conform to the horse's anatomical requirements.

Apart from the adequate length of the cheek pieces, the throat latch should be long enough to easily fit one hand's width between the jaw bone and the throat latch when fastened. When the bridle is fastened in this way, one often questions the meaningfulness of this part of the bridle: it would not prohibit the way some Iberian stallions can slip the bridle off due to their more pronounced neck crest, if it is fastened so loosely. Horses that do not have this specific anatomical feature, can potentially be ridden without this strap and, in this way, may not be affected when going on the bit. It is worth mentioning that the double bridles of the Spanish Riding School in Vienna and the Royal Andalusian School in Jerez de la Frontera do not have this little strap and yet, present the art of riding in its highest perfection. (fig.2.3)

An often overlooked attachment is the browband, which is, in many cases, too short and presses painfully on the base of the ear through the tension from the poll piece. This causes problems when the horse is asked to come on the bit. Sensitivity in the poll area and problems putting on the bridle can be indicators that this may be the case. Well-know tack manufacturers have developed bridles with clearance [curved shape to accommodate the ears] at the base of the ears along with adequate padded lining so as not to irritate this sensitive area.

The nose-band must be placed *under* the headpiece of the bridle and depending on what type, fastened accordingly. The widely used and deplorable custom of using a crafty lever hoist system to pull the nose-band even more tight, where the horse cannot even chew anymore, should be left alone according to pure common sense. This treatment would only result in unnecessary pressure on the poll and the relaxed chewing of the horse through an efficient and de-contracted [relaxed] M. masseter would be impaired.

The most commendable nose-band of the popular ones available is the dropped nose-band, for it causes a light pressure on the bridge of the nose when the horse opens its mouth, causing the horse to yield quicker in the poll. Besides, there will be no pinching of the leather between the lips and the bit with this kind of fastening. However, the nose-band should be fastened one hand's width above the nostrils on the bony part so as not to impede the breathing of the horse. (Fig. 7.10)

The cavesson nose-band should be fastened two fingers below the facial crest and is used in combination with the double bridle with curb and bridoon bits. (Fig. 7.12). Any nose-band should always allow for good chewing movement, so that the lower jaw is freely movable, and there should be space for two fingers between the jaw bone and the nose-band. The flash nose-band is a cavesson nose-band with a second strap. This should prevent the horse from opening his mouth too wide without causing restricted breathing.

A technical trick in this context is the crank nose-band which has a pulley action on the turned strap and differs from the flash nose-band in this way. Through this pulley action it is possible for the rider to crank the horse's mouth closed with very little effort [giving a deceptively easy over-tightening of the cavesson].

A further variation on the flash nose-band is the Mexican or grackle nose-band, that is fastened high on the facial crest and crossed over the bridge

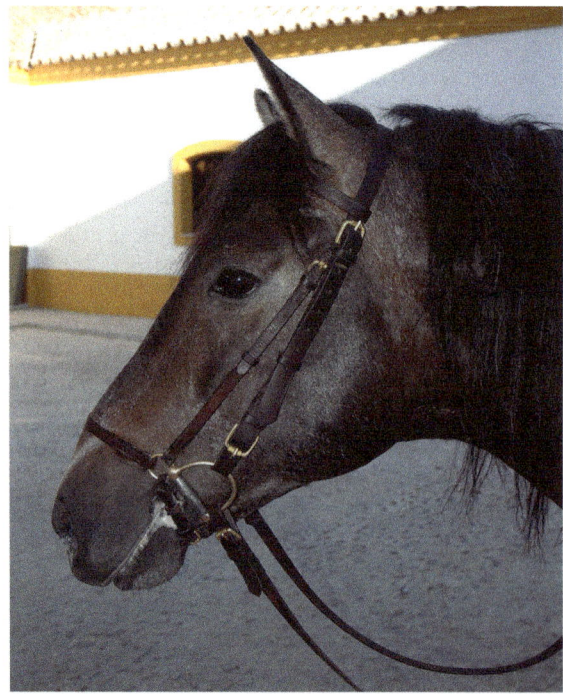

Fig 7.10. Correct fastening of the drop nose band, a D-ring snaffle is used.

of the nose. With this nose-band, a better selective pressure distribution is achieved and the action on the horse's mouth is increased. The breathing is unrestricted due to the high fastening. This is very popular in eventing.

Young horses and horses that have trouble coming on the bit, can in the beginning, be ridden in the combination of bridle and cavesson with four reins. The cavesson must then be fastened much like a drop nose-band and will work through soft pressure on the nose, and the horse can learn to yield easier in his poll. This, however, will only work when the cavesson has a ring-shaped attachment and not a square one on the chin strap. Only in this way can the chin strap be fastened in proper form under the bridle. In this way, the sensitive mouth of the horse can be preserved and it will soon be clear to the horse what the trainer wants from him as he will already have understood the action of the cavesson.

7.2.2. Criteria for choosing the correct bit.

Choosing the correct bit is more often a question of faith than a subsequent functional solution—for ultimately the bit is only as soft or as useful as the hand of the rider at the other end of the rein permits.

As anatomical benchmarks, the morphology and anatomy of the horse's mouth needs to be drawn upon. The width and thickness of the bars of the mouth, the nature of the tongue, and the form of the palate all need to be considered. When a curb bit is chosen, the depth of the bars of the mouth must also be considered, for that is also a contributory factor to the length of the side bars and the height of the port.

The bars of the mouth of a normal light warm-blood type horse is normally not more than 4.5cm, and with the choice of a double broken bit the following arises: when the movable parts of the bit are too long, the lips will be pinched on the side as soon as the reins are taken up, and the articulated mouthpiece will be more or less heavily positioned on the lips. The tongue will be pinched in the process. According to radiographic studies done, the single broken snaffles do not push into the palate as is commonly thought, but rather, pinches the tongue increasingly in the middle. With double broken bits the middle piece must not be wider than the lips since the tongue will be pinched on the side when the reins are taken up.

A similar situation is observed with too wide a curb bit or when its port is too high. Overly wide bits slide around awkwardly in the mouth and pinch the edges of the tongue between the lips and the port, and head shaking will often be the result of the pain felt in the mouth.

The sense of touch of the tongue allows the horse to feel fine differences in the surfaces of the bits and it is for this reason that copper inserts, rollers and gaps etc can be very stimulating as bits to play with. In the same way most horses accept the double broken snaffles with the flat French mouthpiece or the mouthpieces that are rounded at various angles, all of which should defuse the harshness of the bits.

In this context, the Dr. Bristol bit is worth mentioning; it has a double broken mouthpiece and a 45 degree angle to the tongue, but the harshness is aggravated, as the piece in between has smooth edges and is not curved.

Waterford bits with several links as well as chain have a much stronger and inaccurate action despite the many links, and should—just like most of the sharp-edged and painful acting constructions—not be used at all.

The straight bits without leverage should be mentioned. These snaffles are often gladly accepted by many horses, as they lie entirely on the tongue and in this way do not have the nutcracker effect. They are milder than the simple broken snaffle.

Materials that stimulate saliva formation, such as silver and copper in various combinations are better accepted by most horses, as opposed to the nickel alloys that tend to flake off with use. There are ever more horses that show an allergy to metal alloys, which make the alloys an important concern when choosing a bit.

Rubber bits tend to have an eraser-like feeling and should not be used for this reason. Apart from the taste, who wants to have part of the tire of a car in the mouth?

The much-loved burnished sweet iron, used in western riding and with the Spanish horses, stimulates the production of saliva through the natural oxidation processes, but easily looks soiled due to rust when it is not maintained regularly.

The snaffle bit, apart from the mouthpiece, also has the rings to which the reins and the cheek pieces are attached.

The most common rings are the movable round rings of the loose ring snaffle, which allows good free movement, but can cause pinching of the lips when they are worn out.

The egg butt snaffle is somewhat softened by the transition of the olive from of the ring and is less movable. It lies quietly on the margins of the lips and is mostly pleasant in the mouth of the horse.

D-rings, as their name suggests, have D-shaped rings that allow a very pleasant fit in the corners of the mouth and through the light pressure on the opposite side makes it easier for the horses to turn (fig. 7.10). This construction will also prevent the bit from being pulled through the mouth. It can be used in the phase of rehabilitation with all bits and is used for training young horses in the Royal Andalusian Riding school in Jerez.

The Fulmer snaffle has upper and lower cheeks on the rings, that assist when turning and placing the horse. The cheeks should be attached to the cheek pieces with leather straps, called fulmer keepers to keep it from tilting to the front. This type of bit, with movable rings, is used in the Spanish Riding School in Vienna. This bit is also used in phases of rehabilitation with various bits as it lies very comfortably in the horse's mouth.

An unusual form of the side pieces is found in the so-called Fillis or Baucher bit that have an upper cheek next to the ring where the cheek pieces of the bridle gets attached. This setting has the bit hanging free in the mouth, that is liked by horses with a thicker tongue, and allows a better positioning of the horse through the influence of the upper cheeks on the cheeks of the horse. The Fillis bit is also good to be used as a bridoon in a double bridle.

Gags and Dutch gags as well as various other bit constructions are not suitable for everyday use and should only be employed by professionals for a short time when needed for correction purposes.

The bit should lie in the mouth without pulling the lips up too high, and not beat against the incisors. In the ideal situation they should form two creases on the commissura labialis and always lie one finger above the canine teeth in stallions, and with mares one finger above the prospective stallion teeth.

The thickness of the bit should be chosen so it is pleasant for both the horse and the rider. A bit that is too thick will tempt the horse to lean on the hand more than a thin one, however, this is all relative. An expert can also ride on the "rusted key of the front door," as the proverb says.

The thickness of the bit depends in the first place on how "fleshy" the lips are and the length of the mouth. When thick, fleshy lips are combined with a short mouth (ponies) it is better to use a thinner mouth piece. English Thoroughbreds with sharp-edged mandibles and longer mouths should have thicker bits, in this way also avoiding panic reactions that can be caused by sharper bits.

It is often observed that horses who tend to panic will be handled better with softer bits than with sharper bits, as the additional pain will intensify panic and flight reactions and stimulate the horse to pull and run off even more.

The Curb Bit

In discussing the curb bit, one refers to a bit that utilizes leverage to its advantage. It helps to get the horse on the bit and is composed of the following:

The mouth piece of the curb bit is rigid or mobile, but still a bar. This can be straight, arched or tiled forward slightly. All curb bits have a bigger or smaller elevation called the port. (fig.7.11)

This allows pressure on the tongue to be relieved and more pressure put on the bars or the roof of the mouth. The higher the port, the stronger the bit. The height and width of the port is dependent on the depth of the bars of the mouth and is measured from the deepest point of the chin groove to the bars.

When these details are taken into account, there will be much less problems in choosing the mouth piece. Many horses do not like too thick curb bits or snaffles, for they have too much iron in their mouths when the mouth is too short. It is for this reason that the bits should only be chosen as thick as necessary. Under normal circumstances 16cm will be sufficient.

The length of the top shank will indicate how much pressure will be exerted on the poll. Normally a top shank should not be longer than 5cm [2 inches] (standard is 4cm [1.57 inches]). When the top shank is too short, the bit will fail when the chin chain is adjusted normally. The cheek rings, where the cheek pieces of the bridle are attached, should always have a slight curvature to the outside so as not to put pressure on the lips.

The lower shank should, under normal circumstances be twice the length of the top shank (8cm [3.25 inches]) or shorter, which would then lessen the leverage. Shorter shanks act more immediately, but with less strength, whereas longer shanks need more time for the effect to begin, which and is much stronger when it does begin.

In today's dressage sport, the straight shanks mostly come in to use. It is very seldom that one sees the s-shaped shanks used by the army, which had the purpose of the horse not being able to catch the shanks. These curb bits are still being used in the Spanish Riding School in Vienna.

In Western riding, the diversity of the lever shapes and the deviation from the straight shape will additionally increase or decrease the effect. A softer action is achieved by the shanks that are bent backwards, as is seen in Grazer bits. However, when the shanks are in front of the axis, the smallest touch on the reins will already have a very strong impact.

The length of the chin chain is also important and should not reach the top of the mouthpiece, as it will then be necessary to fasten the chain too tight in order to achieve the appropriate angle of 45 degrees [of the shank with the line of the horse's lips when the chain is brought into contact with the chin]. Unfortunately the chin chains are still manufactured as a confection size and the result is often a large number of loose links dangling on the side of the chain hooks. An old rule of thumb says the chin chain should be 3-4 links longer than the width of the bit, so as to reach the best symmetrical pressure possible in the chin groove. Single chin chains have a stronger effect than double chains. The chin chains that were thicker in the middle have unfortunately fallen into oblivion; these chains were very agreeable for the horse to wear due to the better distribution of pressure. Underlays or chain covers for the chin chain, made of leather, rubber or gel can serve as a protection for the sensitive area of the chin groove, especially in Thoroughbred-type horses.

The position of the curb bit should be on the same height as the chin groove, but at least one finger above the stallion tooth. When the chin chain is fastened, the angle between the shank and the line of the mouth should not be more than 45 degrees. Chin chains that are fastened too tightly act too strongly and chains that are fastened too loosely hamper the leverage of the bit.

As always, the hand of the rider is the gauge that will dictate the softness or the severity of any bit.

When the shanks can rotate and the mouthpiece is movable, it is called a sliding bit and this should stimulate chewing. Horses try to lift the mouthpiece with their tongues and will keep it there. This action causes the

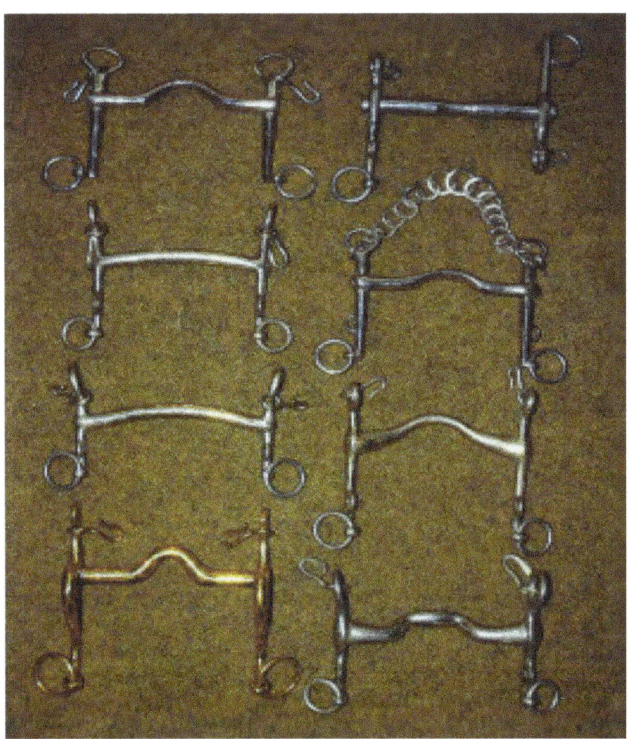

Fig. 7.11
The severity of a curb bit strongly depends on the shanks and the shape of the port of mouthpiece. The longer the shanks and the higher the port, the more severe is the action of the curb bit. Bits from top to bottom and left to right: A curb with mobile shanks, Banbury curb, mors l'Hotte, sliding cheek curb, French mouthpiece and short shanks, German Weymouth with large and broad port, S-shank curb with high port, kk Weymouth bit with short shanks.

relaxation of the muscles of the hyoid bone.

Movable shanks without the pumping effect of the mouthpiece allows for an extra positioning action and is willingly accepted by the horse (Fig. 7.12) Mouthpieces with rollers and keys can activate saliva production, but should only be used as correction for a short period of time.

Ultimately it is the way of training that creates a horse that is pleasant in the hand or not. It is for this reason that the choice of a bit should be well considered.

The thinner bridoon should not pull the edge of the mouth up into more than two wrinkles [at the corners of the horse's mouth].

One should not ignore the fact that the head of the horse, mostly around 40-45cm long, also functions as a lever, and will multiply all the force coming from the rider's hand. Therefore, the rein aids should always be administered thoughtfully and with feeling.

Of course, all of the above applies in the same scope for driving, western and other special ways of riding.

The Pelham

A Pelham is almost a curb bit, with either a broken or a straight mouthpiece, where the existence of a second ring on the height of the mouthpiece that combines the effect of the snaffle with the lever action of the curb in one bit.

In this way, one can habituate a young horse, or horses that are resentful of the curb, to accept a bit with a bar again. Horses with short mouths accept a Pelham easier than a curb and bridoon combination since, with the Pelham, they have less material in their mouths.

Furthermore, the possibility for bending is even better due to the movable shanks than with a curb bit with fixed shanks. Broken Pelhams should be rejected due to their inaccurate function and the increase in the nutcracker action.

Pelham bits with a sliding mouthpiece, copper rollers (*coscojero*, Hanoverian) or simple ports (Hartwell Pelham) are very recommendable bits and can be used to refine the aids, especially in the rehabilitation phase.

A Pelham should always be ridden with two reins in order to achieve a differentiated action.

Pelham roundings, [a strap of leather] that join the two rings [on the same side], does not actually join these rings and is very confusing for the horse as far as the action goes.

The Kimblewick bit or Spanish jumping bit has a special position in the Pelham family. This is a bit with big D-shaped rings and a short upper shank. With the use of the D-ring it is possible to accentuate the lever action or the bar action of this soft bit, according to how the rein is used.

The Uxeter Kimblewick [or Kimberwick] has two slits integrated in the D-rings, making a stronger lever action possible all the time.

The bit-less bridle

The bit-less bridle is any headpiece that controls the horse via pressure on the bridge of the nose and the poll. This includes the hackamore, bosal and various types of cavessons like the Pluvinel and Scawbrig bridle.

All of these bridles have in common that the lever action and therefore the braking action is exploited on the bridge of the nose and chin groove.

The mechanical hackamore is relatively strong and should only be used in professional hands. The nose iron should always lie on the bony foundation of the nasal bone otherwise it can suppress the breathing or even break the nasal bone. The hackamore is nevertheless an excellent aid to show horses with problems with contact or young horses the way to lower their heads. Many horses accept this bridle very well and will even start to chew due to the relaxation of the hyoid apparatus.

The bosal or the classical hackamore more often find use in basic training and Western riding and should keep the mouth of the very young horses soft. The classical hackamore is a leather or horse hair plaited ring that goes around the nose and mandible to end in a special knot at the bottom. Both

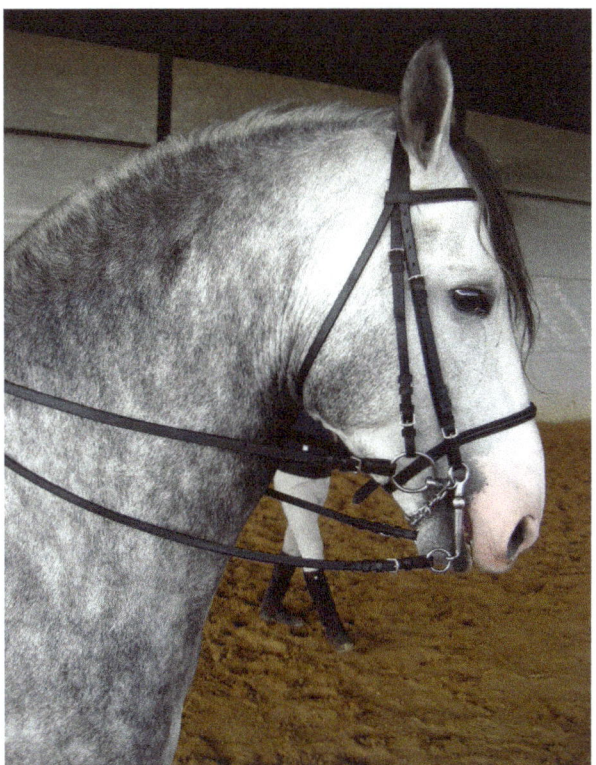

Fig.7.12. In classical dressage the combination of snaffles that cause both elevation and flexion of the neck and poll, the so-called bradoon and the Weymouth bits are used. The goal is to find a fine way to influence the horse. In this photo there is a curb with movable shanks, allowing a better influence in the sideways positioning of the horse.

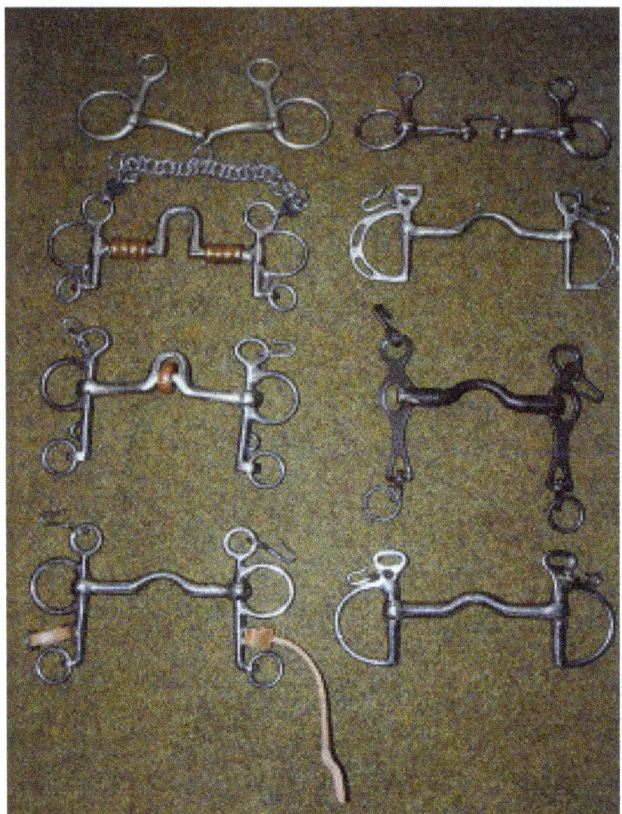

Fig. 7.13
Different pelham bits. From top to bottom, left: Baucher snaffle, Fillis snaffle, Hanoverian pelham, Uxeter-Kimblewick,. Right: pelham with movable coscojero mouthpiece, Portuguese curb, Hartwell pelham with shear belt, Kimblewick pelham (jump curb).

reins are therefore united in one point under the branches of the mandible. Turning is initiated through "neck reining," where the rein from the opposite side is put against the neck, along with shifting the weight aids of the rider.

Basic western training considers the change of dentition and therefore starts the young horses with the aid of the hackamore.

The cavesson variation already mentioned before can be used alone or with a bit. This will diffuse the action of the bit, seeing that the horse has learned to accept the pressure on the nose and relax. The cavesson should never be used to force the horse into a certain position. When two reins are attached to the movable rings on the side, it can be specifically used to position the horse.

The Scawbrig bridle is somewhat unfamiliar English variation of the bit-less bridle and consists of a leather covered metal arch with two rings, and crossed over leather loops that run under the jaw. This causes a rather constant pressure on the nose when the reins are taken up and should prevent the horse from taking his head up and pulling. This construction does not allow for differentiated action. This kind of bridle is also mentioned for completion of the list.

> **Note:** *None of these bit-less or leverage-exploiting bridles should be used with training reins such as the martingale or running reins, as this can cause maximum pressure in the horse's poll and mouth, and result in great pain and damage (pressure on the bars of the mouth, irritation of the periosteum on the bridge of the nose and the lower jaw)*

7.2.3 Influence the bit on movement disorders of the horse and the rider's hands

The bit is simply the extension of the rider's hands. Sense and nonsense regarding such an instrument always depends on the user. Every rider should get in the habit of using the lightest contact possible. Studies measuring the pulling forces have revealed that side reins reach a maximum of 0.5-2.0kg, [1-4 pounds] whereas the contact of a good rider's hand can reach 5-50kg. [10-100 pounds].

The results according to the physical law of leverage is the following: most warm-blood horses have about a 40cm long head and a lever on the poll (4cm) will influence this. When the rider pulls with an average force of 25 kg, the pressure load on the horse's poll will reach 1000kg. This pressure load can be multiplied many times with the use of the longer levers with curb bits and the use of running reins.

Horses try to escape this painful pressure with counter pressure, and are capable of exactly such peak pressure, even if they have a much shorter lever in the poll. Osteopathic lesions of the vertebrae will be the logical result. The neck muscles, especially the M. brachiocephalicus and the M. splenius hypertrophy and make it very difficult and even impossible for the horse to come on the bit. In the same way chronic inflammation of the bursa occipitalis and on the insertion of the nuchal ligament are the products of this kind of riding. As a consequence problems with contact, loss of rhythm and bridle lameness arise which can disappear again with a sensitive rider and soft bit.

Bits that are too big can chafe the bars of the mouth (curbs), tilt in the mouth and provoke tongue faults as well as contact problems. Snaffles that are too big can squash the bars of the mouth due to the nutcracker effect, provoking horses into thrusting the head up. This will cause the horse to loose the arch of the top line and then he cannot put his hind legs under him properly, and the collection greatly suffers. (fig.7.14)

Bits that are too narrow can squash the sensitive lips and can cause an unmotivated tossing up of the head, which is often falsely interpreted as head shaking.

When the mouthpiece is too thin, combined with consistent, never-releasing contact, pressure on the lips and insensitivity in the mouth can be

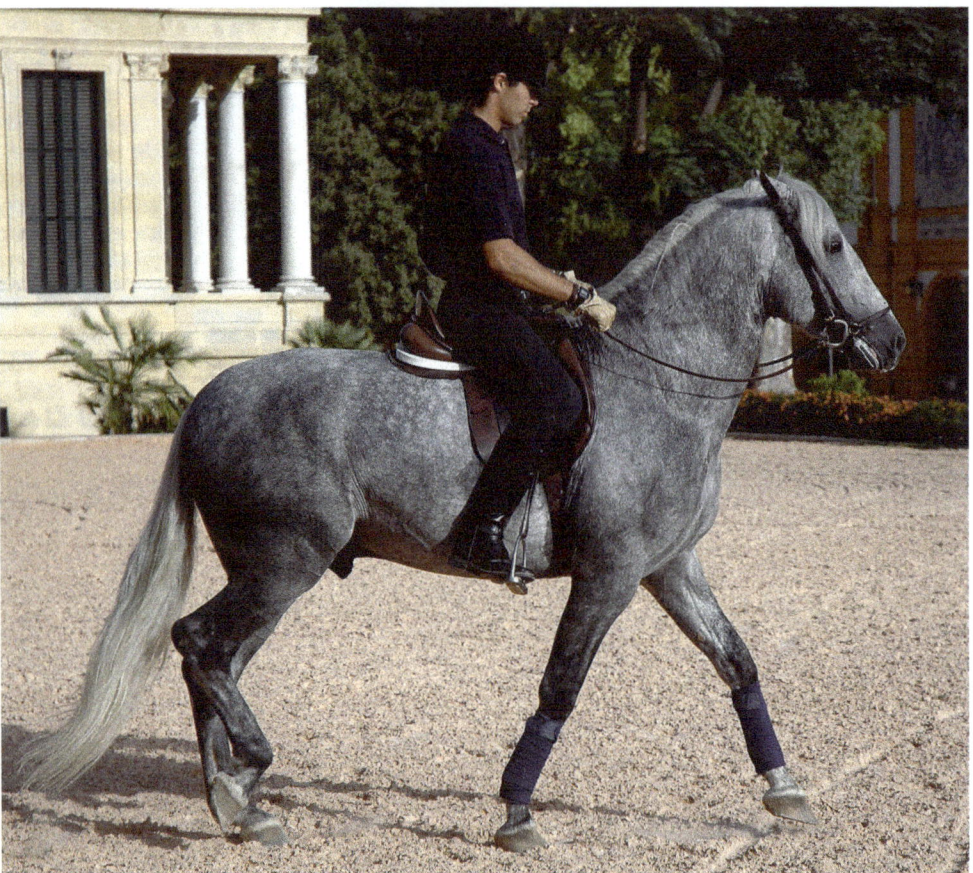

Fig.7.14 A horse lacking the quality that makes him co-operative and easy to handle, can become this way not only from incorrect training. It can also be due to teeth problems and/or ill-fitting equipment. The horse will try to escape the influence of the rider by throwing his head up and hollowing his back, making any type of collected work impossible. The horse in the picture is a young stallion without much experience under saddle.

seen. These horses accept half-halts poorly and the action of the front legs becomes dull.

Subsequently, it should be mentioned that the best bit will not achieve anything in the wrong hands.

The old French masters, who were famous for the lightness in their art of riding, coined the phrase: "hands without legs and legs without hands," which is unfortunately often wrongly interpreted. This should explain that a simultaneous "breaking" and "stepping on the gas" can only mean halt, whereas this statement does not imply that it completes the task of contact. It merely aims to explain that a soft, giving hand awaits the forward impulse from the driving legs and that they do not restrain the action by active influence.

On the basis of the neuro-vegetative reflex arc, it is, due to practical reasons, not possible for the brain to process two equally important pieces of information at the same time. It is for this reason that a soft, light, giving hand is indispensable for every form of art in riding and in rehabilitation, as pressure will always generate pressure and tension.

7.2.4 The teeth of the horse and the bit

Another very important ingredient of an integral therapeutic concept is the health of the teeth. Bad teeth can have a severe influence on the whole body, not only because toothaches can cause behavioral changes, but also because every tooth can be assigned to an organ and interactions can therefore take place.

Ulcerous tips of the root is extensively known in human medicine to cause cardiac problems. They also lead to serious health damage in the horse.

Problems are often found in young horses that are starting their training at the age of 3 years, as the change in dentition starts at 2.5 years and is only complete at 5 years. This will inevitably cause problems with the horse's co-operation and bring resistances due to painful irritation of the gums. During this phase it is therefore important to regularly control for impacted caps, canines that have not yet broken through and wolf teeth.

Dental checks every 6 months to one year is recommended in order to prevent faults in the bite. Faults in the bite or hooks on the teeth can lead to incorrect position of the jaw joint, making coming on the bit difficult [or impossible] and can result in problems with movement.

Adult horses should be checked on a yearly basis. In this way, fissures and fractures can be recognized as possible portals of entry for bacteria and can be treated in time.

The modern way of feeding concentrated feed (mixed grains, mash) and too little roughage (at least 1kg of hay per 100kg) creates the development of ramps on the inside and outside of the molars, as horses often do too few grinding movements with their teeth. The softer feeding ingredients will often not produce sufficient saliva, are poorly chewed and immediately swallowed, whereby the higher incidence of stomach ulcers can be explained if it is not caused by stress, due to the acid buffering action of the saliva in the stomach being reduced.

Physiological feeding dictates that horses should have roughage fed at least 60 minutes before they are fed their concentrates in order to prepare the stomach for the "acid" concentrates. This simple procedure is unfortunately only seldom kept in stables due to lack of staff and time.

Treatment of teeth should only be done through sedation by a veterinarian, with the aid of a mouth speculum, a headlamp, and different rasps that are adapted to the inclination of the row of teeth.

The sedation of the horse guarantees a safe and complete inspection and exploration of the mouth that can only be done by sight, using a speculum and dental head collar.

Many horses have wounds the size of finger nails on the mucous membranes on the inside of the cheeks, caused by too narrow cheek pieces and nose-bands in association with the sharp ramps of the upper molars.

Difficulties with contact and unwillingness to accept the hand of the rider is thus clear and obvious in the truest sense of the word. These changes heal quickly when the horse is allowed to work for a few days without a bit.

Avulsion[7] of the bone is the result of pitiful riding and is unfortunately still seen in practice. In this case, the owner of the horse should be thoroughly integrated in the concept of rehabilitation therapy, so that a satisfying solution can be found for the horse.

Gags and pulling the tongue out of the mouth should be a thing of the past as that only allows for inadequate views into the mouth and can injure the horses (tearing the tongue, chipping a tooth, etc)

The horses should be ridden without a bit for a few days after a dental treatment in order to soothe possible irritation of the mucous membranes, ensuring faster healing for any possible wounds. In such cases the bit-less bridles are most suitable.

7.2.5. Nose-bands and their impact on acupressure points on the horse's head

This Chapter may seem somewhat unusual at the first glance, however the energetic connections should not be underestimated, especially in rehabilitative medicine.

According to the classical Chinese opinions, pain is just a cry for energy flow. Based on this concept, all rehabilitation measures should be classified as mandatory medicine, as the improvement of circulation can be seen as one of the main goals for the attainment or restoration of the body's own integrity. The horse has six meridian origins or endings in the head alone. Additionally to the six paired meridians, there are also the endings of the unpaired Ren-Mai and Du-Mai vessels. (Fig: 7.15)

In the area of the poll, one finds important points such as the Bl 10 and Gb 20, and their course can significantly influence the flexibility of the poll as

---
7 An injury in which a body structure is forcibly detached from its normal point of insertion by either trauma or surgery

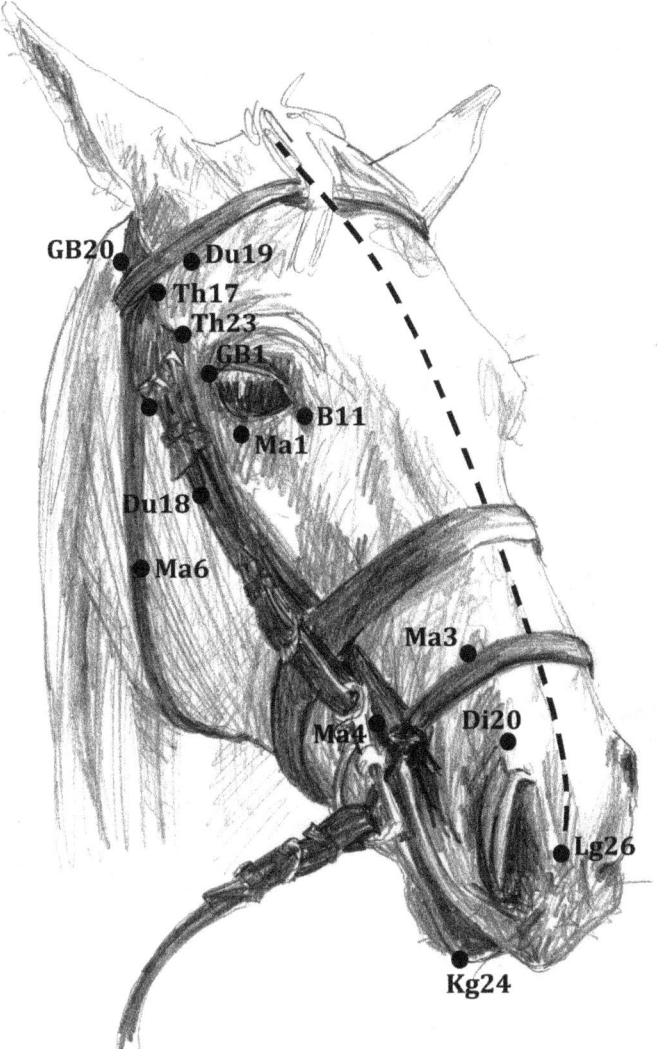

Fig.7.15 On the horse's head are important acupuncture points, which can be strongly affected by the type and fastening of the noseband. A Hanoverian noseband, buckled too tightly, stimulates respiratory points such as z. B. Bi shu, causing problems with the large intestine meridian, and may affect respiratory frequency.

well as the activity of the back and the amount of collection.

In the browband area, at the base of the ears, one not only finds the traditional Chinese point Kai jin zhui that has a strong influence on the temporal-mandibular joint and the sacroiliac joint, but also important points of the bladder, gall bladder, triple heater and the small intestine meridians that influence the action of the front and hind legs depending on the smooth flow of energy.

When a nose-band is fitted too tightly, not only does it block the unpaired meridians, but also influences the large intestine and stomach meridians that run on the side of the horse's head. The former affects the breathing and the latter, the readiness of flexibility in the haunches.

The TCM points Bi Shu and Xue tang are only stimulated when a drop nose-band is fitted too deep and too tight. This will have a negative influence on breathing via the acupuncture points, not to mention the mechanical restriction of the airways.

The cavesson nose-band that is normally fitted two finger's width below the cheek bone, will just disrupt the stomach and large intestine meridians. In this area one will only find the traditional Chinese acupuncture points such as Kai guan. This influences the chewing activity and is used to treat facial paralysis and tetanus.

The Mexican/grackle and the flash nose-band will stimulate the Ma4 and Sou kou points when fitted too tight.

In summary, it should be said that basically correct nose-bands—not fitted too deep or too tight—can be used without a problem, for the actual effect of the nose-band lies in the protection of the horse's mouth, for every action from the hand to lightly open the mouth in a relaxing way will be transferred to the bridge of the nose.

Nose-bands should never be used to prevent a horse from opening its mouth when the hand of the rider is too harsh and causes the horse pain.

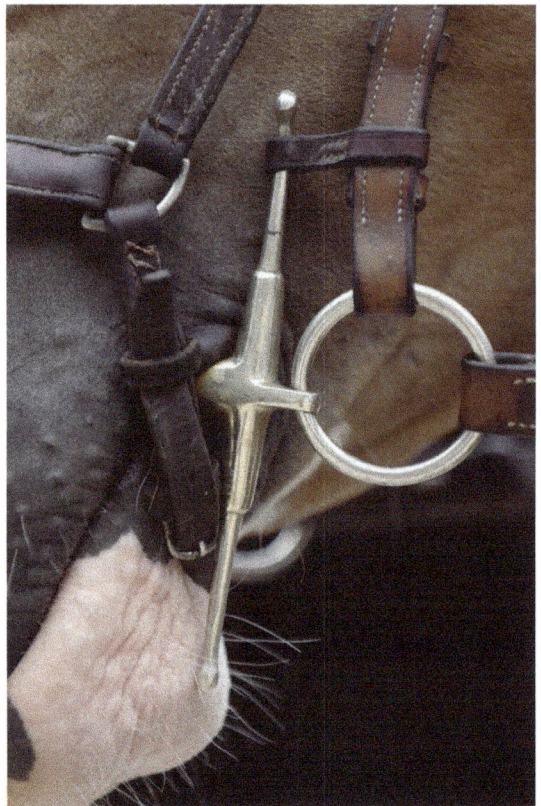

Fig. 7.16 a.
Fulmer [or full-cheek] snaffle with leather Fulmer keepers ensure that the bit lies quiet in the mouth. The shanks support the young horse in the lateral bending.

[Correct arrangement of dropped (also called a Hannoverian)nose band with a full cheek snaffle bit. Note the keepers at the top end of the full cheek of the bit attached to the headstall of the bridle. —Editor's note.]

Fig. 7.16. b.
The hannoverian noseband should lie on the boney part of the nose and should allow enough room to let the horse chew which is only possible when there is 2 fingers' space between the nose and the noseband.

[Allow two finger's clearance under the drop nose band when fully 'tightened'. This is the correct fastening. The nose band should not be used to prevent the horse from opening its mouth.—Editor's note.]

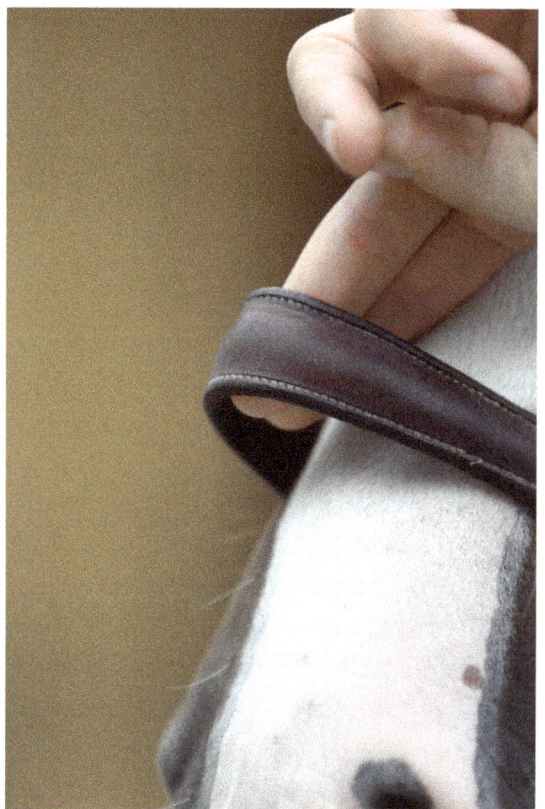

8. Developing the Training

8.1. Prevention and fitness

Prevention and fitness are major factors in equine practice today. The prevention of lameness represents an important theme, not only because of the loss of time but also due to financial aspects.

Studies in the USA show that lamenesses in racing stables were significantly reduced when targeted preventative measures were used, such as thermography, physiotherapy, acupuncture, and osteopathy. In spite of the extra financial cost, there was a considerable reduction recorded in the total price of treatment and loss of races.

The very early detection of problems with training or tension in the competitive athlete, in this case the horse, can lead to better performance with the use of a sensible and individual training plan by the rider. A horse that is tense is much more prone to stress and less willing to perform and often provides the rider with additional dissatisfaction and unnecessary fights.

With the use of thermography (see Chapter 16.4), one can detect changes in the heat pattern as much as two weeks before the clinical manifestation of tendinitis, and take preventative measures such as cooling. This has been proven by studies in the USA.

Regular mobilization techniques and acupressure can increase the subjective well-being of the horse, making them more powerful in their performances. This, in combination with a systematic and logically planned training concept with the added bonus of a sympathetic and patient rider, can lead to a successful performance, much better than the push-and-pull methods.

In modern sport horse medicine, not only is it important to have a healthy, sound horse, but also a mentally fit horse that will be able to withstand a demanding training program.

Definition: *Fitness, apart from the basic physical requirements to perform, includes mental readiness in a calm and happy way, which requires an ability to be motivated by both the therapist and the rider.*

Many dressage horses manage their jobs in a proficient manner, but never exhibit the splendor, the lightness, and brilliance of others. An inner willingness, paired with the correct physical prerequisites, systematic training and physiotherapy, can produce more elasticity and range of movement, certain to impact scores in competition.

8.2. Basic Training Fundamentals

Many papers have been written on training philosophies. A more detailed analysis would go beyond the framework here. However, the points of a logically thought-out program for a young horse before he is a riding horse should at least be touched upon.

Basic training is indeed similar to rehabilitation, but is designed for a perfectly healthy horse who can specialize in any direction after completing this approximately two-year-long program. Much consideration should be given to the myelogenous basics discussed earlier, because the muscle composition (slow twitch, fast twitch) of a dressage horse differs from a three-day-eventer. This direction should be set up at the beginning of the specialization phase as it can be very difficult to change later.

The three essential phases of training are:
1. Adaptation
2. Strength training
3. Endurance training

In the first phase (adaptation), the young horse comes in from the pasture and gets accustomed to many new environmental influences such as the stable, riding school, and lunge arena. During this time, the digestive tract has to adjust to changes in eating and movement habits. The young horse also has to come to terms with new patterns of movement (circles on the lunge) and different ground surfaces, making muscular and tendinous adaptations to the new load ratio. Through this process, a resilient foundation is created. In this phase the horse is only moved forward in a long and low manner. He must find his own rhythm, swing and inner release.

In the second phase (strength training), the thrusting power that was previously developed is now utilized and converted into carrying capacity. The muscle building phase includes work in-hand, and commencing the work under the rider, varying the gaits, lateral work, riding uphill. This is done to obtain supple muscles in the horse. In this phase, the shoulder-in is valuable, for not only does it help straighten the horse, it also helps develop carrying capacity in the haunches and improves freedom of the shoulders. The main gait of this phase is the trot. This strength training requires several months, depending on the situation. Significant growth in muscle mass cannot be expected in less than three months.

In the third phase (endurance training) the cardiovascular system should be adapted to the changed muscular and training environment. For this, longer canter phases are required to improve ventilation. Regular checks of the pulse and respiratory rates are necessary to be sure not to over-train the horse. Horses should never be returned to the stable in an exhausted state or with high pulse and respiratory rates. Interval training and hill-work can be useful to support these stages. The length of training should be judged sensibly. The wise trainer should realize when the horse needs a rest period. Proper warm-up and cool-down of at least ten minutes should be planned into every training session.

> **In Practice:** *The concentration of a horse has reached its maximum after 20 minutes, and will lead to resistance when excessive demands are made after this time elapses.*

8.3 Correct warm-up and cool-down of a horse

As with every normal sportsman, it is important to warm-up the muscles and joints properly before they are worked. This will prevent any muscle or tendon tearing due to a cold start. Warming up should be done for at least 10 minutes at a free walk on a loose rein. Apart from physical relaxation, the horse also gets a chance to stretch outside of the confined stall dimensions—if he is stabled or paddocked—and to supply more oxygen to his muscles without any tension.

> **In Practice:** *The warm-up should not be less than 10 minutes, for that is exactly the amount of time the synovial liquid needs to spread evenly in the joints and offer the cartilaginous structures maximum protection during movement. The same goes for horses from the paddock, for movement in the paddock is not sufficient to lubricate the joints.*

After 10 minutes of walk, horses that are already trained can loosen up through lateral movements and half-turns, making the horse easier to ride. Trotting the horse "for hours" in a straight line only uses up energy and strength, the horse gets worn out and bored.

After this short loosening up phase the horses can be worked according to their level of training for about 20-25 minutes. Working any longer is not reasonable due to the horse's lack of ability to concentrate. During the training, it is advisable to include short relaxation periods, in order to avoid any preprogrammed resistances due to physical overload.

The last third of any training session should be the "cool-down." This is often forgotten, but for muscle physiology it is very important. A relaxing and rhythmic forward and down trot will circulate waste products out of the muscles and bring the pulse and respiratory rate down to normal again.

> **In Practice:** *The cool-down should end with a relaxed walk on long reins so the horse can end the session on a positive note and not return to the stable tired and exhausted.*

9. Work on the lunge.

9.1 General advice

One should distinguish the different ways of working a horse on the lunge: a) the actual work with a properly equipped and fit horse, b) the initial lungeing of a green horse, c) the correction of a problem horse, and d) the maintenance of elasticity of a well-ridden horse. Just lungeing a horse with a halter has nothing to do with gymnastic work, but can be of advantage in certain circumstances when the automatic response to finding balance in the horse can be triggered when it is correctly applied.

We always speak of "work" on the lunge, thus stressing the fundamental aspect of lunge training.

> **Definition:** *Lunge work is the systematic development of training with the goal to improve the movement of the horse and to stretch the topline. It is not uncontrolled running around in circles.*

The strain of the circle through centrifugal and shearing forces should never be underestimated and, as a result, the footing material, the radius of the circle and the speed are of great importance.

> **Note:** *The goal of every training session on the lunge should be to bring the horse into a relaxed and stretched topline through brisk and rhythmic forward movement. This way the muscles can reach maximum elasticity.*

Work on the lunge also has a place in rehabilitation and in the treatment of back problems. The standard method of lungeing places the person in one spot in the middle of the circle in order to obtain constant contact with the horse. However, in the preferred way of lungeing for rehabilitation, the person moves with the horse, thus establishing a more flexible and elastic contact.

This does not mean that the lunge line should drag on the ground, but through regular taking and giving should induce a forward and down stretch of the horse, similar to the effective hand of the rider.

When a young, inexperienced horse is to be rehabilitated, it is a good idea to have an extra person to help lead the horse on the inside of the circle while the trainer, doing the actual lungeing, remains in the center of the circle.

Horses to be rehabilitated are those which have had painful experiences or incorrect training that renders them physically and mentally disadvantaged and therefore, not capable of adapting a normal stretched and relaxed topline due to lack of trust in the trainer.

To this end, the use of the voice, either as a calming but activating aid, or at times, also as a reprimand, is beneficial. Vocal communication is always available and can alleviate a horse's fear and inspire confidence.

All harsh and sudden movements should be avoided to help the horse develop trust. The whip should also be carried out purposefully and to the point, because a continuous forward driving influence from the whip or clicking of the tongue can desensitize the horse and does not generate the possibility for refinement of the aids.

Ideally, the horse should lower his croup [when moving] when the lunge whip is pointed in the direction of the pelvis, while the trainer moves in a triangle behind the horse. When the trainer wants to restrain the horse, he should move the triangle to the front of the horse. This optical barrier will reduce the forward movement of the horse.

Every small gesture of the horse that tends in the direction of forward and downward stretching should be praised and rewarded by yielding the lunge line. Otherwise the desired learning by the horse will be achieved insufficiently or not at all. In this context, horses should always be lunged with a cavesson to preserve the softness of his mouth, even when the horse wears a bridle. Nothing is as confusing to a horse as a command to stretch down that is counteracted by an unyielding and harsh hand from the trainer at the moment when he attempts the downward stretch. A horse in this situation cannot understand what he is meant to do.

In the first phase of training, the horse is lunged free without side reins in a round pen or alternatively with double lunge lines of at least 12 meters in length. In the very beginning, double lunge lines would only serve to confuse the horse and tend to interfere with stretching.

Another stipulation is never to let a horse run around in the round pen in an uncontrolled manner, because any number of unpredictable situations can occur to jeopardize the healing process.

Extreme bending to the inside should be abandoned. In addition to the strongly adverse influence it has on the balance of the horse, it also leads to serious tension of the inside neck muscles and overloading of the outside shoulder. When a horse bends himself to the outside it is a sign of lack of balance and fixing the neck, which acts as a balancing pole. Over-bending to the inside is not a solution. Progressive stiffening and problems with bending will result when the position of over-bending is adopted over a long time.

During the work on the lunge, one should always strive to work the horse in a regular, calm, yet diligent pace; this is the only way the horse can find his own rhythm.

Fast running around in circles only causes wear and tear on the joints and a contraction of the long back muscles, which, in turn causes a hollowing of the back, thus preventing the biomechanics of the back from functioning correctly. When referring to the training tree, the horse in rehabilitation is once again at the beginning, where rhythm and freedom are the primary goals forming the foundation for all further progress.

A uniform curve is easily possible with the aid of the big radius of the round pen, for the horse has an optical aid in the form of the round pen and the bend is not forced. When the horse shows signs of problems with the bend, a rest period can be introduced to allow him to stretch-out for a while, and then, once again ask for a slight bend to the inside on the lunge.

In the rehabilitation phase, one should not disregard that the horses are not as mobile due to their physical problems, they have incorrect or protective postures that should be corrected through training.

Doing many transitions between the different gaits will improve the balance and put the horse increasingly on the hindquarters.

The total working time should be a maximum of 30 minutes since the horse's ability to concentrate will have been exhausted and the continuous movement on a circle can overload the tendons and ligaments.

In order to eliminate tension and a bad working environment, it is necessary to work calmly, consistently and plan the work ahead of time.

9.2 Equipment

The equipment needed to lunge a horse includes a bridle with a bit and a padded cavesson with a fixed nose-band and a jowl strap which can be fastened at more or less eye level. Very useful is the slightly padded kind of cavesson that is used on the Iberian peninsula.

The cavesson should have three rings and should be fastened about one hand's width above the nostrils, under the bridle, similar to a dropped nose-band. The eyelets for the chin strap should be round and not angular to make fastening under the bridle easier and to avoid pinching the lips. (Fig.9.1)

This way of fitting has the advantage that the horse learns very quickly to yield to the pressure on the nose and to stretch down easily. Furthermore, the horse is more sensitive in this area and the trainer does not need a lot of strength to influence the bridge of the nose, as would be the case with the more padded varieties that are fastened like a cavesson nose-band.

The ring in the middle must be mobile. The lunge line is attached to this ring. The two rings on either side can be used to attach reins when the horse is first ridden and in this manner one achieves a more refined coordination between the hand of the rider and the horse's mouth.

The action of the cavesson is already known to the horse and the sensitive mouth can be preserved through the effect of the reins, for the horse

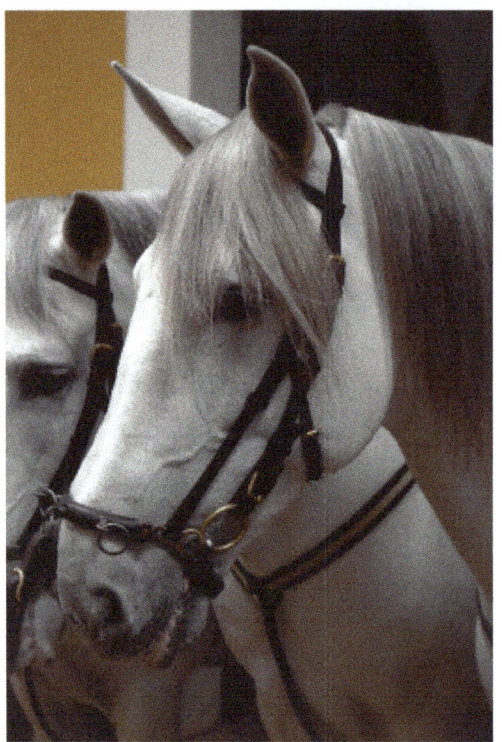

Fig. 9.1. Correctly fitted cavesson fitted over the bridle with a jowl strap that prevents the buckle from sliding into the horse's eye. The round, swiveling ring on the cavesson's noseband allows for a "dropped noseband" to be fitted without pushing the bit up onto the bars.

would rather yield to the pressure on the nose than to a painful pull on the mouth.

> **Note:** *A basic rule: use as little leather as possible! It is for this reason that the browband of the bridle and other extra straps such as the nose-band piece of the bridle are omitted in order not to irritate the horse.*

The best bit to use [for lunging] is either a normal D-ring snaffle or a Fulmer [full cheek] snaffle with loose rings equipped correctly with Fulmer keepers to keep the cheek pieces from jutting forward like the horns of a rhinoceros.

The rumor that more leverage is produced on the poll in this way cannot be comprehended by the author. Both of these bits have the advantage that one cannot pull the bits through the mouth and that they softly press on the side of the mouth when the horse is bent, which makes it easier for the horse to understand when to turn and to yield to a one-sided rein aid.

The bit can have a single or double jointed mouthpiece and the choice will depend on the mouth of the horse and should be chosen accordingly. Bits made from copper or other materials, made to promote chewing on the bit, as well as roller bits can be used to re-activate otherwise inactive mouths.

This said, one should avoid bits with keys. Horses are often encouraged to put the tongue over the bit with them as the keys are usually too low and seem to annoy the horse.

A proper lunge line should be made of cotton, not too heavy and 12 meters long. Leather stoppers sewn onto the lunge line are often awkward and can give way to a loop at the end of the rein. Nylon lunge lines are often uncomfortable in the hand due to the bulky material and should therefore not be used.

Many trainers prefer the use of gloves when lungeing a horse to protect their hands from any abrupt movements. Lungeing in an enclosed circular arena can prevent such situations from happening since the horse cannot break free from the trainer due to the boundary fence.

The lunge whip must be long enough to easily reach the horse with the lash without requiring significant change in position of the trainer. The whip must definitely not be too heavy; it must be well-balanced. A more expensive, but well-balanced whip makes itself appreciated every day. It is more pleasant for the trainer, because the muscles of the trainer's shoulder girdle do not become tense with use.

A lungeing surcingle worth recommending is the padded leather variety with many rings where one can attach a variety of lungeing reins and also the long reins.

The author of this book uses a modified "wooden rider" when doing rehabilitation. This consists of a pad with a metal bracket with 4 eyelets attached on top, where the loops of the breeching for a modified Nelson Pessoa training system can be fastened in order

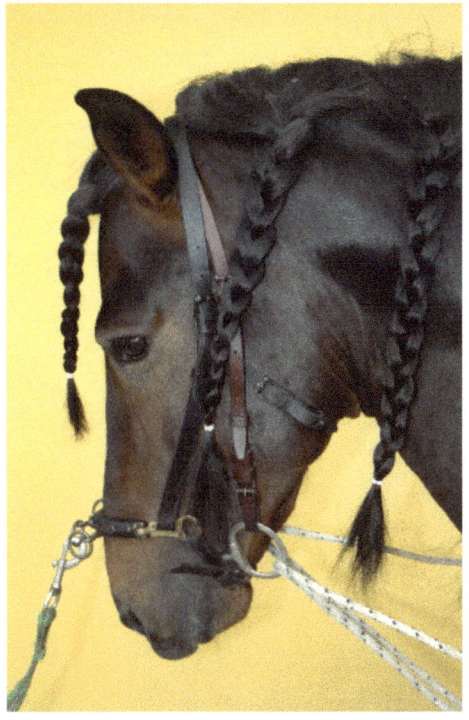

Fig. 9.2 a & b
Detail of the Nelson Pessoa training system set up with a lunging surcingle with loose ring rolling wheels for minimal resistance.

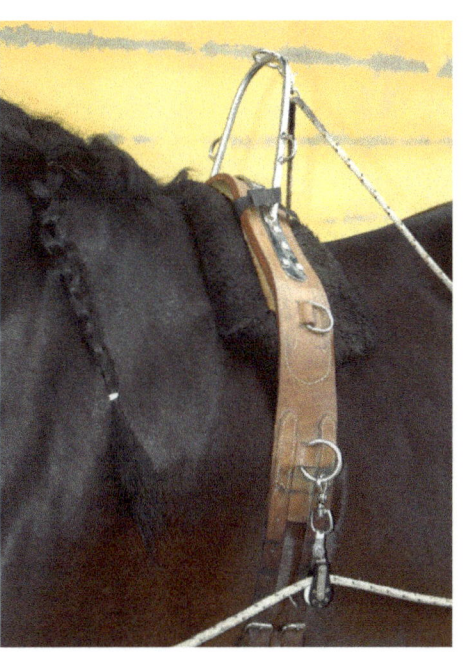

to soften the pull on the hollow above the hocks, in front of the gaskins. There is an extra ring in the middle of the girth to which running side reins or the Pessoa training system can be attached.

Depending on the level of training, when the horse is being lunged, he should wear over-reach and brush boots or working bandages and padding to protect the him from injury, especially in young horses that may not have sufficient balance. Injury occurs when horses accidentally step on the bulbs of their front feet. Hence, young horses should always be lunged with overreach boots.

Weighted boots should only be used in walk and should gradually be adjusted for the horse. Starting with 500gr they can be increased to 750gr. In order to prevent fatigue of the tendons and ligaments, one should limit this work to 10-15 minutes. Weighted boots and weighted shoes that are permanently fitted do more harm than good and should not be used for animal-welfare reasons.

Cantering or allowing a horse with weighted boots to jump around is very dangerous for the joints of the horse, since the added weight has increased centrifugal and shearing forces and can thus strain the joints.

Nevertheless, the sensible use of weighted boots is justified in that it improves the action and muscle development of the limbs.

Subsequently, the wooden balls strung together and tied around the pasterns must be mentioned. These were already used by the old masters to get the horse to improve activity of the forehand. They are 5 wooden balls, linked with a leather band and fitted around the pastern of the front legs. Through the movement, the horse is animated to lift his legs higher whereby the biceps can actively be addressed. In this manner the mobility of the shoulder can be improved in a short time, but after a short while the horse will get used to this method and the specific response will be decreased.

Note: *Trying to improve the action through blistering is no longer allowed according to animal welfare laws.*

9.3. Use of training aids

Lungeing and work in-hand call for the widest application of auxiliary training aids (in the form of various reins). They are used in these types of work to prepare the horse for riding and to help obviate potential problems.

As the term suggests, the reins should be used as an aid for the horse, to help him understand quicker what one wants from him, without actually depriving him of the possibility of trying a new course of action and convincing himself that the movement is possible.

The most appropriate lungeing aid in capable hands is the modified version of the Pessoa training system, as it allows the horse in the deep position to coordinate his impulsion-transmitting hindquarters with the gymnastic extension of his position. This system consists of a type of breeches, covered in wool, that will lie at the height of the buttock. This piece is attached to a ring on the back of the pad with an eyelet. The pieces on the side run parallel to the horse's belly, thread through the rings of the bit and then hooked on to the ring on the girth (fig:9.2a). The modification of the original Pessoa training system lies in the fact that the side traces are taken through a higher or lower attached pulley on the side on the way to the mouth (fig:9.2b) and the breeches are replaced by a leather piece covered in sheepskin. Through this modification, the effect of the breeches remains the same while influencing a bigger surface area behind the buttocks. One also maintains a softer connection to the horse's mouth. To obtain the stretch, the system must be connected in such a way that the nose is slightly in front of the vertical and the head must not be forced into a specific position as this will only provoke unnecessary tension in the horse.

The well thought-out adjustment possibilities of this system makes it plausible to accompany the horse through his whole life of training, from the stretching at the start to the collected elevation, and can be adjusted within a training session to adapt to the requirements in a quick and straightforward manner.

This system is very versatile and useful as a lungeing aid, one which horses accept without problem.

The running side reins should be mentioned for they can be used as a variation of the running reins by fastening them to the girth between the front legs of the horse, to run through the rings of the bit and then attach on the horse's side to the lungeing surcingle.

The advantage of this rein is the imitation of the rider's hand through the lateral boundary of the triangle and, at the same time, facilitating the possibility of stretching forward and down. This quickly makes it clear to the horse what is expected of him in the initial warm-up phase.

Always essential is—and the same goes for all lungeing aids—to attach the reins such that the horse's nose can be slightly in front of the vertical.

Running or draw reins are mostly used when the horse is ridden with knowledgeable hands and this can be a quick solution for a short period of time only. The emphasis here lies on *knowledgeable* and *temporary*, since horses quickly accept that they are pulled down and kept down with this lever system, and the moment the rein is no longer used, the situation deteriorates and the original problem may be multiplied many times over.

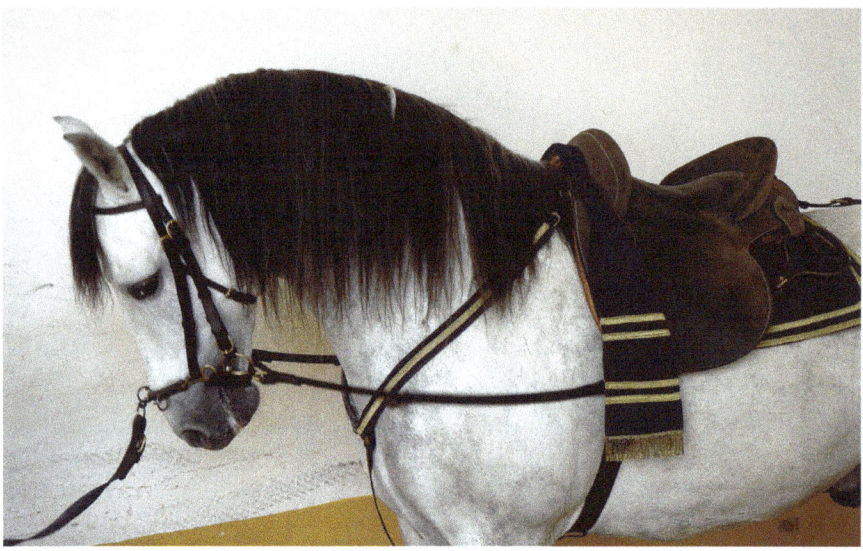

Fig. 9.3. Side reins for work in hand, attached on the sides and without rubber ring inserts to improve the contact. Although the nose could be a little more forward, the contact on the bit is light as the side reins are hanging loose.

In practice: *There are basically two useful variations on the adjustment of running or draw reins, the one being to increase the lateral bending when on the bit. The other is to increase the forward and down stretch. In the first case, the rein is attached on the sides of the horse to the girth, and in the second case, one attaches the rein between the front legs of the horse, the rein then goes through the rings of the bit to the rider's hand.*

Both of these variations should only be ridden with a snaffle and four reins, with the running or draw reins used only as an aid and hanging slightly loose. Forcing the head of the horse down by pulling on the rein and exploiting the lever action should be omitted. This will only bring harm to the horse. Likewise, this rein should never be used with other lungeing aids or bits with a lever action, as this would definitely be classified as cruelty to animals.

Side reins, used in the classical way of training a horse, have a special position. When attached long enough, the horse can outline a bigger or smaller arc, depending on how high the attachment is on the sides of the horse.

Side reins do not allow the necessary forward and down stretching, which calls into question the sense of their use when lungeing a green horse. In later training, the side rein can provide good service for work in-hand. When this rein is attached too short, the breathing of the horse is constricted and the development of the muscles that would later work against the hand of the rider is promoted. The horses are then indeed in a very elevated position, but cannot work properly through the back, so the side reins need to be attached long enough in proportion to every horse. (Fig:9.3) When the side reins are correctly attached, they should be of equal length and the nose of the horse should be in front of the vertical. The bend of the horse is achieved by the trainer turning the fist of his hand holding the lunge line. Not by the widespread bad habit of shortening the inside side rein to enforce the bend. This will only compromise the balance of the horse and force him into a neck position that favors blocked vertebrae and tension. In addition, this way of attaching the reins can restrict the inside shoulder and impede its range of movement.

Both the chambon and the Gogue are lungeing aids that will put pressure on the poll and the bars of the mouth when the horse takes his head up through the use of a special poll piece. Through keeping the lateral movement possibilities, the horse will be encouraged to carry his head deeper. The cords of the Gogue run through the rings of the bit back to the martingale piece. The chambon is attached to the rings of the bit via two pulleys.

The basic idea is a good one, but some horses cannot tolerate increased pressure on the poll due to the aforementioned reasons, and these horses do not accept it well. Apart from that, many horses do not like the direct pull of the bit against their first premolars; therefore, further tension can develop.

When a horse accepts these systems, it can be a good short-term solution although the horse cannot really find a light contact, due to the way the reins are designed since there is no available lateral boundary. These systems are also used in cavaletti work on the lunge and under the rider in the U.S.A. in order to ensure the rounding of the horse's back.

The *"halsverlängerer"* that, in recent years, has become ever more popular, made from elastic rubber, is not recommended for rehabilitation work. It combines the disadvantages of the side reins with the poll-influencing expandable reins, and encourages the horse to lean on the hand of the rider. It is for this reason that this auxiliary rein should not be used.

In all cases, it is most important that the reins are attached long enough in order to reach a stretched posture without difficulty, for if not, the basic principle of "pressure always generates counter pressure" will come into effect, hence rapidly canceling out all the relaxation work.

9.4. Round pen

A round pen is a lungeing arena and is most definitely one of the best inventions to show the horse, in a stress-free way, what bending his body implies, all the while being able to focus the horse on the trainer because of the two meter high enclosure. The surrounding wall should be at least this height so that the horse cannot look over the barrier, even when he lifts his head.

Ideally this area should have a diameter of 20 meters in order not to force the bend of the horse excessively and not to overload of the legs and joints due to too small a circle. The circular working surface will prevent remedial horses, psychologically speaking, from hiding in a corner and from taking on a defensive attitude. The orbit will be more inviting to the horses, despite steady contact, to find their own rhythm against the optical boundary, which would not be as easy to achieve in a rectangular manège or open riding arena with corners. Furthermore, the round pen facilitates corrections in the balancing phase, for the horse can find an optical contact as well. When the horse is worked free, it is also easier for the trainer to use his body language, since the area is a much more manageable size.

Ideally, the lunge arena is covered and made winter-proof so that one can train the horses even in the coldest time of the year. The footing should be nonslip and not too deep (5cm=2 inches). Deeper footing will only deprive the horse of his energy and take away the impulsion. The entry to the lunge ring should also be level with the rest of the boundary or wall and not have a step [or change in elevation] where the horses can hurt themselves.

In the rehabilitation phase, horses should not be allowed to run around in an uncontrolled way on the lunge line. It is possible to jeopardize therapy if a horse breaks into an unexpected sudden sprint.

9.5. Communication with the horse on the lunge

Generally speaking, the trainer's voice, the influence of his body position, the hand aid on the lunge line, and the lunge whip are at the disposal of the trainer.

The voice is the first means of communication a person has with a foal or a green horse. An agreeable deep tone can be calming to the animal, while a lively click of the tongue or a higher pitch can stimulate the horse. A well-directed click of the tongue can help the horse find his rhythm. However, this should not become a clicking concert, for the horse will only become indifferent to that aid. All potential influences should be as discreet and as minimal as possible—only in this manner is it conceivable to prepare the horse to become fine tuned to his eventual rider. The more imperceptible the aids, the more complete the contact between horse and rider.

The position of the trainer lungeing the horse can achieve the following: if the trainer stands on the same spot, at the height of the thorax and forms a triangle with the lunge line and the lunge whip to the horse, it has a neutral and gait maintaining influence on the horse. When the trainer is in a more pointed angle and behind the horse, he can drive the horse in front of him. The opposite happens when the trainer moves forward towards the head of the horse, it has a decelerating effect.

Correct and purposeful application of the lunge whip, which must be practiced ahead of time, can influence the horse in different ways by tapping him with the whip. When a horse barges to the inside of the circle, the trainer can tap him on the shoulder to indicate to move to the outside again. When the lash touches the area where the rider's leg would be, it will be similar to the driving leg aid, whereas the whip held in front of the chest has a braking effect.

The lunge whip can also be used to influence the activity of the hindquarters in correspondence to the reflex points. The hand on the lunge line has a similar function to the rider's hand, yielding, positioning and giving half-halts. Lightly vibrating the lunge line can increase attention before a transition. Slightly turning the hand in, supported by the whip on the area of the rider's legs, will bring about a bend when there are side reins attached which are of equal length. A quick jerk on the cavesson can be seen as punishment and produce obedience once again. Nevertheless one should always endeavor to get along with light and friendly actions in order for the horse to remain finely tuned under the rider later on. A horse that has already been dulled on the lunge, will be very difficult to change into a sensitive dancer under a light hand.

9.6. Starting the green horse on the lunge – Problems and their solutions

The first time a green horse comes into contact with the circular movement wearing a lungeing cavesson, it is always a good idea to have this initial experience inside the 20 meter diameter round pen with an extra person to lend a hand. The trainer has the lunge line in his hand. The helper must first walk with the horse on the perimeter of the circle in order to get him acquainted with the circular path of travel. If the horse stops, the helper can touch him with the whip that he carries to drive him forward. Little by little the helper increases the distance between himself and the horse by moving back, toward the middle of the circle all the while using the whip to drive the horse forward. The lungeing cavesson must fit well and the lunge line should be slightly taut.

All young horses initially have difficulty moving on a circle in different gaits. The majority of horses look to the outside and then fall into the circle over their inside shoulder in one direction. (Fig. 9.4a) Touching the shoulder with the lash of the whip will soon convince the horse to stay out on the perimeter of the circle around the trainer.

In the other direction, most horses become "hollow" by putting their heads more to the inside and then moving their croup outwards. This kind of asymmetry, which is completely normal, should be compensated by correct training under saddle.

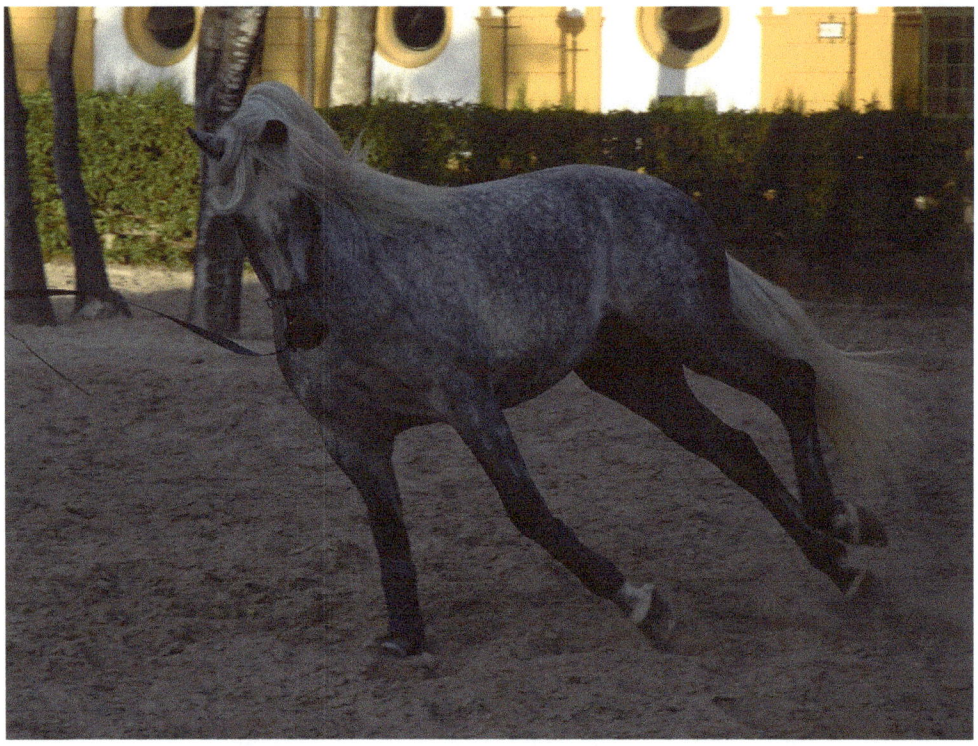

Fig:9.4a. A green horse on the lunge rein before he finds his balance

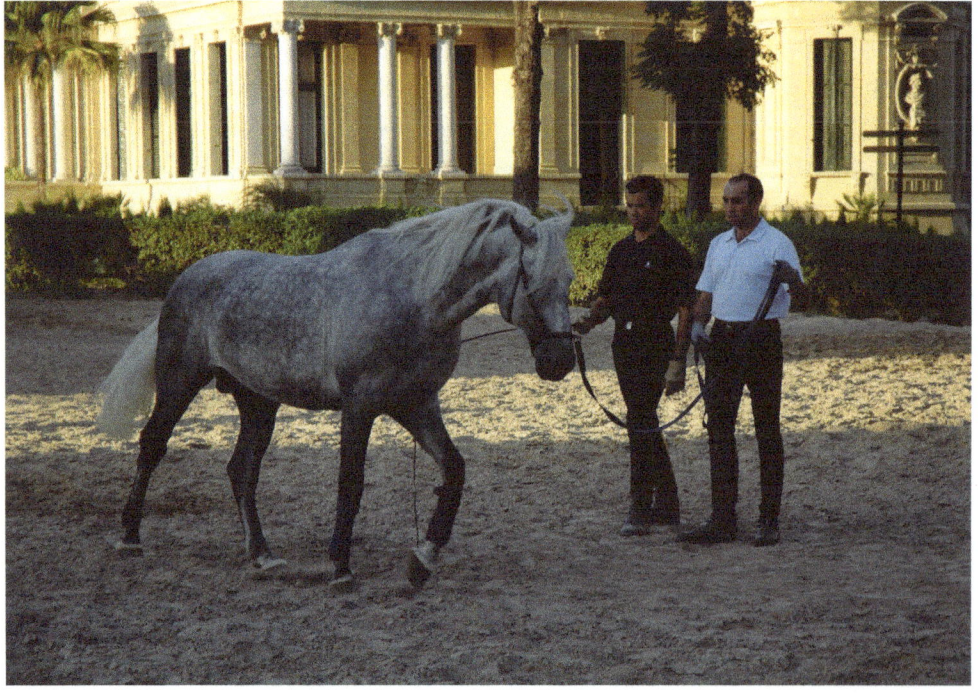

Fig: 9.4b. After he found his balance

> **Definition:** *In order to make it easier for the horse to balance himself at first, it is better to lunge him without any side reins. This is called "auto-equilibration."*

This will ensure that the horse learns how to use his body and his neck as a balancing beam. Relatively quickly, he will find his own center of gravity and his own rhythm by stretching forward and down. (Fig. 9.4b)

> **Note:** *When the error is committed where the horse is forced into a shape by the use of gadgets, the horse will always have problems with temporary loss of rhythm later on, for he will not have learned to balance himself and to use his body effectively.*

Once this initial phase is successfully completed, a bridle and lungeing surcingle is put on the horse, so the horse can become acquainted with the pressure of a girth around his belly. Many young horses try to escape from this pressure by bucking, but they learn quickly that nothing bad happens to them.

Once the young horse moves forward freely and in rhythm, it is time to add one of the training aids in order to support the horse in learning the forward and down stretched posture. A good system is the sliding side reins or the Pessoa Training system, so that the horse can stretch down with equal lateral boundaries.

In the beginning these reins should be attached very long, so as not to trigger any kind of panic reaction.

> **Note:** *In the first few days of learning this, the horse should not be lunged for more than 15 minutes, including many changes of rein, for the under-developed muscles will tire quickly and start to become painful.*

With increased training, the reins can be shortened, such they are of equal length and the nose of the horse remains in front of the vertical. This is very important, as the horse should present the inside bend on the request of the rider's hand and whip and not by means of shortening the inside rein in which case the inside shoulder would bear the weight and reduce the forward impulsion.

The main gait of developing the green horse should be the trot, for it is the easiest gait for the young horse to find his own rhythm and move freely and with contact. The two beat rhythm of the trot makes it easier to compensate for problems in balance than in the canter. The canter is much faster and due to lack of carrying ability, the horse will fall into a disunited canter to keep his balance. It is therefore especially important in the training of young horses on the lunge to have the radius of the circle as large as possible. It is more difficult for a horse with balance problems to move on a circle and he will endure more wear and tear on smaller circles and at fast gaits. Frequent transitions from walk to trot and to halt, as well as some lengthening of the strides will improve the balance and the ability to use the hindquarters in a carrying capacity.

Once the horse is capable of doing these exercises without difficulty, one can begin the canter, once around the circle to begin with to keep the topline activated. The work at the trot should cultivate lateral flexibility while the canter work should activate the arching of the back.

A horse that has been prepared correctly with the voice aids and body language will not have significant problems starting under a rider, for he has learned to trust the trainer.

When the horse is ridden, he must first find his balance with the additional weight of the rider on top of him, without any extra reins, and he must find the connection to the rider's hand.

Once the horse can move with confidence in all three gaits when ridden on the lunge line in the round pen, one can start to ride without the lunge line in the round pen under the observation of a competent person. When the horse accepts this arrangement, one can move to a bigger arena with a built boundary that serves as an optical perimeter. The horse will soon learn to implement the combination of voice and leg aids as these demands have already been learned and are familiar to him from the work on the lunge. A short whip can sometimes help to support the driving leg aids that may not yet be properly understood.

Note: *Once the horse works under the rider, he should still not be put under too much mental or physical strain, as it will only cause great resistance, and may have an unfavorable outcome for the rider, since the horse at this stage is mostly uncontrollable. For this reason it is advised to do many short training sessions per day as opposed to one long marathon session.*

This recommendation cannot always be followed by all our clients due to their professional activities, but every rider must personally interpret his horse's weight carrying capacity. A green horse should be allocated a maximum of 20 minutes work on both reins. The rule of "less is more" should be followed.

9.7. Lunge work and the ridden horse

The goal with lungeing a riding horse should be to work the horse once or twice a week in a relaxed, stretched outline without any weight on his back to eliminate all tension. Once again, it is essential that the systematic build-up of transitions, lengthened strides, and halts are incorporated to make the horse attentive and focused on the trainer.

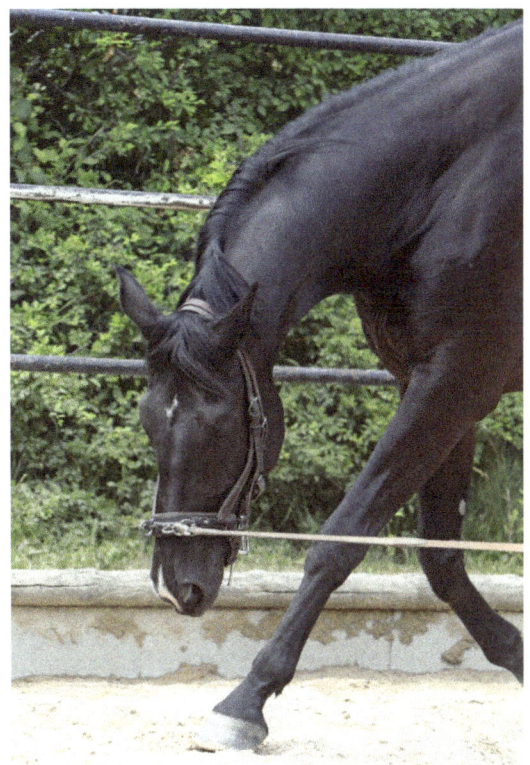

Fig. 9.5. Foreward downward on the cavesson on the lunge. The horse seeks a good contact with the lunge line which enables him to stretch his topline.

[It is is extremely useful to develop the skill of teaching the horse to stretch forward and down, keeping the forehead in front of the vertical after the lunge work has been completed. This helps relax and stretch the back after the contraction of collection work and develops strength of the abdominal carrying muscles.
- Editor's note]

Acceptable rein aids are sliding side reins or the Pessoa system because the best stretching results can be achieved with these auxiliary aids. Side reins adjusted to the correct length can be of use with the riding horse when the horse is worked in-hand before being lunged when a certain degree of elevation is required.

Referring back to the previous Chapter, cavalettis and small gymnastic jumps can be included to cultivate mobility and motivation. Small in-and-out jumps make the hindquarters more powerful and improve carrying capacity and bounce.

Ridden horses should not be lunged for more than 30 minutes, as the circular movement can lead to overloading. Regular changes of rein every 5-7 minutes boosts the flexibility and avoids the horse getting stiff on one side.

Making the circle smaller and bigger cultivates balance and flexibility of the spine. Regular transitions within the gaits and changes of tempo improve the horse's ability for collection through the interplay of balance and the transformation between pushing and carrying.

> **Note:** *Never forget that none of the above mentioned training possibilities can replace correct riding and training of the horse under saddle.*

9.8. Double lunge

Double lungeing is a very useful tool when the horses have reached a certain level of training (at least elementary to medium), as this way of working can improve the rhythm and skill for collection, however, when used improperly can also over-strain the horse.

> **Definition:** *Double lungeing uses a system of reins that is about 25m long, that should be round and stitched at the end in order to slide easily through the metal loops that are fixed on both sides of the lungeing surcingle.*

This system intensifies the leverage that the trainer has on the bit and should be used with great care and caution; horses can rear and even flip over when the action on the mouth is too strong.

When no pulley system is used, the D-rings on the lungeing roller can be used instead to thread the rein through to act on the horse's mouth without any strong kind of leverage. In this way the horses can be prepared for the work without being disturbed in the mouth.

> **Note:** *Despite the high gymnastic value of double lungeing, it is best used only by experts since the possibility of doing more harm than good is very high.*

Nevertheless, in the right hands, double lungeing can be profitable and can have high gymnastic value. It engages the hindquarters and prompts the loin area to round itself. In the same way as with riding, the yielding of the rein is a faster way of rewarding the horse than with any of the other training aids such as side reins. Horses can be bent and positioned without being ridden, which can improve their suppleness immensely.

Carriage horses with back or hindquarter problems can really be helped with this training system, since they are already familiar with the system.

When the trainer is extremely skilled, the horse can also be jumped in this system, and doing cavalettis and gymnastic jumping is also possible. A similar influence to that of the rider can be achieved; horses can be loosened both to the inside or the outside, depending on what is required.

Likewise, lateral work, piaffe and passage as preparation for work under saddle can be done with long reining [or double lungeing] and suppleness can be perfected.

10. The Training Scale

Definition: *Under the title,* The Science and Art of Riding in Lightness, *the training scale is a structured system understandable by the horse and adapted to equine anatomy and biomechanics. The goal is to foster longevity of the equine sports partner while simultaneously maintaining his health with respect to the animal's intended use.*

In return, however, this coherent and specified training system can, based on the limits of biomechanics, also be implemented as correction and rehabilitation in order to get the corresponding muscle sections to respond more accurately and becoming more involved in the training, thus resulting in improvement in the movements.

Definition: *By gymnasticizing we mean a logically constructed gymnastic type of training designed to keep the body elastic and flexible in order to become and remain capable of high performance.*

All the exercises of classical riding only have positive gymnastic effects on the horse provided they are developed gradually. An exercise that is removed from the training context and just taught without a gymnastic foundation is not only damaging to the horse's health—for he cannot use his body completely—but it often looks ridiculous and makes the horse lose his dignity.

The training scale is the foundation of all training that is appropriate for the species, for not only is it considerate to the physical, but also to the mental development of the horse.

The core pieces of the training scale in order of succession are:

Definitions:

Rhythm *is the spatial and chronological symmetry of all footfalls, strides and jumps in the sense of an even repetition of footfalls in the motion sequence.*
Looseness *is the state of physical and mental serenity, that forms the basis of all further stress-free (free of tension) training.*
Contact *is the soft, elastic and even connection of the "expectant" hand of the rider to the mouth of the horse. The horse must seek this connection and it must not come primarily from the hand of the rider.*
Impulsion *is the transmission of the controlled and energetic impulse from the hindquarters on the overall forward movement of the horse in all gaits and has nothing to do with the speed of the movement.*
Straightness *describes the accurate tracking on both straight and curved lines,*

> *taking place in the adjustment of the longitudinal axis of the horse's body to the school figures.*
>
> **Collection** *is seen as the quintessential position, where the horse brings both his and the rider's body in such a state of harmony, that the weight distribution of both has the tendency to be more distributed on the hind legs of the horse, making the topline of the horse look shorter and because the base of support of the horse becomes shorter and therefore more stable, it is easier for the rider to influence the horse with less effort. The horse thereby becomes easier to direct and turn.*

The training scale that is distributed by the F.N. [German Equestrian Federation] as guidelines for the correct and specifically safeguarded training of riding horses, was not developed out of the fickleness of the riding masters. It arose as a logical consequence of the anatomical and biomechanical connections in the body of the horse.

This system includes the military service regulations 12 of 1912 of the cavalry school in Hanover as its foundation [*H. Dv. 12 Cavalry Manual on the Training of Horse and Rider*, Xenophon Press 2014], which is based on the doctrines of the old masters, combined with the revolutionary (at that time) jumping style and cross-country work of the Italians. Due to the necessity for horses in the cavalry to be kept healthy and fit for a long period of time, this system of training established itself and is still applied within the guidelines of the German Equestrian Federation.

This system takes into account not only the physical but also the mental development of the horse, which lies at the foundation of all inner looseness—a prerequisite to being able to work in a useful and constructive way with a horse. When it is applied correctly, with feeling and understanding, it will safeguard the horse and the rider from excessive demands and unwanted resistances, which are often due to mental and physical overstraining.

It is through the training scale that the dogma "from easy to difficult" becomes useful in the rehabilitation of horses. It is especially in physiotherapy that the scheduled programs for movement occupy a large space; not least because of the measures used in physiotherapy to prepare muscle groups, these muscles must then, according to their biological function, move in order to improve. The musculo-skeletal system of the flight animal lives from movement, and gets damaged when there is a lack of use. Muscles and bones atrophy and are no longer capable to comply to the full scope of their activities.

> **Note:** *It is especially important in rehabilitation to keep the rest periods as short as possible. Lack of movement can cause an unnecessary delay in the healing process due to reduced circulation and therefore poor supply of nutrients to the damaged tissues. Breaking down progresses faster than building up.*

Nonetheless, every rehabilitation program must be individually tailored to the specific indications of the patient.

These points are fundamental for every kind of useful muscular training to be done in terms of the important physiological training principles.

A horse can only relax (looseness) in a calm even pace **(rhythm)** and through that develop muscle in the forward and down stretching posture **(contact).** When the horse does not have inner looseness or he travels slower then faster in an uncoordinated way, he cannot achieve sufficient muscular activity to allow a complete stretch followed by maximum contraction.

When the first three phases are reached, one will see that the basis of a reasonable and efficient workout structure has already been established. The controlled development of thrust of the hindquarters **(impulsion)** makes it easier for the horse to bring his hind legs under his center of gravity, whereby he can round and stretch his loin area. This can simplify problem solving when riding to correct crookedness and bend **(straightness)** and affords us the necessary basis for an easy-to-ride, balanced horse **(collection).**

> **Note:** *Due to the process of muscular development in the young horse and for the horse in rehabilitation, these points cannot be arbitrarily mixed; each point can only exist or be achieved once the preceding point has been confirmed.*

Viewed physiologically, training has three more pillars than can be compatible with the training scale and thus improves the understanding and the requirements of the system. The first three points: rhythm, looseness and contact are assigned to the development of thrusting power; the horse must first and foremost move forward easily and diligently before he can be expected to advance to the next stages of training. This thrusting power will be converted into carrying power in the course of the development of momentum and in the increased bending for straightness. This will pave the way to viable collection. When further training continues to sculpt the carrying power, so that the horse is capable of pausing in an extended bending phase, the steps will become more elevated and cadenced, and the suspension will develop.

Now the training scale should be brought in connection with the anatomical conditions of the riding horse, from which the following consequences must arise for the training.

In the first phase, **(rhythm)** one respects the pureness of the gaits, both in the green horse and in the rehabilitation horse. Disturbance within the rhythm, meaning quickening of steps, nodding and incorrect movement sequences, for example the tendency to amble, are justified in many cases by strong tension of the M. longissimus dorsi, often caused by a too strong and arrhythmical influence of the hand, the bad seat of the rider or a poorly fitting saddle. In the beginning, each horse must be allowed to find his own individual rhythm and be capable of keeping it for short periods of time already early in the training.

When the rider forces the forward movement too severely, tense steps with a tight back and tension in the shoulders will result and the horses do not react well to the rein aids and become difficult to steer.

In the rhythm phase, the initial goal for the horse should be to find his own balance and then the balance with the added weight of the rider. In addition, all the muscles responsible for impulsion, for example the M. semi-membranosus and M. semi-tendinosus, are being stressed. When too much activity is demanded in this phase (example: auction horses), physical "tensions" are unavoidable, and these horses are in an almost impossible position to reach the next step, the phase of impulsion. Moreover, these young horses in the adaptation stage (3-5 years), are not prepared for this strong deployment of momentum (extended trot), as the buyers would like to see, and experience early damage in the back and tendon areas. One should always envision that an extended trot has the same maximum load capacity as an elementary jumping test.

When a horse has become accustomed to the weight of a rider in a relatively free posture and trusts his trainer, then he is free from any mental stress. In this phase, the trusting attitude of the horse can be seen when dealing with his rider and a content chewing on the bit is an unmistakable sign of a para-sympathetic effect.

Only completely relaxed muscles are capable of maximum contraction and of supplying themselves with sufficient nutrients. By the same token, a muscle capable of full contraction and relaxation is capable of transporting lactic acid and other metabolic waste products away faster, whereas a permanently tense muscle can never achieve its full performance capacity.

In the looseness phase, the horse begins to stretch down with his neck and to arch his back, whereby the supraspinous ligament stretches, the M. longissimus dorsi relaxes and the stomach muscles can be really active for the first time.

The spinous processes of the thoracic and lumbar vertebrae will thus be freed on top and the back will begin to swing rhythmically and effectively. This good back activity can be recognized by the regular and rhythmic contraction and relaxation of the lumbar area and the fact that the horses start to happily chew and snort as a sign of relaxation.

In this phase, the horse should search for the contact in a forward and down manner and not a forward-backwards manner (deep and behind the vertical).

The correct seeking of the contact will cause a stretched posture of the neck muscles and, in the process, reconstructing the muscles that have become painful can be relaxed during the activity.

The balance situation both the horse and the rider, that has been changed due to the lengthening of the neck of the horse, which acts as a balancing pole, must also be reconsidered, for the horse must first find a new balance. Once this phase is completed, the horse can always, when he has too much stress in training, return to these basics, for he has also learned how to relax under tension. In the **contact** phase and even later on, the horse must time and again be given the possibility to change the position of his neck, for on the one hand he is not used to a longer and consistent position of the neck and on the other hand the overworked muscles can induce tension in the area of the poll.

In practice: *One should attempt a certain degree of being on the bit and try to remain there for a few minutes. After just a short while one will start to notice a strong pull and tension, similar to the appearance of fatigue which appears in the muscles of the horse's neck. Horses react to this situation by trying to pluck the reins out of the rider's hand, in order to free themselves from this tension. A few rounds in walk on a long rein can readily dissolve these problems during the activity.*

In the contact phase, besides the relatively rectangular posture, the beginning of being "on the bit" takes effect. The horse starts to adopt the pleasing head carriage, because he has learned to use the neck as a lever arm against the weight of the rider and to support the activity of the back in this way. It is far too early to encourage the horse to keep his poll as the highest point at this stage, for the carrying power of the hindquarters have not yet been fully developed. In many horses, especially stallions, this demand is not possible due to the bulk of the neck, and despite the correct activity of the back and the hindquarters, they go slightly behind the bit or with a broken neck, which is definitely not the same as the broken neck forced by hand action that is too strong.

Once the horse has found a good contact with the hand of the rider, the rider can demand more forward impulsion, as the horse will now be in the position to balance both himself and the rider in unison.

Frequent changes in the pace and lengthened strides can be used like an accordion to lengthen and shorten the horse, not only to make him better to ride, but also to improve the activity of his back.

The **development of momentum** as basis and preliminary stage for collection leads us now to speak of the straight horse, for this horse is more capable of carrying weight on the hindquarters whereby the gluteal-, quadriceps and the hamstring muscles can be further developed.

In the phase of **straightening,** the shoulder-in serves as the foundation of the lateral gaits. It is not without reason that the greatest Portuguese master of all time, Nuno Oliveira, called it "the aspirin for riding" (see Chapter 11.2.1). It improves the carrying power, promotes the freedom of the shoulder and the horse can be controlled better by the rider, for it allows for the understanding of the interplay between the leg and hand aids.

Once the horse is steady and straight in all three gaits, in the transitions and in the lateral movements, one can begin the next phase, namely, **collection**. Collected exercises include, for example, piaffe in-hand, pirouettes and flying changes. The horse has learned to understand the interplay between tension and relaxation and does not fear the new lessons, for he has had adequate mental and physical preparation.

It is only a horse that has been trained in this way, due to inner serenity and contentment, that can deliver the image of the joyful collaborator, with true lightness so often demanded. These horses will always give the rider and the audience the impression of harmonious unity and their performance will always be a pleasure to watch.

10.1. Rhythm—The quality of the basic gaits

Definition: *Rhythm is the chronological and spatial symmetry of the movement of the horse.*

Rhythm only describes the beat of a movement sequence, that can be slow or fast, and does not give any information about the quality thereof. The young horse or even the spoiled horse must nevertheless be capable of finding his own rhythm in order to establish a working way of going, because a calm and regular way, together with a fearless inner attitude, leads to muscular looseness. Muscular relaxation is essential for every useful form of training.

Rhythm and looseness provides the basis of a high quality sequence of movement that is improved by correct contact and impulsion. Therefore, it is useless to have uncontrolled development of impulsion without rhythm and looseness, for it only serves to promote wear and tear and causes tension in the horse's back and neck. Faults in the rhythm of a specific gait are visible in various irregularities in the sequence of movement, for example shortened steps, ambling, contact problems, and the rounded, regular sequence of movement is greatly influenced. The walk will often show ambling-type of movement due to the tension in the back, this is frequently caused by too strong influence of the hand when the horse is asked to go in collected walk and it blocks the movement from going through the long muscles of the back.

A young horse whose balance has not been fully developed can also have problems with finding his rhythm. Because the muscles of the horse are not yet adequately trained, he is not yet capable of moving in a balanced way in a circle under the rider, and he cannot keep a regular pace on the curved line in a specific gait. On the lunge he will every now and again loose his balance due to the speed in which he tries to move on the circular line. The horse is only at the beginning of his training and the development of bend is the 5th point on the training scale.

These circumstances should not be ignored with the "back users" that are to be rehabilitated. The ever changing center of gravity makes the horses sometimes go slower and sometimes go faster in the circle, and when referring to the definition of rhythm, it can be perfectly correct. This is why looseness in connection with rhythm is of great importance, for only these combined attributes offer the horse the possibility of employing his muscles efficiently within the meaning of the training scale and to continue the training.

In the beginning, young horses will have the tendency to move more on the forehand in their rhythm since finding the center of gravity on a circular line in a specific gait is an acquired skill. The neck will serve as a balancing rod and must therefore not be locked in with any lungeing aids. The tendency to be more on the forehand will be improved by itself in the course of training once the horse has found its balance and confidence. Only after this automatic balancing has taken place can auxiliary lungeing aids be added on the lunge, and only after that the horse is capable of finding his balance under the rider. Everything else would be premature and not beneficial for the development of the muscles or the skeleton.

In this Chapter the quality of the basic gaits are discussed; faulty patterns of movement such as ambling, bridle lameness, disturbance in the rhythm and their possible causes will be addressed later.

> **Note:** *In principle, all basic gaits (walk, trot and canter) should be rhythmic, cadenced and full of impulsion. In all gaits the beat must be clear and recognizable.*

In extension, horses must only expand their top-lines to lengthen the strides, without becoming hurried or faster, whereas the collected gaits are not merely becoming slower or without impulsion but in such a way increase the will to go that the measure of the gait can be shortened (piaffe).

The purity of the basic gaits is especially important in dressage tests, because loss of rhythm will be penalized.

The **walk** is to be viewed as the most important gait, for it almost not possible to improve its basic quality and in the event of tension in the back, especially in the more collected levels, it will easily be inclined to defects and temporary loss of rhythm.

The **trot** serves as the working gait and due to its double beat, can be improved and developed the most. Even horses with no spectacular expression can reach considerable extended trots when enough time is allowed for them in their training to develop appropriately strengthened hindquarters.

The **canter** can only be slightly improved upon and is characterized in the basic quality through expressive jumps in a forward and upwards manner.

When a horse is said to have a "sufficient" walk and canter due to his conformation, it means he over-tracks well, and it will be possible to improve the quality of his trot with correct and systematic training.

> **Note:** *All gaits can be subdivided into different degrees of collection, high school airs (highest collection), collected, working, medium, extended and racing gallop.*

The horse should always be allowed to fill the rectangular shape when he extends his position or does extensions. An extension with a short, extremely elevated neck obstructs the free and unconstrained activity of the back and thus blocks the hindquarters. Horses that extend in this way, mostly do it with considerably angled hocks, but without the relevant bending of the haunches, whereby the movement becomes that of a dazzler, the so-called "leg mover" (using only the legs in a flashy way, not using the back in a natural way) and should be classified as inferior quality, in comparison to the movement of a horse that is complete in itself, with a rhythmic extension that, due to lacking carrying power, is not yet spectacular. This should especially be considered in the young horse acceptance tests, for the horses presented here are mostly green horses that lack the strength to carry themselves in an extension.

This classification within the gaits is very important during training; changes within the pace are essential to improve the balance and straightness of the horse.

10.1.1 The walk

The walk is the slowest of all gaits and has four distinct beats. One can easily count clearly a defined 1-2-3-4 footfall; in a correct rhythmic walk one should not find any temporary loss of rhythm. The free walk must be ground covering, long and clearly defined. One of the criteria would be the triangle seen between the forward stepping hind foot and the lifting of the front foot. When this triangle can be seen clearly, it means the horse strides with sufficient energy and far enough under his own center of gravity. In the process, the horse should step far ahead of the footprint of the front foot in order to secure the rhythm later on in the collected paces.

When the horse tenses his back due to too much influence from the hand, especially in the collected walk, the horse will produce a pacing rhythm. That means that the legs on the same side will move forward at the same time, rendering the walk without impulsion, fluctuating and without rhythm. The horses lean on the hand and the collected walk is marred. It is for this reason that it is important to use the interplay between medium, "working"[8] and free walk—the last of these has the length of stride corresponding to that of the extended walk—in the training periods and use the collected walk only in tests in order to avoid faults in the rhythm.

The footfall sequence of the walk is divided into eight sequences of movement:

1. Left hind, left front, right front
2. Two diagonal legs—right hind, left front
3. Left front, right hind, right front
4. Right hind, right front
5. Left hind, right hind, right front
6. Left hind, right front
7. Right front, left hind, left front
8. Left hind, left front

The natural free walk of a horse should be of a correct rhythm and even, in which the horizontally carried neck may produce a nodding movement. This is labeled as a good walk and serves to balance the horse. Very well and highly trained horses also perform this nodding movement, but in a milder form as they are already in a better balance.

In the walk, one distinguishes between the walk of young horses and the "working" walk, normally used in training (to warm-up) which has a requirement that the horse steps with his hind foot into or over the footprint of the front hoof. The position of the horse is longer than in collected walk; the horse has a long rectangular form. The collected walk, due to the high degree of collection, will have shortened steps; the horse has a shorter outline and the movement becomes higher instead of longer.

The school walk can be the culmination of the collected walk, which is only seldom ridden today. The steps become higher and shorter with the four beat rhythm remaining intact.

In the medium walk, the horse should step clearly over the imprint of the front hoof and his topline is also extended. The horse should seek the contact of the bit through lengthening his neck, the nodding motion may become stronger.

---

8   The author specifies five distinctly different walks: medium, working, free, extended and collected.—Editor's note.

In the extended walk, the walk will reach maximum length of stride, without significantly incorporating more speed. This kind of walk should correspond to the free walk purely from the length of the stride, however with contact and a definite tendency to the forward and down stretch.

The so-called Spanish walk, where the front legs are alternatively and calmly stretched horizontally, does not only have a show effect, it is a wonderful way to improve the freedom of the shoulder, although many purists do not qualify it as classical. When stallions fight one sees this pattern as a prompt to play or fight. The action of the foreleg is clearly improved through this lesson. Horses that have difficulty in the passage will be well supported with it in the activity of the forelegs.

10.1.2 The trot

The trot is a two beat movement with a moment of suspension between the exchange of the diagonal limb pairs. Great importance is attached to the trot at auctions, even though this is the gait that can be most improved upon out of the three basic gaits.

Still, a good trot alone does not make for a good dressage horse. The trot enjoys a very high status in training, for it is the working gait that promotes lateral ability due to the two beat changing rhythm. In this double rhythm it is easier for the horse to find his balance under the rider because every moment of suspension is followed by a limb support sequence, thus making the loss of balance a smaller risk.

De la Guérinière already advocated training the horse in all trot tempos, including piaffe, and only after the horse has enough strength and tendency for collection, to address the canter which is more susceptible to errors.

Today, we know that the canter is at least as important as the trot, for the canter arches the topline and all muscles are thereby trained correspondingly.

Counting the rhythm of the trot, due to the quicker footfalls, is somewhat faster: 1-2-1-2 etc The sequence of the footfalls is as follows:

1. Right hind—left front
2. Moment of suspension
3. Left hind—right front
4. Moment of suspension

The trot must be of a pure rhythm, full of impulsion and cadenced. The rhythm of the trot is significantly influenced by the action of the horse's back and the rider's hand. When the hind-leg contacts the ground too early or the front foot leaves the ground too early, it can be the result of an unyielding hand or tension in the horse's back and accordingly the lumbar part of the back.

The Science and Art of Riding in Lightness

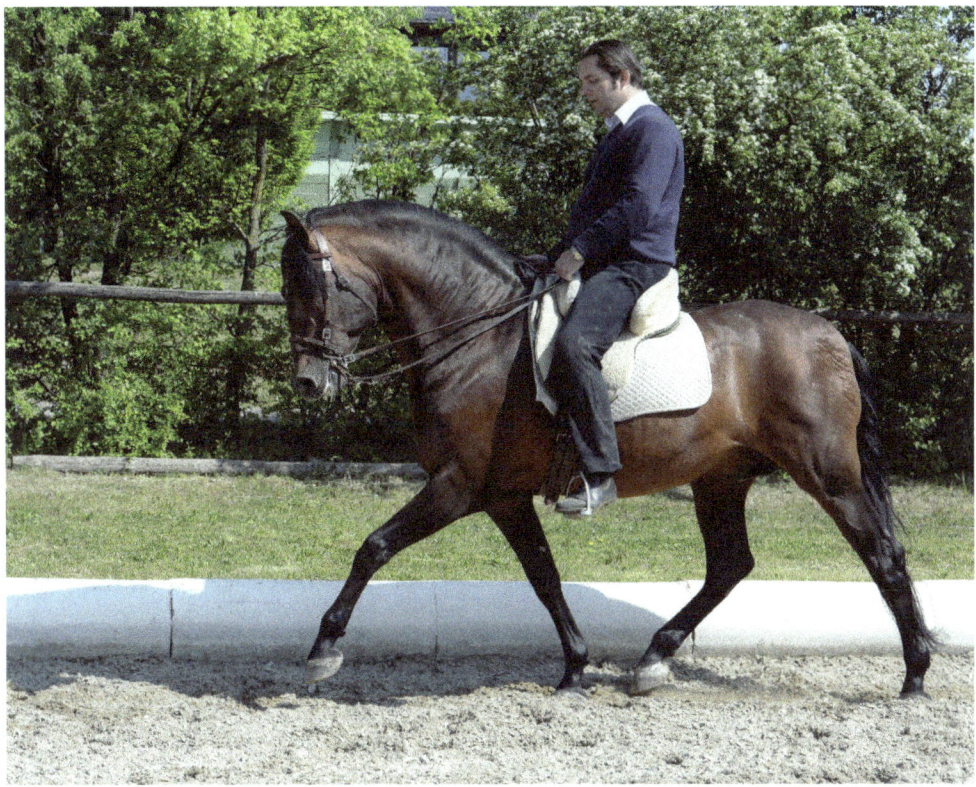

Fig. 10.1. Trot
a. The extensions in the gaits, especially in the trot must be developed from a collected horse which is able to bend the haunches. only such an extension will maintain the horse's health and will allow the rider sit comfortabley because the horse's back is also swinging and working.

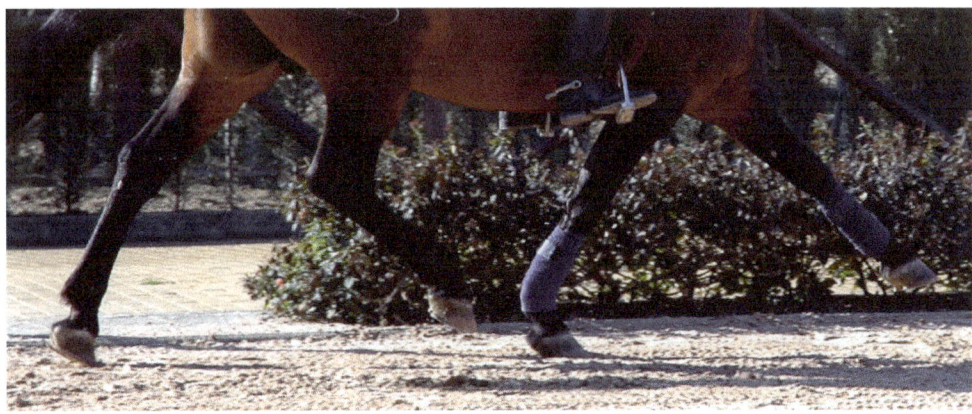

b. Extended trot - the canon bone of the back leg and that of the diagonal front leg are parallel to each other, the horse steps to where his foot points - "back user"

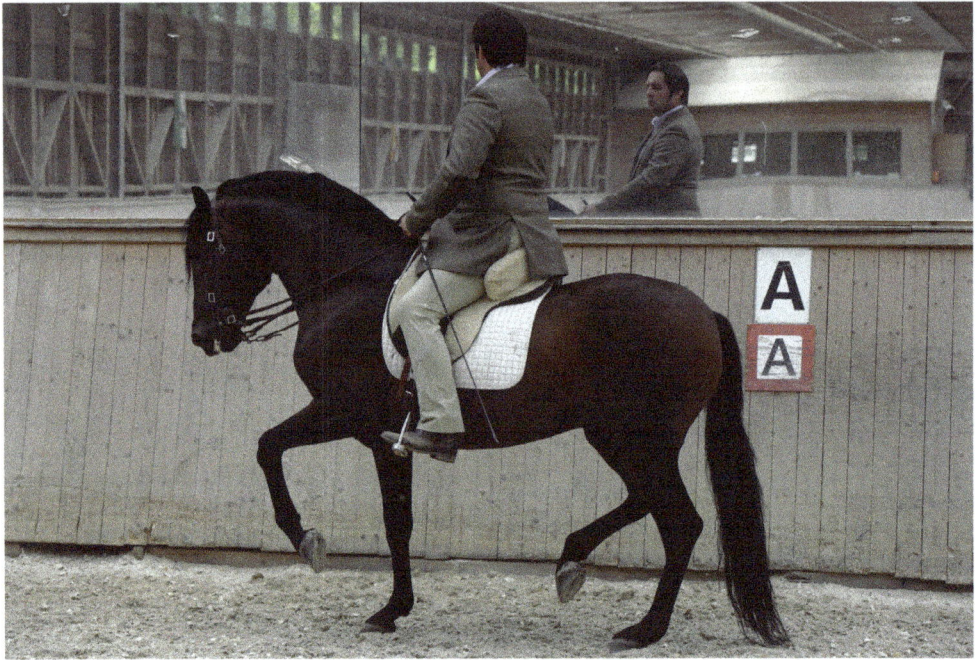

10.1 c. School trot—Wonderful balance and cadence in the piaffe. Here you can see the concentration of the forces in the horse's middle by maintaining a light contact in the hand. The author sits relaxed and has lowered his hands and legs so that the horse can work independently.

Horses that are not balanced or that do not have carrying ability to keep them on the hindquarters and control the forward impulsion, will rush after their center of gravity that always falls forward, causing a hurried basic rhythm. These horses are heavy in the mouth, and lie on the rider's hand in order to find something to support them in their lack of strength, the hindquarters look lighter, the forehand becomes heavier because the horses drop their heads.

We distinguish between: piaffe, passage, school trot, working trot, collected trot, medium trot, extended trot and racing trot.

In the working trot, the horse moves forward free and effortlessly in a longer outline with a moderate stride length—at least stepping into the imprint made by the front hoof—is required (fig.10.1a)

Medium trot demands longer strides and then reaches its maximum length in extended trot (fig.10.1b) without increasing the speed. It is only in the racing trot where the reach is extreme, the horses carry their necks very high, are often held that way with the aid of an over-check, and resulting is a tremendously tense back with a powerful increase in speed of up to 40 km/h. In this gait the hind legs will step wider in order to pass the front legs, since if they don't 'straddle' the front feet, they will always injure themselves by interfering.

The school trot (fig. 10.1c) as the shortest, most collected trot, makes the horses seem shorter with a cadenced, elevated movement that reaches perfection in piaffe (trot on the spot) or in passage. (fig.12.1) Cadence is the prolongation of the bending phase, the steps become more elevated, powerful and elastic.

The length of the stride is shortened in the more collected types of trot, whereby the moment of suspension seems to become prolonged (maximum prolongation of the moment of suspension is in the passage).

In contrast to the Spanish walk, the Spanish trot, which is the alternate stretching of the front legs in a horizontal position in passage rhythm, is not of real value for training of the back; most horses do not have enough action in the hindquarters and an extremely exaggerated action in the front legs which "causes them to stay stuck in their backs or be broken there." The horses must be completely elevated, disrupting the action of the back and dragging the hindquarters behind the outstretched fore legs.

In order to assess the quality of the trot movement, it is important to have a picture in one's mind of the regularity of the movement where the hindquarters are of crucial significance. The shoulder mobility should be elastic, light and ground covering, free of tension and without disturbance in rhythm. Horses that only trot out in front, the so-called dazzlers, due to insufficient activity of the hindquarters, also have inadequate activity and tension will appear in a relatively short time. In an extended trot, the canon bone of the hind leg should be parallel to the forearm of the diagonally opposite front leg. Only then can one speak of a calm and regular rhythm in the trot.

This indication secures a rounded and harmonious picture of the movement. The hind feet of the horse should at least step into the footprint of the front foot. In the collected trot this description will no longer fit, due to the increased elevation and because the haunches are more bent.

10.1.3 The canter

The canter is the fastest gait of a horse and is characterized by three beats with a moment of suspension.

The three beat can be observed as a rhythmic 1-2-3-1-2-3, almost like a waltz. The horse must move forward with leaping strides full of impulsion with a definite uphill tendency. A four beat canter—often found in racing gallop and sometimes in an incorrect school canter—is faulty from the classical viewpoint. A four beat canter is the result of too strong hand activity during the diagonal phase [second beat of the canter] or too much tension in the kidney area. Different tempos and degrees of collection will determine the gait as well: school canter, collected canter, working canter, medium canter, and extended canter as well as the racing gallop.

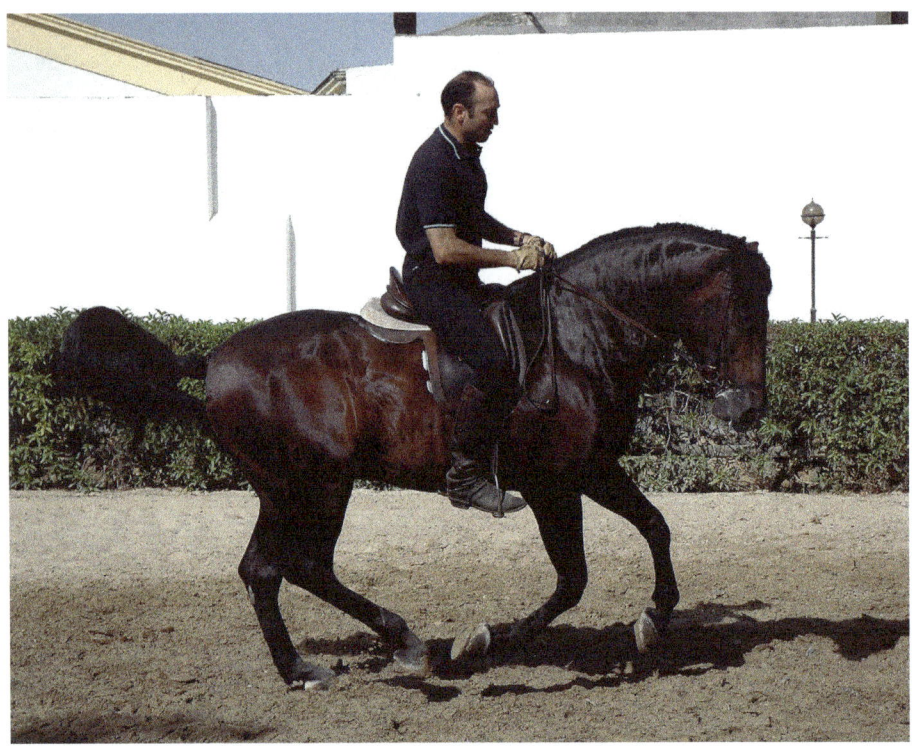

Fig.10.2. Right canter a. Working canter

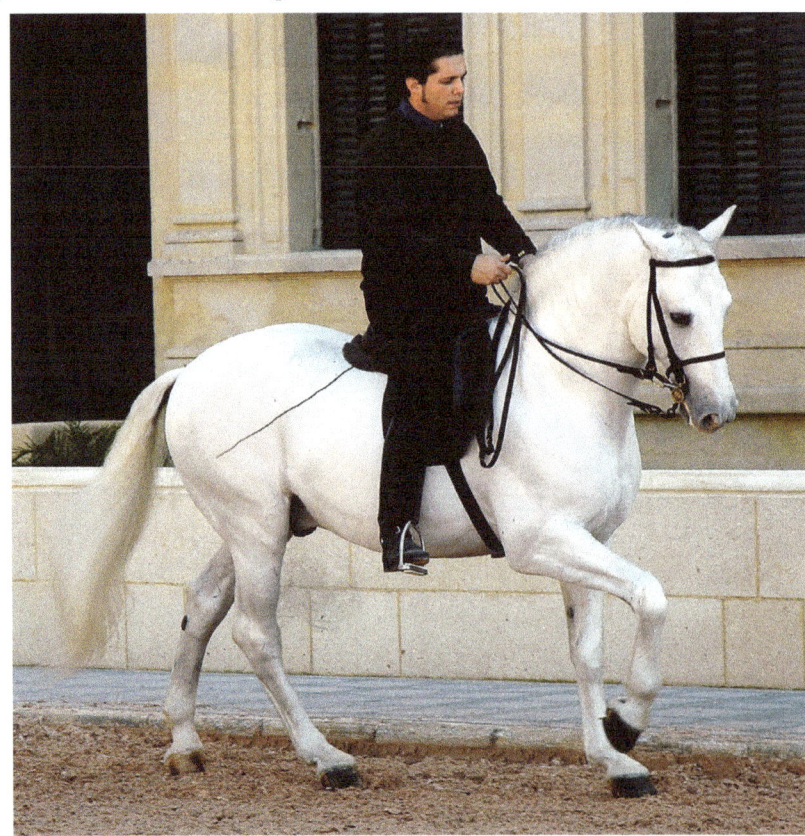

b: Collected canter. Note the good self carriage of the horse with loose reins

Left and right lead canter can be distinguished, where the inside foreleg that reaches further forward is the leg responsible for the term. The footfall sequence of the right canter is as follows: (fig.10.2)

1. Left hind
2. Left hind, right hind and left front (as diagonal pair)
3. Right front
4. Moment of suspension

The left canter is a mirror of the right canter where the horse strikes off with his right hind-leg.

The working canter is when the horse moves forward freely and easily with a strong tendency to round his back (fig.10.2 a).

The collected (fig.10.2b) and school canter can only be worked by the powerful arching of the loin area and with calm, rhythmic, cadenced leaps. Maximum lengthening of the topline is found in the extended canter, without a significant increase in speed. The horse must fill out the rectangular frame, and this is only possible when the neck is clearly stretched to the front. When horses are restricted in the jowl it can lead to temporary loss of rhythm and a four beat canter.

Medium canter is the intermediate gait between the working and the extended canter.

The racing gallop is actually a four beat gait, since the diagonal phase is interrupted; the inside hind-leg hits the ground before the diagonally opposite foreleg strikes the ground; this is due to the speed. The gallop also has a moment of suspension, where the all of the limbs are swung forward during the strong arching of the topline. When the school canter is too collected, this can also become a four beat canter, something the old masters saw as desirable, but in the competition world today it is seen as a big fault as the canter should always stay in a clear three beat rhythm with a moment of suspension following it. This four beat canter seems to favor many representatives of the ever popular Baroque horses with their compact physique and action-packed forehand, for the horses canter very spectacularly in the front but seem to drag their hind legs in an almost trot like form. The problems only make themselves known in further progress of the work when flying changes become a stumbling block; restoring the basic quality of the canter can be very time-consuming.

The *terre a terre* is a two beat movement, where the horse lifts both front legs simultaneously, while the hind legs simultaneously contact the ground. Through this repetition, small double beat jumps are generated; they were used in the Renaissance and Baroque times to improve maneuverability and as preparation for the *capriole*. Although the *terre a terre* is very similar to the canter work, it has not much to with it due to the lack of the three beat and is therefore an independent lesson that is an intermediate training step between the airs on the ground and the airs above the ground.

A further two beat canter will be the *redopp*, where the front legs jump forward simultaneously, followed by the hind legs that are laterally displaced.

This is still practiced at the major schools of the art of riding (Vienna, Jerez, Lisbon and Saumur) as preparation for the capriole, but it has no real value in leisure riding nor in competition riding.

10.2 Looseness

> **Definition:** *Looseness is the further development from the basic ease the horse carries within himself.*

Looseness is the foundation for every controlled gait full of impulsion that can be produced by the driving legs of the rider. A horse that is supple and loose will show all the signs of being relaxed and happy, while at the same time moving forward powerfully. A loose, swinging tail, while the loin area releases and contracts rhythmically, is an unmistakable sign. Due to the parasympathetic reflex, the horse is stimulated to relax the muscles of his hyoid (tongue bone) and will start to contently chew on the bit and stretch his neck forward and down, whereby the wither and back in the saddle area will lift up through the pull of the supraspinous ligament on the dorsal spinous processes, opening the spaces between them. The hindquarters will be prompted by the driving leg aids of the rider to step increasingly under the horse's center of gravity.

Swishing of the tail, the noise the penis makes in the sheath and grinding of the teeth are unmistakable signs of lacking or nonexistent looseness, and should be corrected from the start. The expression on the horse's face and the way the ears move reveal a lot and should be included in the assessment of the initial physical state of the horse during the work.

It is through this form of mental and physical relaxation that the working muscles can be efficiently and correctly built up. When the horse has learned to relax under the rider, it is also possible to shorten the warm-up period, instead of riding the horse for hours to "tire" it ostensibly trying to convince it to yield. It is also as important that the horse learns to relax in the rest periods in order to gather strength for the next working sessions.

> **Note:** *Every collected exercise must be followed by a relaxation exercise in order to protect the muscles from lactic acid accumulation and to act according to the physiology of training. Only a totally relaxed muscle can, through complete contraction, put maximum performance in its full spectrum. Looseness must be asked for, and achieved in every level of training.*

Looseness can be seen as the criterion for correct training. In rehabilitation, it has special significance, for many horses have problems with pain because of the way they have been ridden and have lost confidence in the rider and the work and will come to the training completely tensed up. Therefore, it is an essential step to obtain or recover the inherent freedom from constraint again, and to create trust and the foundation for looseness. There is no other way to sensibly and efficiently build the muscles up. This rational quality of looseness is the origin and resilient base for further training.

10.2.1 Inner freedom from constraint—mental relaxation

Waldemar Seunig[9] already used the term inner freedom from constraint to describe the horse's innate characteristic as follows:

> **Definition:** *Inner freedom from constraint should not be confused with looseness for it reflects the mental and physical state of the horse, where the horse will only activate his muscular activity as much as needed in order to move his body while using as little energy as possible.*

Therefore this state describes a rather passive tendency, yet as a prerequisite to obtain the looseness and how it can be influenced by the rider. The horse moves forward rhythmically without any special expression, but remains on the forehand. The inner freedom from constraint as a basic attitude towards work and towards the trainer is crucial, for a horse that fears demands can never move effortlessly and without tension. Tenseness and loss of rhythm can easily disturb his sensitive structure.

10.2.2 The stretched position—forward and downwards

The forward and down stretched position occupies a crucial status in horse training, for it is considerably dependent on the development of real looseness and can only be reached in accordance to this kind of activity in the back.

> **Note:** *In the stretched position it is essential that the topline of the horse, including the neck, is lengthened in a forward and down fashion (fig. 10.3) and not as is often seen in a down and back manner, for these horses are behind the bit and influence from the rider is difficult to effect.*

---

9 Waldemar Seunig, (born August 8, 1887; † 25 December 1976 in Munich) was an Austrian officer, sport rider, horse trainer and author. Best know for his book, *Horsemanship: A Comprehensive Book on Training the Horse and Its Rider.*

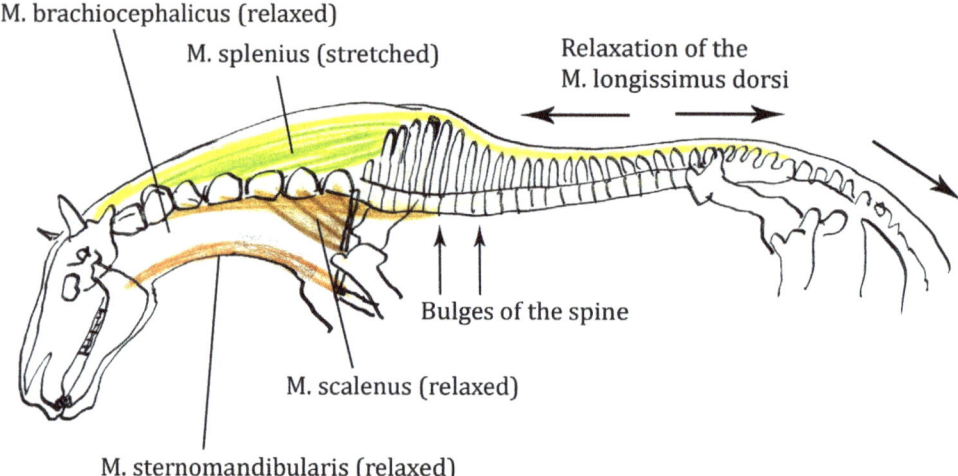

Fig. 10.4 Forward and down results in a stretch of the top muscles in both the neck and back while, at the same time causing the lower neck muscles to relax.

The angle between the jowl, atlas and throat must be increased and the horse's forehead should be in front of the vertical. The stretch in this position will cause, among other things, an extension of the mm. splenii, longissimi cervicii, trapezii, serrati cervicii, rectus capitii and all of the muscles of the topline of the horse's neck and back (Mm. longissimus dorsi and ileocostalis) (Fig.10.4) Besides the stretching of the topline, the lower muscles of the neck will relax and have a substantial influence on the freedom and mobility of the front legs. The M. brachiocephalicus and the muscles of the hyoid bone are significantly involved in this position.

Following the parasympathetic reflex, the relaxed hyoid bone muscles can cause the horse to start mouthing the bit and start foaming. This can even be observed with bit-less bridled horses. Furthermore, on account of the stretched position, there will be an increased pull on the supraspinous ligament and due to the attachment to the spine, it will pull the spinous processes forward in the process. Due to the caudal construction of the first 14 thoracic vertebrae, the withers can be lifted a few centimeters as a result of the leverage, opening the inter-vertebral spaces and counteracting the much feared kissing spine syndrome.

It is essential for patients in need of rehabilitation of the back that this stretched position is achieved through a calm and rhythmic tempo. Because the last thoracic vertebrae and the lumbar vertebrae point cranially and the sacrum then again points caudally, the static of the vertebrae will be supported. The lowering of the head will cause a slight lift in the area of the saddle. As was mentioned already in the anatomical perspective in part 1, it is also important to strengthen the back and stomach muscles in order for the skeleton not to be damaged by the weight of the rider. Supporting the fact that an arched back is more viable than a sagging back, it is important for a correctly trained horse to go into the stretched position at a moment's notice.

Podhajsky already said: *"even a completely trained horse should at any time be in a position to immediately take on the form of a young horse."* With this statement, he was in accordance with the biomechanical point of view on the correctness of the stretched posture.

The lumbar area must be lifted through increased driving of the legs in order to get the hindquarters more active. The psoas muscle is of great importance here as the main muscle to tilt the pelvis. It is only when the M. longissimus dorsi and M. ileocostalis rhythmically tenses and relaxes where one can see it in the play of muscle behind the saddle, and the tail swings rhythmically from side to side, that the back is active.

The second and last third of the neck muscles must also rhythmically tense and relax with each movement. This action of the neck muscles will lead to a beautifully curved topline and reduce the unwanted lower neck, making it easier for the horse to carry his neck with ease when the head is elevated and the horse will not need to lean on the hand of the rider.

Nonetheless one should be warned against the sudden, too deep, yanking the reins from the rider's hands action, for this has nothing to do with the biomechanically correct stretched posture. Maximum opening of the intervertebral spaces is, on one hand, restricted by the bodies of the vertebrae and, on the other hand, dependent on the position of how the neck comes out of the horse's body. In most horses this point lies approximately on the same height as the shoulder joint or a few centimeters below that. When the horse carries his neck too low, he can experience balance problems. The angle the neck makes to the body becomes too great and impedes the movement of his front legs. In the beginning, horses that have not yet found their balance, will move in this exaggerated position on the forehand. However, this should not be judged as incorrect for it will be a transitional stage only, seeing that contact is required before the development of impulsion and that should be achieved first in this attitude. Later on, when collection and elevation is required, the horse should still have the tendency to want to search for the hand of the rider, thus resulting in the free and easy movement by itself. From a biomechanical point of view, this is also the only position where the face joints are in such a position that they can allow for a lateral flexion of the neck while using the lever mechanism to its best advantage. When the horse's neck is very elevated, the angle of the facet joints are too steep and only a minimal lateral position of the head can be

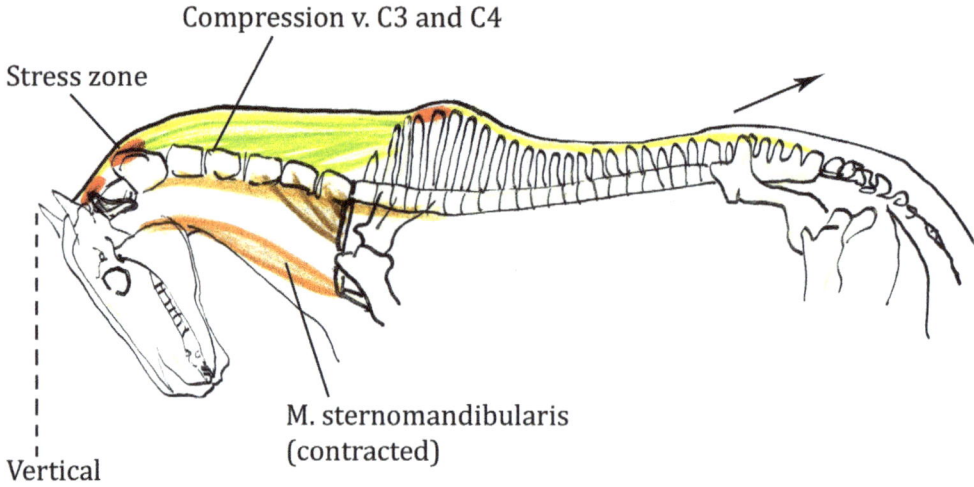

Fig. 10.5. Hyperflexion of the neck instead of a correct forwards and down can have a damaging impact on the neck vertebrae, joints, muscles and bursa. In this position the neck looses its function as lever and an elastic, useful activity of the back is hardly possible. The pull on the supraspinous ligament is already interrupted between C2 and C3 and can therefore only slightly be of aid in lifting the back.

achieved. This relates especially to the facet joints of the third and fourth neck vertebrae, which will almost point in a right angle to the ground. A bend to the side is not possible in this position. The angle of the jowl also plays a role; it will bump against the wings of the atlas and by squashing the parotid gland, cause a lot of pain to the horse.

Faulty and damaging in principle is the forward and back or a deep rolling in of the horse's neck (fig.10.5). When the pull on the supraspinous ligament is not uniformly to the front, but weakened by the development of a broken neck, it is not possible to lift the withers and the back in the so-desired and biomechanically correct form. Due to this contracted posture it leads to compression of the third and fourth neck vertebrae, furthermore causing osteopathic lesions and tension in the mm. splenius rectus capitis and longissimus cervicus with simultaneous shortening of the M. brachiocephalicus.

Through the correct forward and down stretched posture, one reaches a light traction on the neck vertebrae and the result is better mobility. It is due to this fact that one can understand that tension in the neck can be the result of bad riding. The extremely deep and rolled in posture robs the horse of all sight and the horse will always try and push against the hand in order to partake in his surroundings. Through this, pressure peaks of several hundred kilograms can be exerted on the poll, especially when draw reins are used to obtain this posture. The backs and croups of these horses stay relatively straight, the hind legs can only be driven under the center of gravity with effort and the horse goes on the forehand. The horse looks as if it has been split in two, as if the hind legs are working backwards instead of moving forward under the weight of the body. Tension of he psoas muscles and osteopathic lesions in the sacroiliac area can be part of this incorrect work. The correct building of resilient back muscles is not possible with these horses. The lack of activity in the hindquarters and the fact that the topline does not arch, only feeds the kissing spine syndrome possibility.

10.3 Contact

Definition: *Contact is the light, even connection of the mouth of the horse with the hand of the rider that occurs when the horse searches and stretches forward for the bit.*

It is extremely important to have a correct understanding of contact. Often, it is thought that contact is the position of the horse's head through the influence of the rider's hand, but the opposite is true. A horse that is relaxed and in a rhythmic tempo can be prompted to stretch forward and down when

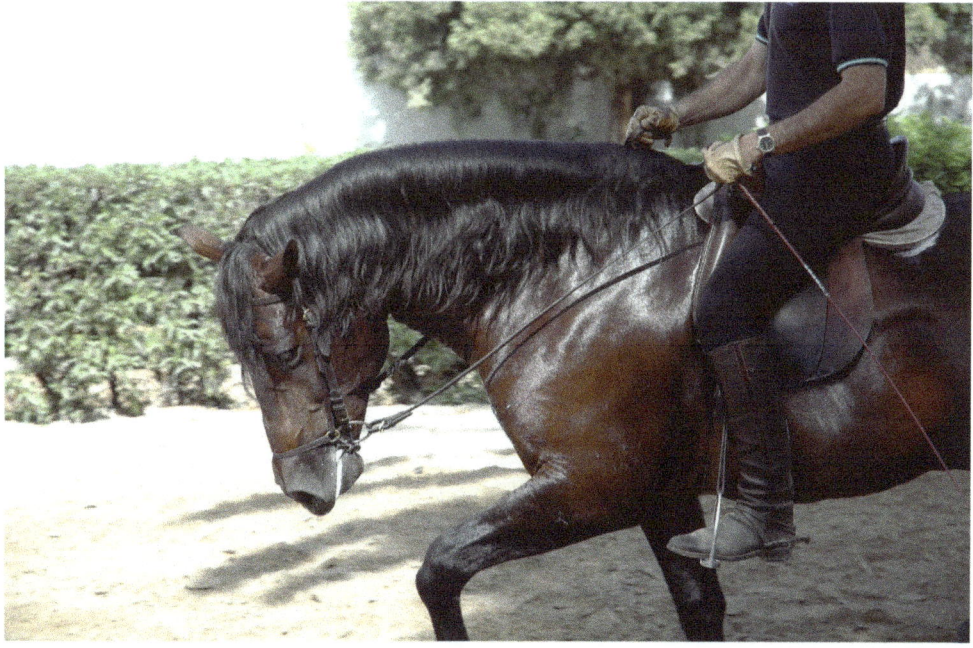

Fig.10.6 The horse searches trustingly for the contact to the soft and sensitive hand of the rider. The horse mouths the bit contently and has his full attention on the rider.

the rider asks for more activity from the hindquarters. Through this effort, it is the horse that searches the contact on the bit, and not the rider who forces the horse into the position by pulling on the reins.

A horse that has contact should stretch forward onto the bit with his neck as horizontal as possible, while moving forward freely in a trusting and satisfied manner and without elevation of the neck. Elevation is achieved only later through further training. (fig.10.6). Many young horses can be seen lifting their necks when canter is asked because they still do not possess sufficient balance, and by using their necks will try to obtain the necessary impulsion to canter. This compensating motion can be tolerated at this stage of the training for it should disappear when the hindquarters are strong enough and the aids are more refined as training continues.

10.3.1 On the bit

Definition: *Being on the bit (ramener) is the direct longitudinal flexion of the horse's head and neck.*

The poll should be the highest point—something that is often not possible in the Iberian horses due to the extreme development of the neck and anatomical reasons—and the profile [forehead] should be slightly in front of the vertical. This position can, at any time, be achieved at the halt by keeping the hand still. It is directly governed by the flexion of the atlanto-occpital joint and its surrounding muscles. The horse should subsequently relax the temporomandibler joint, the M. masseter and the muscles of the hyoid bone and begin gently mouthing the bit. However, being on the bit, by definition, has nothing to do with collection or contact, but is only an action that accompanies active hindquarters and a supple back where the soft and waiting hand of the rider receives the impulse.

10.4 Impulsion

Definition: *Impulsion is the controlled forward impulse that is generated from the hindquarters to sustain the movement of the horse. The forward movement is the soul of the art of riding (Louis Seeger) for without the forward thrust, no exercise will be of profit to the horse.*

Impulsion is generated by the influence from the rider's back and leg aids. In young horses that do not yet know the interaction of these aids, the use of the voice or a whip can be advantageous to make the forward drive of the legs more understandable. Impulsion is the foundation of getting a horse straight

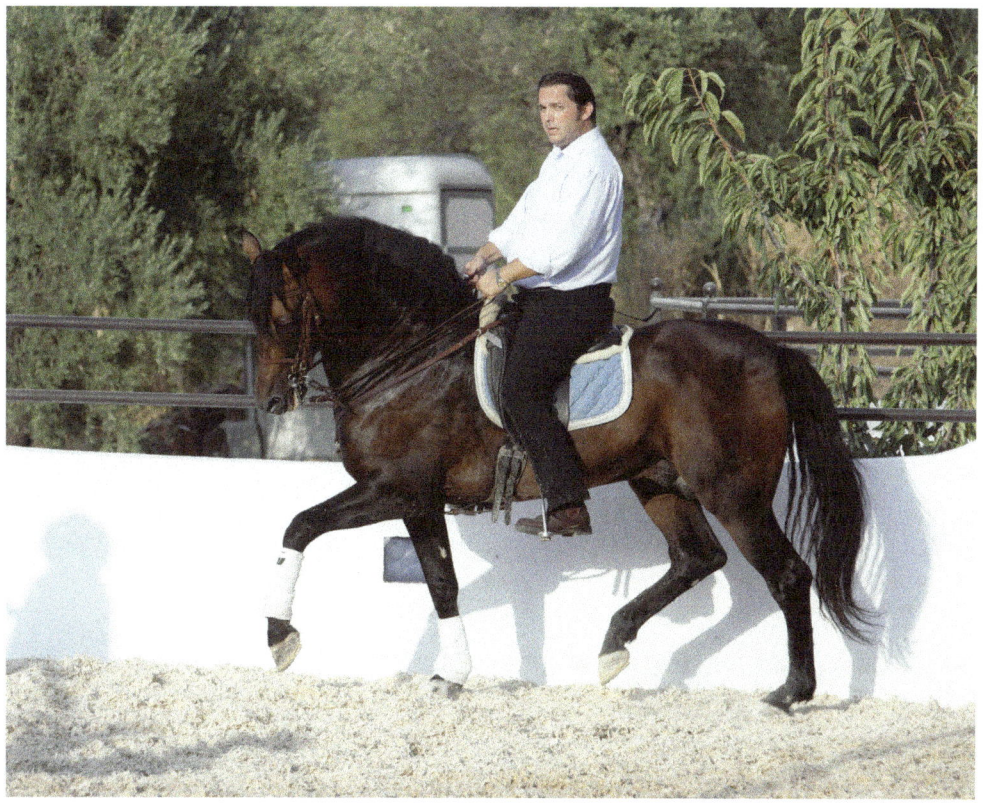

The author in a very well-balanced seat and low hand passing through the corner. every corner is a quarter of a circle of 6meters in diameter and one step of shoulder-in! Never forget the corners—there are four of them in the manege and there is quiet a lot of gymnastics in them. The shoulder-in on the straight track is nothing more than passing one corner, maintaining the same lateral bend position and ending in the next corner.

[Here the rider has and exemplary contact, offering the bit forward. The horse seeks the bit in a casual, carefree, easy way in which to communicate with his rider. The horse carries himself in 'self-carriage' as does the rider. Both are free of 'holding on' to each other through the reins. The rider does not pull back to 'take' the contact but instead, offers the contact forward in a progressive way as he and the horse move together forward through space. The rider sits in balance. The reins drape and rest in a soft curve on the horse's neck when not needed at any particular moment for feedback between the two partners. The contact of the rider's seat and thighs with the horse's back is continuous but not tight. This smooth and seamless connection mitigates the need for excessive rein use.]—Editor's note.

and is ultimately necessary for collection, for a horse without impulsion can never lower his haunches and actively perform collected exercises. The activity of the hindquarters must still be at the heart of every exercise. Only when a horse has surpassed the first three steps of the training scale and is therefore balanced, can the possibility exist that he develop a controlled push based on the correct contact. The controlled development of the pushing power is essential. The horse must never just hurry forward for this will result in fundamental training problems and lack of balance.

The energy created by suspension of the back in the movement develops from an energetic stepping, well-tilted hindquarters; simultaneously one should pursue that the horse steps at least into the footprint of his front hooves when in a working tempo. Through the increased bending of the haunches, while riding "in position"[10] and straight, the inside hip will lower even more, the angle between the big joints become smaller and from the forward thrusting power one can develop the strength to carry weight.

10.4.1 Controlled forward impulsion vs. speed

> **Note:** *One should ensure that the horse does not go faster, hastier or start running when his position is extended in the development of suspension. This often incorrect release of impulsion is the result of lack of strength to carry weight and insufficient elasticity of the back.*

In order to step forward in a controlled way full of impulsion, the horse must allow the movement from the hindquarters to swing forward with an elastic and supple back, all of which is softly received in the hand of the rider and only possible with a horse that is horizontally balanced. The horse should fill the rectangular form[11] in the lengthening of the topline through the generated forward movement as well. The center of gravity lies in the transition between the first and second third of the horse's body. Driving with

---

10   The horse is 'in position' if he is in balance—meaning that the horse should go in the *ramener* [see Chapter 2] position with a supple back and a harmonious distribution of the weight. If he is out of this position, he lacks balance and is either running after his center of gravity [falling forward] or if he is 'behind,' he overloads his hindquarters, if he is skewed or crooked, he runs to the side, usually through one shoulder.

11   'Rectangular form'—By this I mean that the horse should have the tendency to slightly lengthen the topline so that he can fill up the reins with his topline but without leaning on the hand. The horse's topline should become elongated and should not become shortened in the extensions—today one sees many incorrect examples of horses running faster in the extended trot and becoming very short in the neck.

the legs brings the hindquarters further under the center of gravity, whereby the body of the horse can experience better support and becomes more stable. The back will be arched and the horse tries to keep his balance in the deep position. Horses that have been actively supported with the hand are not capable of this and will tend to fall on their forehand due to the driving impulse of the legs, because the sagging back will prevent the hindquarters from being shifted under the center of gravity. It is for this reason that horses that have been routinely supported by the hand become even heavier in the hand and more on the forehand, for they have not been allowed or taught to keep their own balance. They constantly look for support in the rider's hand to compensate for the lack of balance and strength to carry weight.

A further biomechanical reflex will be the contraction of the M. longissimus dorsi generated by the act of moving, and, due to its job as establisher and extensor of the spinal cord, this contraction will stabilize the spinal cord in any sudden forward movement. This is why horses that run or hurry in extensions are uncomfortable to sit—because their backs do not swing in an elastic way.

This reaction and stiffening of the spinal cord is a component of the flight reflex of the prey animal, and in order to see better, is accompanied by the high head carriage, and that again causes the back to lower and be inaccessible for an elastic and swinging movement. This stress factor will logically produce a higher muscle tone to prepare the muscles for a rapid fleeing sprint. All of this can be observed in horses that are not relaxed.

Consequently one can only take a step back and work on the lacking foundation and in restoring the trust.

10.4.2 Trot extension—an exception?

Specifically the young horse is not physically able to execute a well-positioned extended trot because of the short time he has been in training.

Definition: *The term "lengthening the outline" describes the lengthening of the strides within a gait in the "working posture."*

It is necessary to gently prepare the horse for the interplay between the various tempi within the basic gaits. By moving the center of gravity [back], we can effect the desired increased use of the hindquarters. It is important that the lengthening of the outline be obvious and that the horse should be brought back into the basic working tempo [after each lengthening].

When lengthening the outline, the horse should be allowed to fully fill the rectangular frame of the working gait and the strides and neck should be noticeably lengthened. Though initially only lengthening for a few steps at a time, the horse will gradually to learn to play with his center of gravity and control his balance and the length of the strides. From this basic model comes the foundation of correctly ridden extensions whereby the horse can develop the muscles of his back and hindquarters so that the he can execute a well-positioned extended trot that is, above all, comfortable to sit. Such extensions seem unspectacular at first, but will improve as the strength to carry weight of the hindquarters increases.

Horses that are asked to present extended gaits too early [in their development], without the physical ability that comes with correct training, will perform these with very bent hocks and the support of the rider's hand. The back and haunches will be blocked due to the lacking strength to carry weight, since they are kept elevated by the hand and they give the illusion of a level of training they do not possess. One frequently sees these tensed-up trot movements in three-year-old auction horses, with stiff backs, as they attempt, in vain, to develop thrusting power from their hocks. If these horses are trained further in this manner, without appropriate gymnastic work, early wear and tear on both physical and psychological levels will result.

When one remembers that riding extended trot [on the diagonal] carries the same load on the suspensory ligaments as jumping an entire course of 1.30 meters, it becomes clear that even dressage horses only have a certain number of extensions [available] in their legs. This is especially true if the horse is asked to execute them without the necessary development of required ability to carry weight.

A good quality extended trot is characterized by the fact that the horse lengthens his outline and his strides, but does not increase his speed. The canon bone of the hind-leg should be parallel to the canon bone of the diagonally opposite front leg. The hindquarters should be pushed together like an accordion in order to powerfully push off. This [correct thrusting] will ensure that the hindquarters develop enough carrying and pushing power, and the front legs will not just be [incorrectly] lifted and elongated by active raising of the neck. It is also important that each front foot steps directly into the trajectory of where it points when it is fully extended [and not drop to the ground falling short of that location]. All of this constitutes the quality of a good extended trot.

The so-called "dazzlers" that show extreme activity in the forelegs but do not offer enough support in the hindquarters are marked down in dressage tests, and are merely "leg movers." The desired "back mover" moves with the use of his entire body and an elastic back. The [incorrect] "dazzler" horse looks military-like in their movement and often have very highly positioned necks.

10.5 Straightness

> **Definition:** *Straightness is the orientation of the longitudinal axis of the horse on a straight line, so that the lowering of the inside hip results in the inside hind leg stepping increasingly under the horse's center of gravity, making the inside shorter and stretching the outside. The shoulders of the horse are brought ever-so slightly fore, in front of the hind-legs.*

This way of training horses stems from the innate one-sidedness of the horses. Horses, like people, are also left or right handed which causes a preference to move in one direction more than the other. Limited by the conical form, the forward movement of the wider hindquarters mostly arrives crookedly to the front and the horse tends to track sideways to the inside [with the haunches to one side]. This phenomenon is understood as "natural crookedness," and it is assumed that this congenital unilateral shortening of the muscles comes about through the position of the foal in the womb.

At the beginning of their training, the majority of horses are hollow on the left side and prefer to move on this direction and can accomplish that without balance problems. The goal of the training is to ensure an equilateral development of the muscles to make sure that the horse can move equally well in the lessons in both directions.

By stretching the short side of the horse, one can work on straightening him. All straightening is preceded by riding the horse "in position." The neck is used as a balancing pole to transfer the center of gravity to the outside. The horse is prompted by a slight positioning of the head to the inside to move his shoulders to the middle. Supporting this rein action will be the rider's inside leg driving at the girth, that on the one hand keeps the forward impulsion and on the other hand is softly driving sideways to get the croup out and counteract the crookedness.

> **Definition:** *If the shoulder comes more to the inside, so the outside ear of the horse is in a line with the inside shoulder, one speaks of shoulder-fore or plié, which is the preparation for the shoulder-in on three or four tracks.*

The shoulder-fore can activate the inside hind-leg and induce flexion and carrying capacity, making the horse lighter on the inside rein and stretching towards the outside rein. The restricting outside rein assumes a key position in straightening and bending, for the contact should follow automatically from generating the rounding and rotating of the spinal column by the driving inside leg. This should all lead to longitudinal bending. The stretched forward and down position in combination with the lowering of the inside hip improves the stretching of the outside M. braciocephalicus and the mobility of the outside shoulder.

Because the rider has the tendency to put more weight on his inside seat-bone to maintain the longitudinal bending, the horse is given the possibility to stretch the outside M. longissimus dorsi and M.iliocostalis.

This effect is strengthened by working the horse on three tracks in the shoulder-in. Decreasing the circle and increasing the size of the circle will help develop the strength to carry weight and the reaction to the sideways restricting and driving leg aids. Further development to accept the sideways driving and thus straightening leg aid will be accomplished by the turn on the forehand and the turn on the haunches; the former has more of a loosening effect and the latter has more of a collecting effect.

All collection and bending exercises must be used cautiously and in the right dosage because the lateral gaits demand more balance, strength to carry weight and coordination. In order not to tire the horses too much, it is recommended to do short but good iterations of the exercises on a regular basis and then return to a break in order for the horse to process what was learned. This [short interval training] will prevent too much lactic acid from building up in the muscles and will also prevent over-stretching and will help keep the horse motivated and interested.

10.5.1 Natural asymmetry

> **Definition:** *Natural asymmetry is the crooked [off-set] propulsion of the hind legs that causes them to step to one side of the hoof prints of front hooves. The cause of this asymmetry could stem from the way the foal lies in the womb of the mare along with the 'triangular' shape of the riding horse [narrower in front and wider behind] causing it to move crooked when ridden.*

The more muscled hindquarters will push more than they carry, and the forehand will try to evade the impulse from the haunches by stepping to the outside. It is for this reason that one can often observe young horses when they are first ridden, trying to orient themselves by finding contact with the wall with their outside shoulder so as to keep their balance.

The natural asymmetry is one of the reasons why a horse must first learn to track correctly by aligning the shoulders [with the haunches by bringing them toward] the middle of the school as a prerequisite to beginning collection. When one views green horses moving freely on the lunge, one will quickly find out that on the one rein they will look out of the circle and fall to the inside with the shoulders, but in the other direction, they will look to the inside of the circle as their hindquarters drift to the outside. These are the first attempts of the horse to find its balance in all the gaits on the unfamiliar path of the circle. The capacity of the horse to keep an even bend demands straightening work to establish the curved path of travel and the development of strength to carry weight to maintain it. The horse must first find balance in the movement by means of 'auto-equilibration,' free and without any restricting aids, because any kind of reins will force the horse into a predetermined posture, making finding his balance more difficult.

'Auto-equilibration' is also important in the rehabilitation of horses. They have to return to the basics before they can build up again in a sensible progression. Omitting this step would subject the already overloaded forehand to stresses which would permanently harm the horse. The goal of training should be to make the horse supple such that both sides become approximately equal and so that he can perform the exercises as mirror images.

10.5.2 Paths to straightness

The major goal is to align the shoulders with the hindquarters or the other way around in order to create a horse that moves straight in his tracks. Seen from the front, the observer should only see the front legs because the hind legs follow in the exact same track as the front legs. The shoulders can be put in shoulder-fore or *plié* to align them with the hind legs. Shoulder-fore is the first exercise in riding that forms the basis of shoulder-in, which was considered the "aspirin for riding" by Nuno Oliveira, and serves to straighten the horse.

> **Note:** *One has to warn against premature attempts to straighten the horse with the use of shoulder-in since the young horse lacks sufficient strength to carry weight on the haunches and cannot cope with increased bending of the haunches over longer intervals.*

Insubordination and tension can be two consequences, therefore careful use of the *plié* and later on, the shoulder-in is advisable so as not to force premature loading of the hindquarters. The result would be a leg aid that drives the horse sideways without any bend or any worthy gymnastic value. Working the horse with the opposite bend [to the outside] can work wonders and should not be forgotten in this context.

Correctly riding through the corners should be the same as riding a quarter volte, where the inside hind leg is encouraged to step more under the body by the inside leg aid of the rider. Above all, the execution of school figures are of particular help in improving the ability to influence the horse and should not be dismissed as unnecessary nor as burdensome. When correctly executed, the exercises <u>often emerge</u> as complete lessons lesson plans. Concentric reduction and increasing of the size of the circle will improve the acceptance of the leg aids, and will improve the ability to guide the croup or the shoulders in any direction. Leg-yielding should be the basic exercise to teach sideways driving aids and should not be undervalued, for the horse learns to move sideways independent of the sometimes over-taxing longitudinal bend. This will improve the efficiency of the reaction to the leg aids.

In the correct execution of the turn on the forehand lies the key to success, for there are two possible ways to execute this exercise. The first and easier exercise positions the horse against the direction of movement of the hindquarters and then the driving leg aid facilitates the sidestep of the hindquarters around the forehand. The shoulders should move in a tiny circle in a regular walk rhythm. The turn on the forehand in renvers [haunches-out] positions the horse in the direction of movement of the hindquarters, this requires a greater degree of suppleness from the horse and more feeling and preparation in the execution. Nevertheless it is of great value, for a horse that is prepared in this way with a flowing execution of the exercise becomes less tense with each repetition of the movement and thus easier to ride.

The converse exercise, the turn on the haunches, positions and bends the horse in the direction of the movement and is a collection exercise. The horse should make steps in a tiny circle with the hindquarters without losing the forward movement, while the forehand moves around in a larger circular path. The full turn on the haunches begins and ends with a halt whereas the half-turn on the haunches begins from the movement [gait]. A half-turn on the haunches can be ridden in all three gaits and becomes a half-pirouette in trot or canter. Walk pirouettes can be ridden as quarter, half and full turns and serve as a means to improve the coordination of the interplay between the inside leg and the outside rein.

In none of the aforementioned exercises is pulling on the inside rein allowed, because the forward tendency would then be lost. Almost without exception, when contact or impulsion is lost, one should ride straight forward in an energetic way. As is evident from this exercise's physical arrangements, the goal is the mobilization of the forehand and the hindquarters with the aid of the legs, rendering a positive influence and serves to straighten the horse almost automatically, because the horse learns to move away from pressure of the leg and to fill up and stretch into the outside rein contact.

10.5.3 Riding with bend—limits and possibilities of bend in the ribcage

In the classical art of riding the demand for bend in the ribs, produced by the inside leg aid, is always demonstrated. When one views the thorax from a biomechanical point of view, it is evident that the first eight true ribs, which

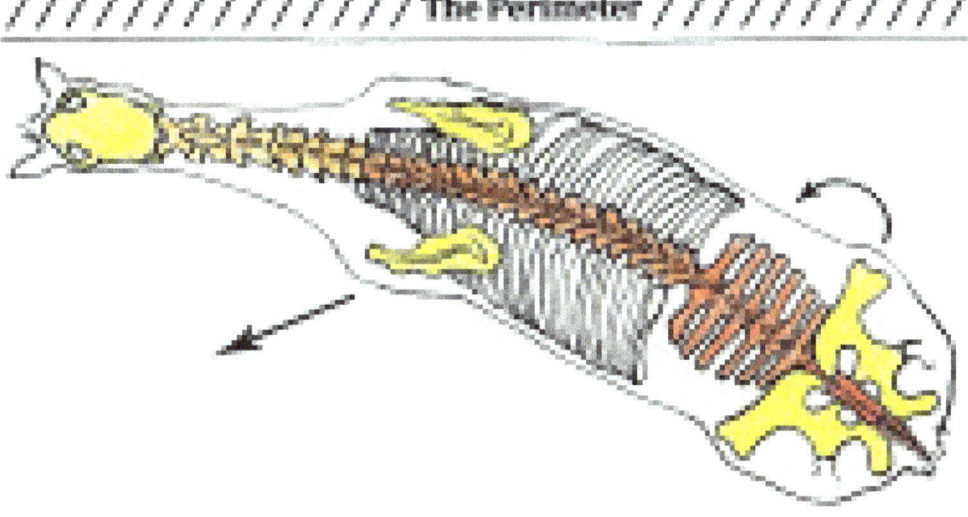

Fig.10.7 Travers—a genuine bend around the leg is not possible due to the rigid construction of the thorax.

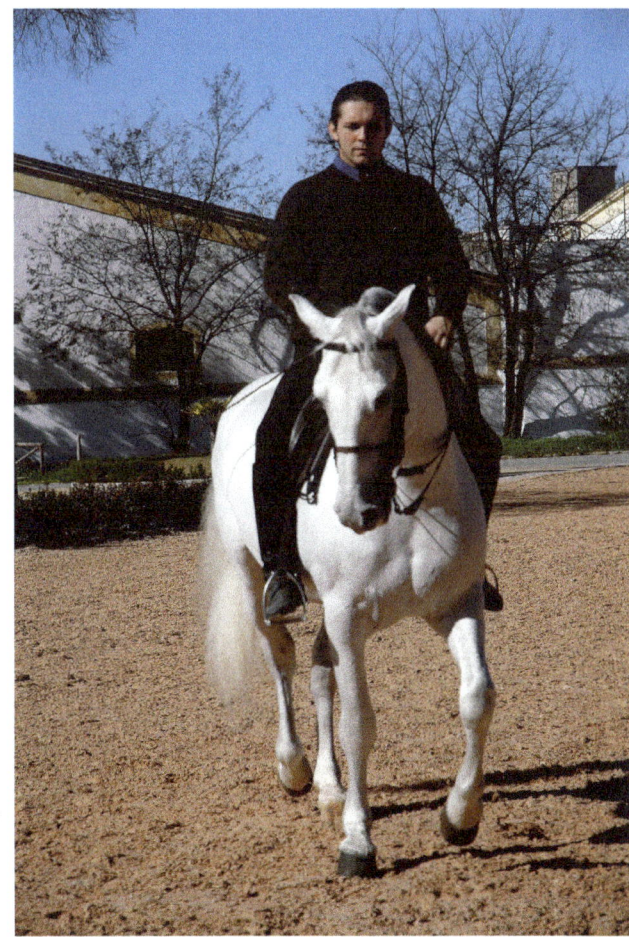

Fig.10.8 The apparent bend (in the ribs) around the inside leg in lateral gaits (renvers) is obtained by arching and rotation of the thoracolumbar area and the position of the neck.

are connected to the sternum, does not allow for any sideways bend. The rest of the ribs that are connected with cartilage and function as breathing aids cannot offer much more in sideways bend seeing that the width of the ribs and the space between them are limiting factors. The ribs that are pressed together on one side must be stretched apart on the other side. The muscles between the ribs also have to occupy space, which makes a maximum bend of 2-3cm possible in the ribs. (Fig. 10.7)

Nevertheless, horses appear to be bent around the leg in the lateral movements. (fig.10.8) This is the result of arching and rotation of the thoraculumbar area behind the saddle. This area is very mobile and does not have any ventral support from bone. The rotation in the lumbar part can also cause the croup to "overtake" in the half-pass when the shoulders are not properly aligned in the front. For this reason, the demand for bend in the ribs is just as little achievable as keeping an even circular line from the poll to the tail. Through the circular movement the inside shoulder and inside hip come closer to each other, while the outside legs go further apart or open. Only the neck vertebrae are mobile enough to participate in almost all lateral movements. Nevertheless, it should be cautioned not to bend the neck too much to the inside, for the forward impulsion will be lost by the heaviness on the inside shoulder.

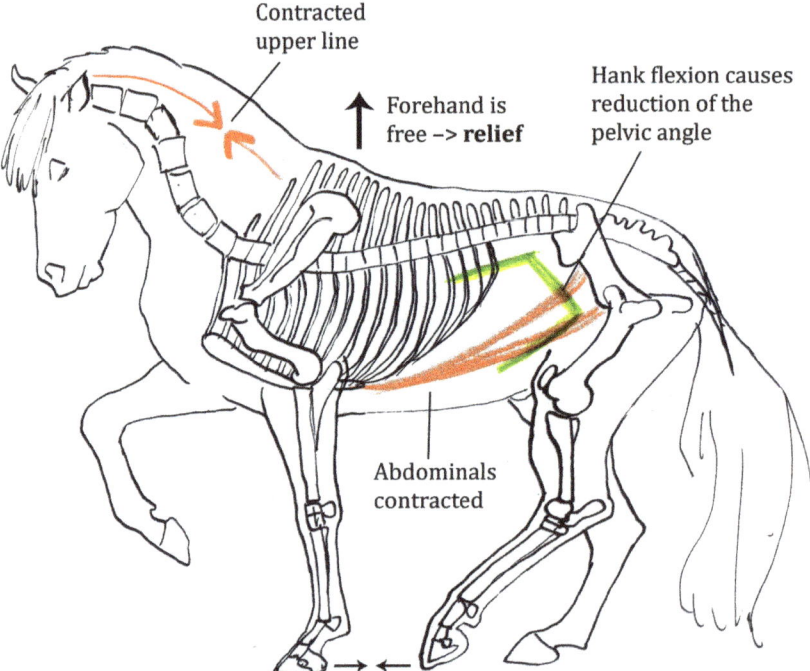

Fig. 10.9.a The horse in good selfcarriage, with elevated and rounded neck, steps more under the center of gravity and enabling greater suppleness and range of motion in the shoulders.

All sideways bending exercises should maintain a harmonious symmetry when possible, and avoid over bending and pulling, as the meaningfulness of lateral work is nullified when the forward impulsion is lost and thus has no gymnastic merit anymore. One should bear this in mind when the complete length of a fully grown warm-blood is 3 meters, then the possible total bend of the spinal cord amounts to 15cm.

10.6 Collection

> **Definition**: *Collection is the last step in the training scale of the F.N.. I prefer to use the word, "rassembler," because the concentration of the forces in the horse's body allows us the coordinated use of its resources making it even possible to ride. For this author, "rassembler" is the means necessary to ride and not just an abstract goal. Furthermore there are three additional degrees of [longitudinal] bending that are possible in the haunches. Whether a horse achieves this additional level of engagement of the haunches is highly depend on a) what the horse's individual conformation will allow and b) the gymnastic preparation that the horse has had. These additional three degrees of bending of the haunches is not achievable by all horses because it requires a great deal of strength and balance, and very elastic muscles and joints. In this sense, it is be better to use the German word, versammlung, [gathering] to refer to the concentration of forces necessary to ride. This last point on the training scale depends on the capacity of haunches to bend and on the elasticity and flexibility of the horse's back.*

The horse needs to become so powerful and balanced through his muscular development, that he is able, with the added weight of the rider, to reduce his base of support by bringing his hind legs further under his body and moving evenly with rhythmic and cadenced steps. In this last step of the training scale, the horse must developed the so-called "springing force" of the impulsion and the strength to carry weight. The reduced angles of the haunches, caused by the contraction of the abdominal and psoas muscles and lowering of the croup, makes the horse appear deeper behind and more "seated."

The improved balance gives the horse the capacity to slow down the movement both in the moment of suspension and in the supportive phase, resulting in a majestic picture with an elevated expression. The loins transfer the impulsion to the arched back which, in turn, elevates the neck. The neck is in an extended elevation, making the movement of the forehand freer and lighter. The well set neck in the extended elevation is "in position" with the poll as the highest point, and well-rounded. (fig.10.9.a) The well-developed trapezius and splenius muscles make the stable position of the neck possible without need for any extra adjusting movements.

The M. longissimus dorsi and the M. iliocostalis which are responsible for maintaining the longitudinal flexion, must swing elastically in order to allow the movement to come from the hindquarters moving forward uninterrupted into the mouth of the horse. By virtue of the reduced base of support and shifting back the center of gravity, it is possible for the rider to affect the balance with minimal changes of his weight and give almost invisible aids that induce the horse to perform the exercises.

Following the guiding principle "from easy to difficult" one must never forget that a true collection can never be reached without relaxation, so the adherence to the consecutive construction of the training scale comes full circle.

The degree of collection will vary depending on the horse's age and level of training. Only a collected horse can be ridden and well-controlled in dangerous situations. Furthermore, collection is indispensable for the health of the horse on the grounds of the gymnastic effect, which is proved by the longevity of the horses in the Spanish Riding School in Vienna. Horses at an age of 20 to 25 partake in the performances regularly. Slow, purposeful, systematic training can make longevity a perfectly realistic goal for the normal horse.

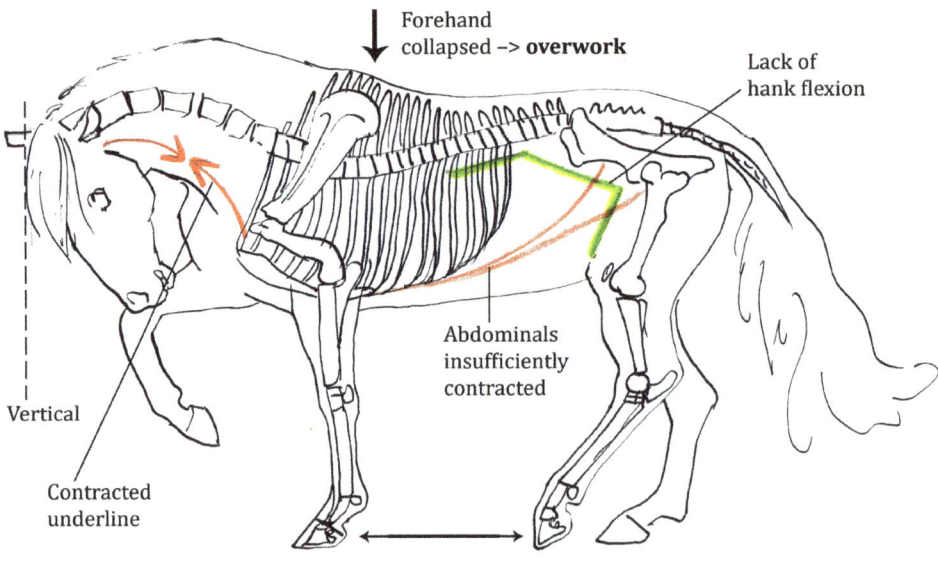

Fig. 10.9.b An improperly adjusted horse. If the horse is too deep in his head position, he is unable to free his shoulders; because of the excessive weight shifted to the front end, the shoulders are overloaded instead of being freed.

10.6.1 Rein-back

Definition: *Rein-back is movement in which the horse moves backwards using alternate diagonal pairs of legs in sequence.*

Although this exercise demands a high degree of collection, suppleness and balance, it is already expected in the tests for young horses. Unsightly displays are all too often seen including pulling on the reins, hollowed backs, dragging of the feet backwards etc

Even though rein-back is of utmost importance to the obedience of the horse, and is of immeasurable value in reviewing suppleness, the horse should, as a prerequisite, be able to comply with the first five points of the training scale and only then, can he be brilliant in this difficult collection exercise.

This swing is a characteristic exercise of a well-ridden and supple horse in every Grand Prix test, for this walk exercise where the horse takes 6 steps back, 6 steps forward, 6 steps back and then proceeds forward again, ???offers no possibility to seriously influence the movement sequence.??? All of this should proceed fluently and without hesitation.

Merely walking backwards [in a four-beat rhythm] should be seen as a grave fault and should be corrected immediately, because the horse can hurt his sacroiliac joint through excessive bending. Left uncorrected, this movement could lead to further strain in the psoas and hamstring muscles.

A movement has gymnastic effect only if it is executed in a slow, calm

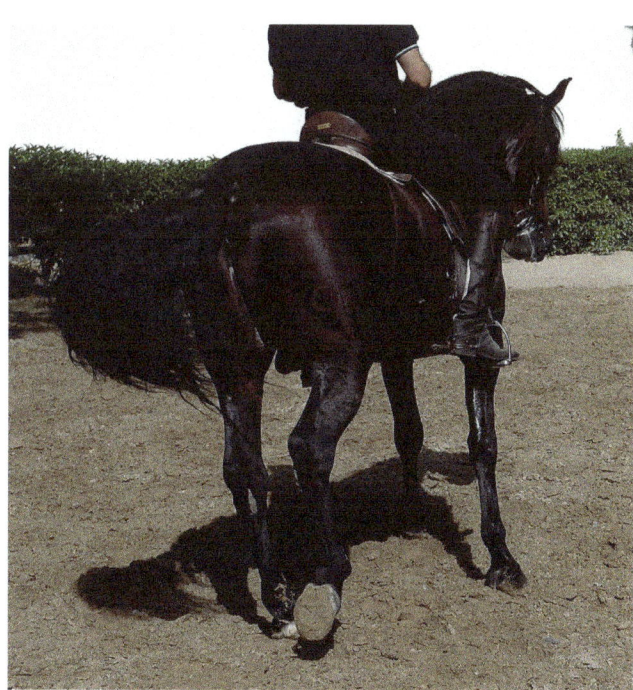

Fig 11.1 Via counter position on the left circle, a shift of balance to the inside occurs. The horse seems to move away from the outside leg aid effortlessly toward the middle of the circle and thus improves the freedom of the inside (left in this picture) shoulder.

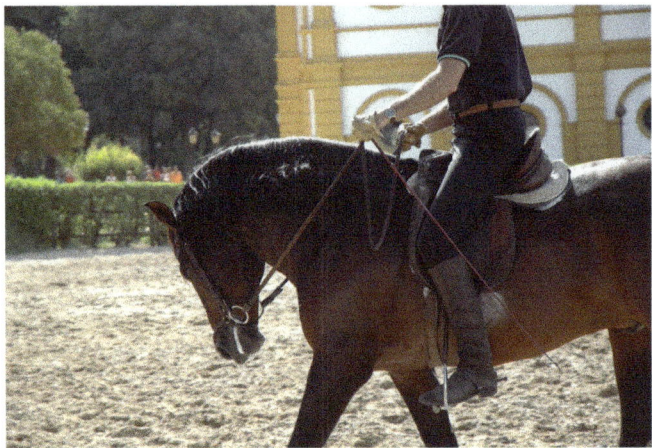

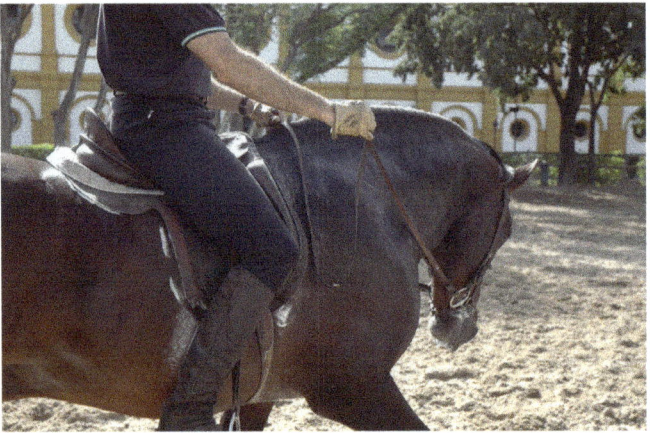

Fig 11.2
a. When riding in the counter position (here on the left rein) the inside leg must act in a supporting manner and keep the bend. This will improve the straightness and the longitudinal bend is preserved.

b. Counter position on the right rein: the inside rein (here, the right rein) must sometimes be used as an openning rein in order to give the inside shoulder some room and to insure a flowing movement.

and coordinated manner. Fast and hectic movements do not help the horse and cause wear and tear.

Rein-back followed by immediate forward movement in walk or trot can help to improve the activity of the hindquarters for piaffe, since the horse prepares the haunches appropriately by lowering his croup. The combination of the forward and backwards movement will improve the urge to move forward since the rein-back represents a strong obedience exercise. The Spanish walk can also be improved by the rein-back. It is important that forward impulsion is not ignored when the rein-back is practiced, for horses can easily learn and gravitate to withdrawing backwards as an evasion which can lead to dangerous and unpredictable situations.

11. Use and benefits of counter position and the lateral exercises.

11.1. Riding in counter position

Although riding in the counter position can be an excellent way to gymnasticize a horse, it is very sparsely discussed in the conventional books on the art of riding. [In this Chapter on counter position, the "inside" is the side of the horse to the inside of the arena (it does not refer to the "inside of the bend"). Correspondingly, the outside refers to the side of the horse that is towards the outside of the circle or the outside of the arena (not the "outside of the bend")].

> **Definition:** The counter position is the position opposite to the direction of movement, or longitudinal bend, of the neck and body. (fig11.1)

By riding in counter position it is possible to stretch the inside neck muscles, so that the inside shoulder can obtain better mobility and improved range of movement (fig.11.2). In addition to this, the outside hind foot is addressed in the same manner as in the half-pass, without having to maintain the longitudinal bend.

This is especially important with young horses, that do not yet posses the necessary strength to carry weight and are not capable of keeping a longitudinal bend for an extended period of time. With more advanced horses, one can achieve an increased lowering of the inside hip and therefore demand that the inside leg carries more weight with the use of a *plié* or shoulder-in. When this exercise is demanded of a horse that is not capable, it can easily lead to tension since the horse will likely find the position unpleasant.

Many young horses with extreme natural crookedness cannot be straightened in the first attempt for they have neither the balance nor the strength to do so. If a rider tries to force the croup to the outside with strong leg aids, it can lead to anxiety and fear of the leg, and the possibility of suppleness is lost.

> **Note:** *Because horses usually carry the head to the outside to find their balance, the natural crookedness can be reinforced by the counter position. The horse quickly learns that the position he offers can become more comfortable if he straightens in the forward movement. We must warn that the counter position should not be produced with an exaggerated bend in the neck to the outside, for the horse would then become blocked in the forward movement.*

By addressing the inside shoulder and the outside hind leg simultaneously the horse will learn to balance himself quicker. Counter shoulder-in [shoulder-out] on the long wall and leg-yielding on the diagonal or down the long side are excellent exercises to improve flexibility and establish balance under the rider. Riding the corners slowly in counter position also helps immensely with the balance. Logically, after every short training session there should be a relaxation phase in the stretched posture to prevent the muscles from tiring.

When the horse is with his head in a deeper position through the stretched posture, the only efficient stretching possibility is through the use of the counter position. When the horse moves in a rhythmic, even tempo, it becomes possible for him to release blockages in the neck vertebrae with the so-called "auto-unblocking."

Riding in the counter position only leads to the desired goal once the horse has found his rhythm and suppleness. Here it is about the targeted use of the shift in equilibrium to the contra-lateral side, and horses are shown an almost playful new possibility of movement. Forcing the counter position according to the mechanical laws only, for example with the aid of extra reins or lever systems, will never have the desired results. Conversely, once the horse has learned to relax with the use of the counter positioning method, it is possible to restore suppleness when momentary lapses occur.

11.2. Lateral work

Definition: *Lateral work includes all movements on multiple tracks (2-4) that have a forward tendency and a sideways crossing of both the front and the hind limbs, asked for by the rider.*

During the sideways movement there should be an even, longitudinal bend through the entire body from poll to tail. Evading the driving leg by stepping only to the side [without a forward component] has no value in gymnastic training and does not serve the rehabilitation process nor does it build muscle.

Note: *The advantages of lateral work when performed correctly lie in the controlled influence on the movement.*

Through calm, rhythmic crossing of the limbs, the muscles have enough time to relax and stretch, loosening tension in the warm-up phase and appropriate use of lateral work shortens the warm-up much more than what would be typically accomplished by just trotting forward for an extended period of time. In the walk the horse can easily learn the interplay between the sideways driving leg and the outside rein, and can quickly stretch into the forward and down posture.

All lateral movements help to improve the relaxation, and promote the building of muscles and foster obedience. The gymnastic benefit is not solely for dressage horses but is also valuable for horses of other disciplines. Through the finely tuned interaction of the balance, the horse learns to concentrate more on the rider and coordinate his body better. Lateral work is invaluable for improving proprioception in the rehabilitation phase.

> **Note:** *An important principal for all lateral movements and exercises is that they should be done with few, but good steps in the beginning, so as not to overstrain the muscles and not to take the joy out of learning something new.*

Horses learn very quickly that this way of moving under the weight of the rider is easier when they can round their backs, thus improving the ability to carry weight of the rider. Calm and rhythmic steps and lifting the feet during the exercise improves not only the concentration but also the coordination and proprioception of the posture and positioning reflexes. In this way, we obtain a horse that is flexible and able to move in an elastic way. Through correct use of lateral work, the horse becomes able to use his body more efficiently due to improved circulation and this, in turn, supports the rehabilitation process.

Lateral work can be taught initially in-hand. In this way, the horse will learn to balance himself in the sideways movements without the added weight of the rider. This prepares the horse for when he attempts to do this under the rider's weight. This preparation will eliminate many unpleasant pictures such as rapping of legs and pulling on the reins that do not help the horse with the general understanding of new lessons. Quite the opposite, horses become frightened and tense by these unrefined means nullifying any potential gymnastic benefit.

> **Note**: *The "even bend" that is demanded has anatomical reasons why it is only possible to a certain extent; although horses appear to be bent around the inside leg, for example, in the half-pass.*

The most flexible part of the spinal cord is the neck hence, it should not—because of the balancing effect—be positioned with too much bend in the lateral exercises, because the one-sided contraction of the M. brachiocephalicus can block the ipsilateral [same side] shoulder. The bend of the neck should, therefore, be kept to a minimum. It is sufficient when the rider can just see the inside eye of the horse. This conservative amount of bend will neither impede the forward movement nor the sideways tendency.

Furthermore, one must warn against pulling on the inside rein in an attempt to bring the neck into an extreme bend, because this will massively disturb the propulsion of the hind legs and puts excessive weight on the ipsilateral [same side] shoulder. The horse will loose his balance and, subsequently will fall over the outside shoulder—instead of freeing it up. This is often seen in an incorrectly ridden shoulder-in, where the rider attempts to keep the bend and position by pulling on the inside rein; the horse clearly suffers from a loss of impulsion and rhythm and the lateral exercise looses all gymnastic value.

The longitudinal bend in the ribs is limited to merely 2-3cm [about one inch] by the width of the ribs and the distance between the ribs, and the true ribs make the thorax seem rigid due to their relative compact connection to the sternum.

The longitudinal bend that impresses the observer is, in actual fact, an upward arch with a simultaneous rotation of the thoracolumbar connection. This causes a one-sided contraction of the psoas muscle, producing a lowering of the inside hip. At the same time, the hind legs are brought more under the body by the adductors that, in turn, leads to greater stepping under on the inside and the appearance of a concave shape. (Fig. 10.8.)

Flexing the horse to the inside only has a limited effect on the longitudinal bend, because a more bent position [in the neck] actually lessens the longitudinal bend [in the entire length of the horse's body] and the collection is lost in favor of the falsely-perceived loosening effect.

A maximum position of 45 degrees to the wall should not be exceeded, because in angles greater than 45 degrees, forward movement is lost in favor of sideways movement.

The most important component is always the forward tendency and it must be present in all exercises. Without the forward tendency, there is no classical riding. It is for this reason that loss of rhythm and impulsion in the lateral movements should be seen as fundamental errors and must be corrected immediately by briskly riding forward; horses can easily learn to evade the influence of the rider with this backwards [lack of forward] tendency. Left uncorrected, horses will begin to go behind the hand of the rider, do not react to the leg aids, leaving the rider helpless due to the loss of control and can lead to dangerous situations.

In all lateral exercises, it is important that the shoulders are slightly in front of the hindquarters so that it is always possible for the horse to step forward with sufficient impulsion. It is only in this position that the horse is able to load the hindquarters, for a croup that passes the front is only able to push and no longer able to carry.

The Science and Art of Riding in Lightness

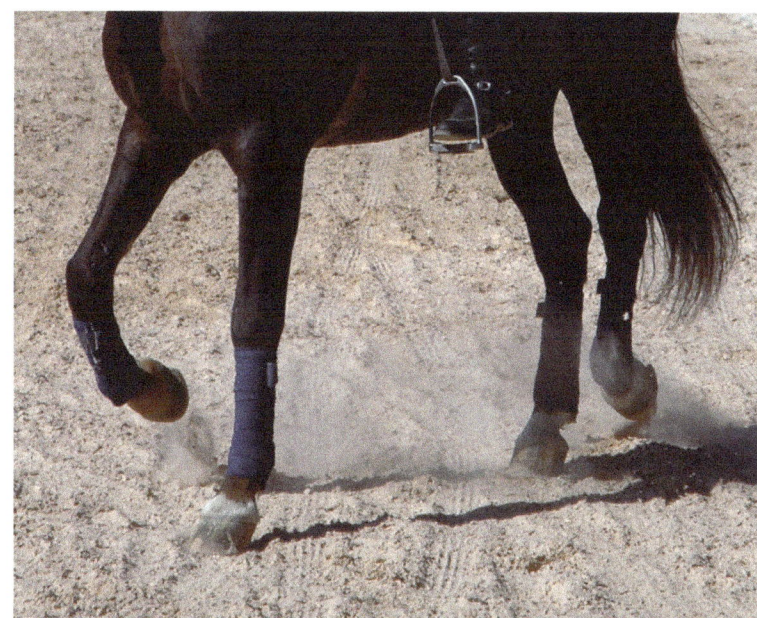

Fig 11.3. Shoulder-in

a. Performed on four tracks, it demands less lateral bend and therefore is more useful to loosen the horse.

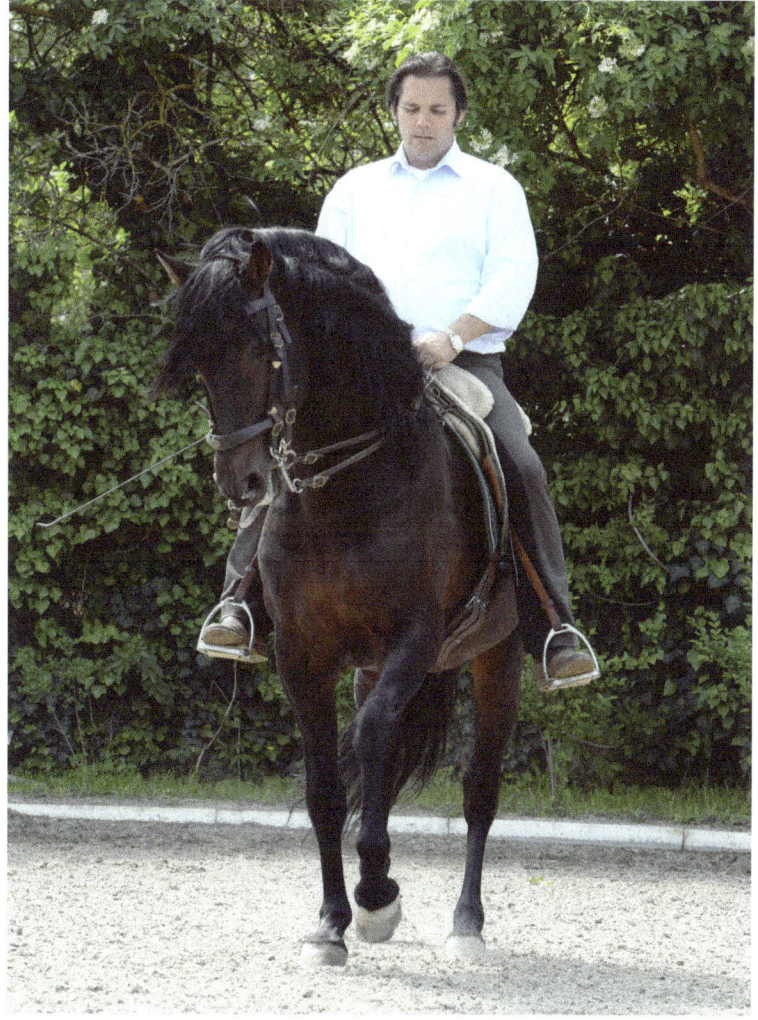

b. Performed on three tracks, the exercise has a stronger tendency toward collection.

Fig 11.4 Execution of the right shoulder in at the moment when the horse crosses the right hind leg; the impact on the muscles, cross-section at L2

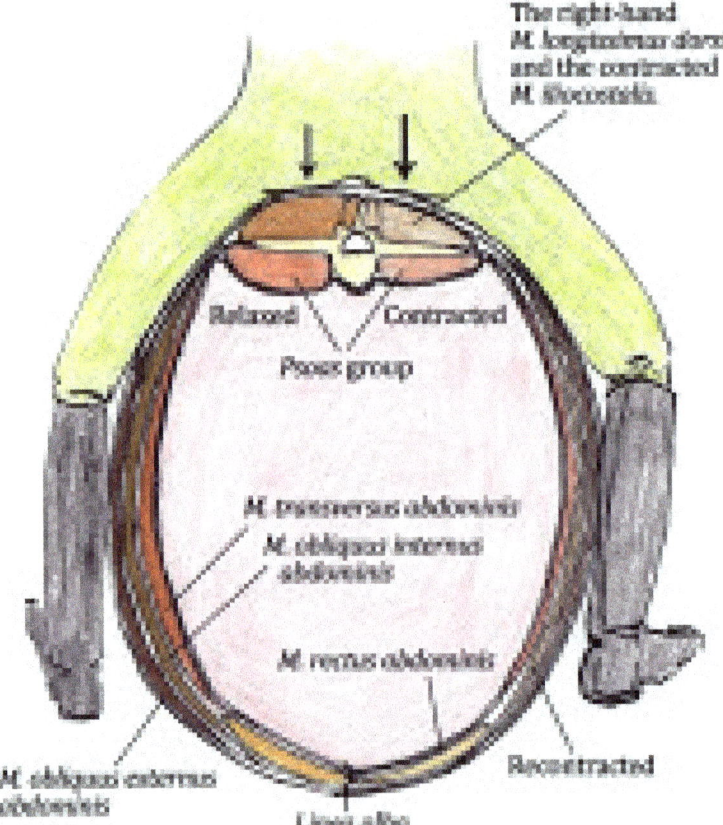

Through correct and regular bending work, one is able to stretch the outside section of the ileocostalis and longissimus dorsi respectively, making the smooth transfer of the *schwung* possible from the hindquarters to the poll. The sideways crossing of the front legs brings with it a beneficial stretching of the triceps in adduction, while the mm. pectoralis and brachiocephalicus are stretched during the abduction. This endeavor improves the action and range of motion of the forehand. Strength to carry weight by the hindquarters can be improved immensely by the crossing of the legs, and this can also solve difficulties with the contact and "heavy mouths" when lateral work is brought into play in a regular, systematic and consistent manner. The interplay between the lateral exercises will hugely promote lateral flexion of the spinal cord and the arching will improve the quality of the basic gaits.

The tendency to pace, which comes from tension in the back, can clearly be improved or even eliminated completely with the use of lateral work.

Nevertheless, whether lateral work is used in rehabilitation or to improve the training, one should never forget the groundbreaking direction of the training scale for every exercise is a process based on basic motion that must comply with certain criteria to be considered good quality and of gymnastic value.

Even the old masters, especially François Robichon de La Guérinière, who was the inventor of the shoulder-in on straight lines, were able to appreciate the value of these exercises and used them as the basis for the collected exercises such as piaffe and pirouettes. The lateral exercises preserve the flexibility and improve relaxation, balance and obedience to the rider, making finer coordination possible between horse and rider. Apart from this finer coordination between the hand and the leg aids of the rider, the horses become more attentive, maneuverable and stronger, due to the fact that these exercises help the muscles adapt to designated use as a riding horse.

The basic lateral exercises are the shoulder-in and haunches-in. They provide the basis for renvers, half-pass, pirouettes, turn on the haunches and turn on the forehand.

11.2.1 Shoulder-in—counter shoulder-in

Shoulder-in was already being considered by the Duke of Newcastle as the "leg-yield on a small circle" and was further cultivated by François Robichon de La Guérinière on the straight line and used for its gymnastic effect. The great Portuguese master, Nuno Oliveira called it "the aspirin of riding" that could resolve everything, which is definitely partly correct.

> **Definition:** *The classical view of the shoulder-in is the sideways movement, where a horse is on four tracks, with the horse positioned to the wall at a 40-45 degree angle, head to the inside, and moving against the direction of the bend. plié or shoulder-fore is the preliminary exercise to the shoulder-in, where the shoulders are only taken imperceptibly to the inside of the school in order to straighten the horse without moving sideways on 3 or 4 tracks.*

The rules of the F.N. call for less positioning and want to see the horse with only his forehand to the inside while moving on three tracks (30-35 degrees) (fig.11.3) The weight of the rider is more on the inside seat-bone in order to relieve the outside back muscle that is required to stretch, while the rider's inside leg drives the horse sideways. The rider's outside leg is behind the girth as a supporting leg and helps keep the bend. (fig.11.4)

Shoulder-in can also be ridden alternately on three or four tracks, where the longitudinal bend is sometimes more emphasized and sometimes pronounced and in so doing, the alertness of the horse is stimulated.

The shoulder-in is the most important lateral exercise so it is taught first to the horse to combat his natural crookedness. In the beginning, ridden only at the walk, it can help tense horses adopt the stretched posture; they can only move sideways in a controlled and coordinated manner. A calm and rhythmic execution is important to reach the desired gymnastic effect.

All merit of the shoulder-in lies in the fact that it causes improved bend of the haunches through the lowering of the inside hip and the resulting freedom of the outside shoulder, seeing that this is supported by the inside hind leg. The stretch in the outside back muscle and the outside M. barachiocephalicus will result in improved willingness to contact the outside rein. The poll becomes freer, the temporal-mandibular joint relaxes, the horse starts to mouth the bit and the horse becomes lighter on the inside rein, assisted by the aiding of inside leg. Depending on the position used, this exercise can sometimes be used more for collection and sometimes more to loosen the horse.

Note: *Shoulder-in must never be achieved by pulling the head to the inside with the inside rein, for this will destroy the mobility of the shoulder and the forward impulsion of the hind legs.*

The inside shoulder will become unnecessarily heavy, the horse will loose his balance and fall sideways over the outside shoulder and will not be able to free up the outside shoulder with the help of the inside hind leg.

An initial positioning to the inside can also improve the piaffe, since the lateral bend helps lower the inside hip and the inside hind foot then has it easier. In the same way, the shoulder-in can be used in the early days of piaffe, for it will improve the strength to carry weight and crookedness will be compensated, the stance phase of the hind legs will be prolonged and more gluteal and hamstring muscles will be built.

One can correct the mistake of the croup leading the shoulders in the half-pass by preceding the half-pass with a shoulder-in. All basic gaits can be improved in their cadence, collection and strength to carry weight when these exercises are effectively combined.

In Practice: *Once the horse has gained more balance and power when he is working in collection, he is able to extend, for example, the trot much more easily when he is extending on the diagonal, yet without rushing or falling on his shoulders. This can be described as the liberation and transformation of the engaged and weight-bearing, flexed haunches transforming the potential energy stored in the flexed, collected, haunches into greater forward expression of impulsion in the extension of the gait. The change between these two modes of using engagement makes the horse more supple, gives the horse better balance and improved back-engagement.*

> **Note:** *In collection, the horse must posses very much controlled energy in order to perform a "slow," cadenced, movement—the forward must always be present in every gait or exercise. Extension is the result of an engaged haunch which is flexed!—not open—this flexion of the haunches enables the horse to maintain his balance and his back-engagement. Merely rushing forward makes the horse lose his balance, the horse falls on the shoulders, overloads the tendons and joints of the forelegs and becomes heavy in the hand. In this situation, the* rassembler *is necessary and the* demi arret *[half-halt] to restore the balance and position in the horse.*

Horses with contact problems can also be convinced to stretch into the outside rein once again with the use of shoulder-in. The horse will follow the reflex to the leg pressure, which contracts the stomach muscles and enables the horse to stretch into the outside rein.

The shoulder-in on four tracks helps horses with a tendency to pace because it improves the coordination of the legs. Once the shoulder-in is understood, it can be utilized in many ways to loosen the horse at the beginning of the work, as well as to straighten and establish obedience. Alternating the position of the bend will promote increased fine-tuning between horse and rider.

Riding shoulder-in on a spiral in on the circle can evolve into a turn on the forehand, making the shoulders freer through the rhythmic steps and the horse learns to accept the sideways driving influence of the inside leg aid better. The result is improved longitudinal bend and contact on the outside rein with less weight on the inside rein. This is a much better way to solve contact problems without the use of any gimmicks or strange bits.

> **In Practice:** *Young horses should be introduced to shoulder-in at a relatively early age, for it is of considerable utility for straightness. When a young horse learns this relaxed way of going under the rider in a trusting atmosphere, the shoulder-in position can be of great value in moments of panic, such that the rider can quickly and effectively re-gain control and coordination of the horse. The attention of the horse can be returned to the rider in a playful way and the power transferred to work, and the positive praise has a cumulative benefit.*

It is worth mentioning the positive influence that the shoulder-in has on straightening a naturally crooked young horse.

> **Definition:** *Counter shoulder-in [shoulder-out] is a shoulder-in where the head is not to the inside of the school, but facing the wall.*

This will make the sideways crossing of the legs easier for the horse. Highly spirited horses with an irrepressible forward drive that refuse to accept the outside rein, can be introduced to this valuable exercise.

When this exercise is practiced on circles or voltes, one can achieve an improved longitudinal bend, and when alternated with haunches-in, can significantly improve the mobility of the spine and deliver a harmonious quality to the transitions. The horse becomes better controlled, since the circle has a calming and bounding effect on him.

A horse on the left rein, bent in counter shoulder-in, is bent to the right. Through this exercise, it is possible to improve the longitudinal bend on one rein, especially when the horse does not yet know quarters in. Furthermore, this exercise is suitable for horses that refuse to accept the outside rein, since the wall offers an optical boundary and the horse is easier to control with the decelerating visual effect of the wall nearby. The sideways driving leg aid can also come to better use when horses tend to run away due to lack of strength to carry weight.

11.2.2. Haunches-in (Travers)

Definition: *Haunches-in is a lateral movement in which the horse has his head positioned in the direction of the movement and his quarters to the inside of the school while moving sideways, usually in a straight line.*

The horse can also be positioned at a 40-45 degree angle to the wall in this exercise. The rider sits more on the side to the direction of the movement on the inside seat bone and drives the horse forward with the inside leg while the outside rein, together with the supporting outside leg that slightly drives the horse sideways, maintain the movement.

This is considered a counter exercise to the shoulder-in; it especially encourages the outside hind leg to carry weight and thus facilitates the forward movement of the inside shoulder. This exercise is ridden on four tracks and noticeably improves the coordination of the horse's legs. Fluid transitions between shoulder-in and haunches-in improve the coordination of the movement and mobilizes the loins and sacroiliac joint. Through the reciprocal lowering of the inside hip one can target specific muscles without having to spend hours training them. Initially horses should always go straight for a few strides between each change [from shoulder-in to haunches-in, and vice versa] in order to prepare the horse for the next movement. Once the horse understands this change in the bend, one can shorten the intervals until the horse can easily perform a fluid change between shoulder-in and haunches-in. This combination makes horses

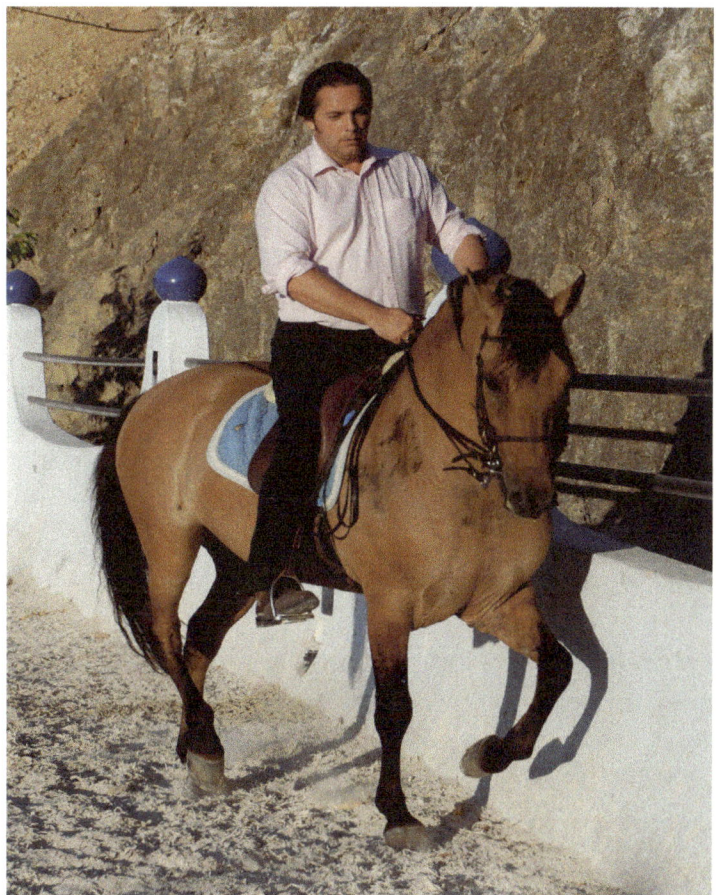

Fig. 11.5. Haunches-in [travers] is the counter exercise to shoulder-in and becomes a renvers when ridden on a free line. Alternating between the different lateral movements has great gymnastic value.

more supple, free, maneuverable and the obedience to the leg is improved immensely.

Haunches-in represents a significant component for all turns on the haunches, pirouettes and the half-passes. When the haunches-in is ridden on an ever decreasing circle, one soon has a lovely pirouette or turn on the haunches, where the horse moves with the hind legs on a tiny circle while the front legs describe a large circle around them.

Through careful and deliberate influencing of the position of the croup when riding a square pattern, it is possible to ride a quarter-turn on the haunches in every corner, meanwhile making the distinction between straight forward and forward and sideways clearer to the horse. This exercise is highly suited for teaching the horse to understand the exchange between straight and sideways.

The sides of the square should be about 5-6 horse lengths and can be used for riding shoulder-in, renvers and haunches-in before the quarter-turn on the haunches. This will improve the attention, obedience and very clearly the use of the haunches, which should always be kept mobile in this exercise. Riding in a square promotes balance and the ability to collect and the exercises can be varied at will.

This short "romping on the spot" in the quarter pirouette as Guérinière already called it, will slowly help the horse to arrive in the more strenuous full pirouette without over-taxing his body and loosing the enthusiasm for the exercise. Through the immediate forward movement after the corner of the square and the preparation for the next corner, the rider has the control of the forward tendency, and the horse should not perform mechanically, which would rob the rider of his influence over the horse. This can happen when pirouettes are mindlessly performed on the same spot and the horse automatically starts to execute the exercise by himself. The best test for this is to immediately ride forward after a few strides of pirouette, to test if the horse anticipates the continuation of the turning movement or if he waits the aids of the rider expectantly.

11.2.3 Haunches-out (Renvers)

> **Definition:** *Renvers is a haunches-in movement on a free line [away from the wall], or a haunches-out movement when ridden on, or near the wall. In the latter example, the croup is toward the outside of the arena and the head and shoulders are on an inside track looking in the direction of movement with the horse bent to the outside of the school. We can also say that the renvers is the travers on the "wrong" side— the renvers takes its reference point from the imaginary wall; on the centerline, one isn't able to determine if we are in travers right or renvers left [for they are same movement on the centerline].*

The rider sits in the direction of the movement, with more weight on the inside seat bone [here, inside refers to the direction of the bend].

This exercise can also be seen as counter exercise to the shoulder-in and can be ridden alternately with the shoulder-in which will greatly improve the mobility of the neck. In order to perform this exercise correctly, the horse must already be perfectly controllable in the previous two exercises [shoulder-in and haunches-out]. Prematurely alternating, before the aids of each exercise are well-understood, may confuse the aids.

When riding a volte in renvers [haunches-out], one can progress to a quarter turn on the forehand at the corners, as the turn becomes tighter.

Alternately changing between haunches-in and renvers [haunches-out] will improve the flexibility and alertness of the horse immensely.

All of the exercises above are more or less stimulating for collection which, in turn, promotes freedom of the shoulders and builds strength to carry weight. They also help develop the rider's soft contact with the mouth of the horse as the horse begins to carry himself.

11.2.4. Half-pass

Definition: *In the half-pass the horse moves in a similar way as in the haunches-in. The difference is that the horse travels on a diagonal line with the forehand slightly in advance of the haunches, not only sideways but also forward. Hence the name "half-pass" (half forward). This results in a forward and sideways movement across the diagonal line with the horse looking and bent in the direction he is moving. (fig.11.6) In the half-pass, the rotation of the pelvis and the chest is fundamental to be of gymnastic value. The freedom of the inside shoulder in the half-pass is the result of a supple back and not the result of speed. Today we see a lot of horses moving sideways on the diagonal without any lateral bending which can potentially harm the coffin joints and the tendons.*

The rider sits in the direction of the movement similar to haunches-in, but, in the half-pass he yields more with the outside rein and provides more driving forward-sideways aids with the inside leg.

The horse should have sufficient longitudinal rounding. The croup may not precede the shoulders as this condition will result in a disturbance of the rhythm. The weight bearing capacity of the haunches (*tragkraft*) will also be diminished if the haunches lead the shoulders in the half-pass because the horse will push more than he carries and the collection benefit of this exercise will be lost. [When the haunches lead, they do not step under the horse's center of gravity but, to the inside of it.]

Note: *Tragkraft (the possibility of bearing more weight on the haunches) is the result of schwungkraft (controlled impulsion in lightness) with engagement of the back. The main idea is to shift the horse's weight back so that the joints of the haunches can be passively bent. The angle at the hip joint should be closed by 5 degrees. The degree of closure of the angle of the hip required is not excessive. Yet this small amount [around 5 degrees] is necessary to enable correct passive engagement of the haunches which the quality that allows us to ride a supple, light and healthy horse.*

In half-pass, similar to the haunches-in, the hamstrings of the outside hind leg will be stretched more and the inside shoulder will become more free. Through abduction and adduction—crossing of the front legs—the pectoral muscles will be addressed alternately with the adductors. The biceps muscles will be strengthened while the triceps will be stretched and the gymnastic effect be effectively adjusted, provided that the horse performs the exercise in a calm and even manner.

Fast sideways running is incorrect and has no gymnastic benefit. The horse must also not be laterally positioned too strongly in the neck, for a twist in the neck in the direction of movement can limit the freedom of the shoulder. The horses will fall on the shoulder due to lack of forward impulsion.

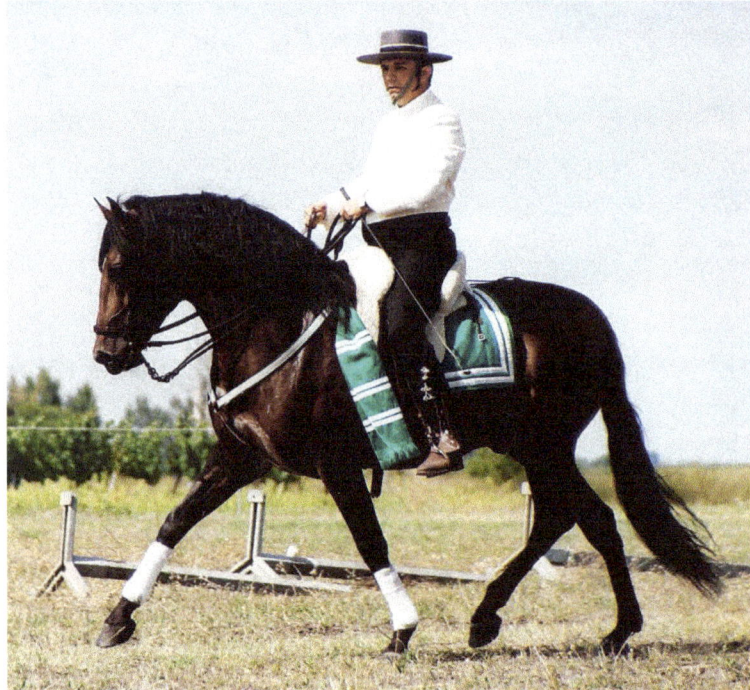

Fig.11.6.
a. Half pass to the right in maximum longitudinal bend and legerté. Note the yielding hand and light contact to the horse's mouth (the author on PRE stallion Camborio)

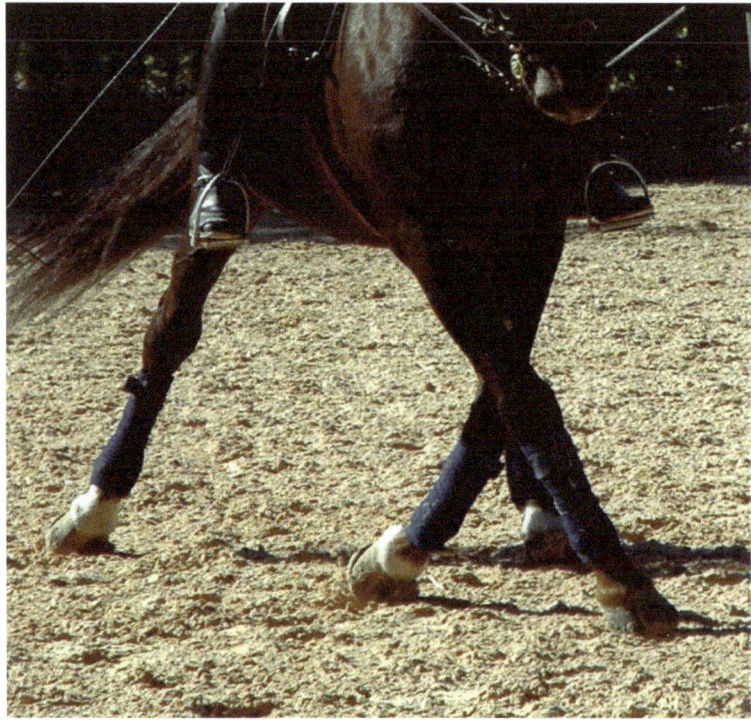

b. In this detailed photograph the sideways crossing of the legs in trot is obvious, this is only possible through systematic gymnastic work (demonstrated by J.M. Sanchez Cobos on Impetigo)

> **In Practice:** *Since the horse does not possess sufficient strength to carry weight and balance himself when this exercise is being first prepared, and therefore, cannot perform the entire length of the diagonal in the desired [half-pass] form, it is best to develop this exercise by alternating a few steps each of straight and then of sideways riding.*

This method will allow for better control and protects the horse from becoming over-taxed and frustrated. The forward tendency is, as always, the highest law. When one has difficulty with the bend, it can be corrected by adjusting the position on every stride, but this should never degenerate into a wanton left and right pulling of the head of the horse. Any change in the head position must be slow and fluid so as to avoid ill-effect; these changes must never be abrupt.

11.2.5 Leg-yield

The only purpose of leg-yielding is to make the un-strengthened horse sensitive to the sideways driving leg aid and to make him cross sideways without longitudinal bend and the collecting effect [of the half-pass].

Leg-yielding can be used as a preliminary exercise to lateral gaits and to improve the freedom of the shoulders. The rider sits on the inside seat bone, the horse is positioned opposite the direction of the movement. The horse here has no longitudinal bend and does not need to have the outside back muscle free to stretch. This opposite loading with the back will push the horse away from the movement, and this counter position of the neck will free the outside shoulder.

> **Definition:** *The "inside" of all lateral movements is the concave side, produced by more or less positioning through the lateral bend.*

This exercise along with the turn on the forehand—which is opposite the direction of movement—only has the effect of improving obedience and has little gymnastic function; the horse in leg-yield does not have the longitudinal bend necessary for the development of strength to carry weight. On the other hand, leg-yielding can improve bending when it is used alternately with the strongly bent lateral movements [shoulder-in, haunches-in, half-pass], for the horses can then move sideways in an unconstrained manner. It is thereby possible to eliminate tension resulting from incorrectly prepared collection exercises.

Naturally, this does not apply to pre-existing osteopathic lesions that should be subject to a separate viewing and analysis.

Robert Stodulka, D.V.M.

12. Application and benefits of the high school exercises of classical dressage

The basic idea of classical dressage is to keep the riding horse healthy for as long as possible through the use of gymnastic exercises that make the horse useful to the rider without any damage to the animal. The horse should become more beautiful, expressive and self-assured through the systematic training. The overall picture is one of a harmoniously built athlete. Xenophon already said that one should ride a horse in the manner that it likes best—meaning as a stallion does when showing off to impress the mares.

According to this challenge the main goal of the art of riding and the physiotherapy is maintaining the health and to recover the abilities of the horse. Overtaxing and impatience, for whatever motive, have no place in classical riding. The training of a dressage horse takes many demanding years and one can then not harvest the fruits when there has been some physical damage once one finally arrives at the goal. Therefore, it should be thought that the journey is the goal, for the moments of perfect accord in the art of riding are naturally only fleeting; it is about a dynamic process and not a static one. A photograph of a beautiful piaffe can be kept in the archives for eternity, but the expression of absolute beauty can only be presented live in the moment. Always improving the sequence of movement and refining the aids in order to achieve more of these moments of perfect accord, can be a consuming but rewarding goal.

Due to the fact that the horse as an athlete is also subject to his physical and mental state on any given day, it becomes logical that one should re-start the next day where one previously left off. This basic concept is just as important in rehabilitation, for it is often attempted to shorten the time of healing through externally created pressure.

> **Note:** *It is equally important to stay in balance even though it constantly changes, where some steps back are also allowed from time to time. A static state of balance yields stagnation and impossibility to develop further, which works against the basic idea of improvement of physical condition.*

The type and degree of this change of balance is individually dependent on age, level of training, health etc. It must be considered freshly for each horse and his specific character.

A frequently observed problem in riding is the amount of wear and tear on the horses in training. Often, reintegration of the horses back into normal course of training is difficult. Sometimes horses do not complete basic training free of lameness due to an incorrect structure of the training. In many cases, commercial pressures, lack of time, and cost of training of a horse are the reasons not very "horse-friendly" practices are adopted. The resulting impact of such short-cuts is often physical and psychological damage.

Many young horses, that are not yet physically and mentally capable, are asked too much, too soon and fall by the wayside. They cannot cope with the high demands made on them in the name of "sport." De Pluvinel said: "The grace of a young horse is like the scent of a flower—once it is gone, it never returns again." With this in mind, the respectful management of the horse is a basic prerequisite for natural dressage, that should also be reflected in the inner attitude of the trainer. It is only the love for the horse, paired with the necessary theoretical knowledge that allows the rider to reach these artistic nuances, making the horse more beautiful and bestowing upon the rider the feeling of exaltation with the horse working with, and for him.

It is for this reason that the exercises of the classical school should not be seen as the end product of some mechanical training;, but rather as the product of systematic training that does not merely subdue the horse and turn him into a puppet on a string. All systems of training that do not respect these nature-given limitations of the horse are to be accurately and critically questioned. To see the horse as an integral functioning organism with a soul must be the rider's priority.

12.1. Piaffe

Piaffe is one of the key exercises of the high school and classical riding of the F.N..

Definition: *In this trot-like movement almost on the spot, the horse combines maximum forward thrust with strength and converts it into the energy of a spring, with an almost imperceptible forward tendency, stepping rhythmically.*

The haunches are bent and shifted so much under the center of gravity, that the croup lowers and the back arches (fig.12.1.a). Through the prolonged stance phase, the rhythmically springy hocks seem to be stepping powerfully, but not in a nervous manner. They support the front limbs that can freely display their action and [the forearm] can even be lifted to a horizontal position. It is important in the piaffe to maintain the rhythm and the cadence. The horse should never have a nervous, expressionless or even back and forth swaying steps, for these incorrect movements undermine the gymnastic value of the exercise.

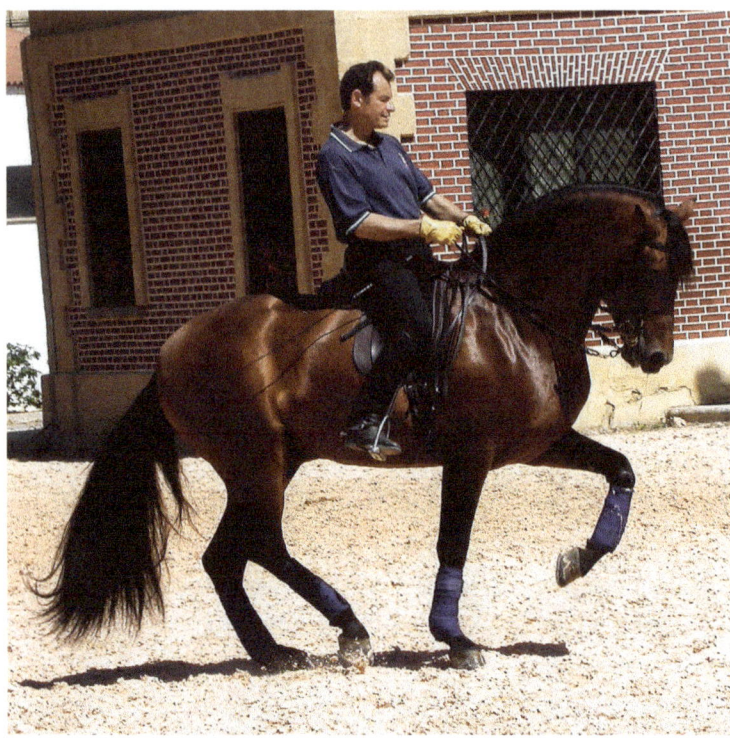

Fig. 12.1.a. A straight piaffe as the result of systematic training. The horse in the photo lifts the diagonal pairs well and seems balanced under the Olympic rider Rafael Soto.

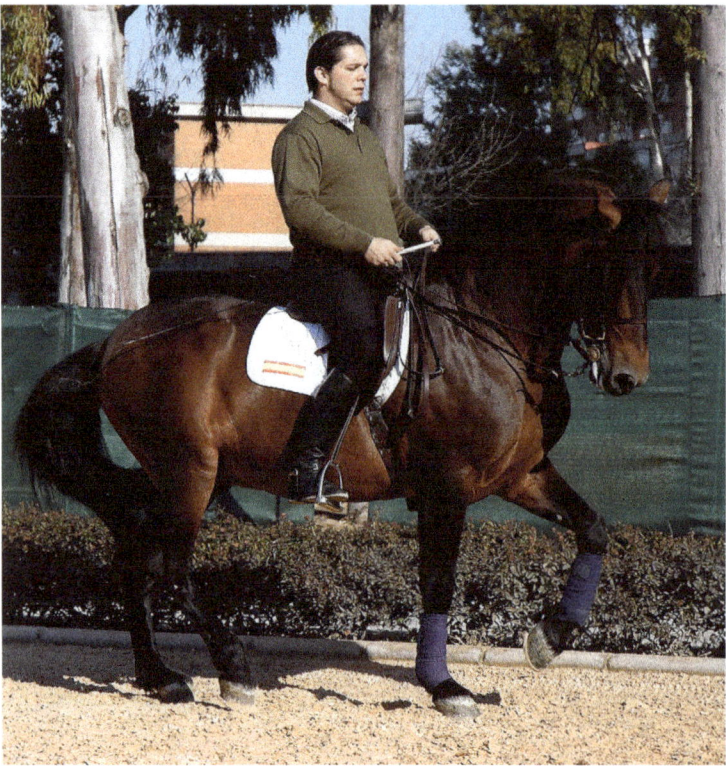

b. To achieve a straight piaffe, the horse must be able to perform the piaffe equally well in both directions. The author demonstrates piaffe to the right on a young PRE stallion. The horse has to bend his inside hind leg more through the position of shoulder-fore. The degree of collection is not as high in this exercise.

The result of this movement is a rhythmic interplay between maximum tension and strength to carry weight with simultaneous and perfect lightness and almost effortless moments of relaxation when the diagonal pairs alternate. The high elevation due to the well-developed strength to carry weight is the result of the active topline and not the influence of the rider's hand. In this exercise, the willingness to go must be increased in such a way that the length of the gait becomes shortened. The steps become more active, shorter and higher, and the forward impulsion achieves more expression.

This exercise will enormously promote balance and the rhythmic carrying ability of the haunches in the exercises approaching it. At the same time the psoas muscles and the abdominal muscles are contracted working antagonistically with the M. longissimus dorsi. The back is arched, the croup is lowered. To the observer the horse will seem shorter. The arching of the loins, produced by the increased stepping under the center of gravity by the hindquarters, will cause enhanced gymnastic activity of the adductors, the hamstrings and the gluteal muscles, all through the flexion of the haunches, which is essential to carry the horse and keep his balance. Asymmetric muscles can in this way be built up correctly.

In Practice: *Addressing the individual hind leg that one wants to lift can be achieved out of the movement or at the beginning, from the halt, which should be easier. When the horse has learned to stand squarely and calmly and chews the bit trustingly, the rider tries to get the horse to move one hind leg with pressure from his legs. The rider's hands remain quiet.*

Through the alternating raising of the hind legs, the horse moves the center of gravity back, making the base of support smaller. Almost by himself, the horse will start to calmly move his legs in diagonal pairs simultaneously, without doing a hectic dance on the spot, for it has been schooled properly with the preliminary exercise.

Initially, one should ask for only a few calm steps; the first goal is not to achieve a perfect piaffe, but the reaction of the hind legs to the leg aids, without actually slowing the horse down with the reins. The half-steps start from behind, the hand awaits the forward impulsion and does not stop the movement. If the hand is used to slow the horse down, the horse will only lose rhythm, tense up and rest his weight on the hand. The positive effect will be lost. When the preparation for piaffe is carried out correctly, the horse will perform the piaffe without tension or influence from the rider's hand, seemingly voluntary looking for the contact, from his heart.

Piaffe gives horses the necessary power for canter pirouettes and the flying changes, both of which demand a great deal of collection, with maximum engagement of the hindquarters. The piaffe will likewise, when ridden in short transitions from trot—passage, collected trot—piaffe and extended trot—passage, considerably improve the cadence and expression of the horse in these lessons.

Learning to take advantage of the longer stance phase will clearly improve the lateral movements as well as the basic gaits. It is essential in this gait to maintain the forward tendency, even when the piaffe is sometimes moved a few steps backwards to improve the seatedness. This method was developed from French equitation, which developed the piaffe from the rein-back, using the reasoning that the diagonal footfalls had already been establish [in the rein-back] and may seem more logical for the horse. This method of using the rein-back also lowers the croup more than when the piaffe is learned from the walk. The method chosen to teach the piaffe should be indicated by the horse. Piaffe should not be made more difficult than necessary for the horse.

In the classical art of riding, one distinguishes between a left and a right piaffe (fig. 12.1.b) before one reaches a straight piaffe (fig. 12.1.a) When one allows a horse to do piaffe from shoulder-in, the inside hind leg will be prompted to step under more due to the shorter distance attained from the bend and the outside hind leg will be encouraged to perform a longer stance phase. This saves the rider having a stronger influence on the inside hind leg and can therefore encourage the horse to step more under the body. In this way, one-sided deficiencies, such as inadequate use of a hind leg, can be corrected.

Through the use of this exercise one can selectively address the flexors and extensors of the hind legs and treat weakness and atrophy better. Once the horse is capable of performing the piaffe in both directions, it is easier to achieve a straight piaffe with uniform loading of the haunches, and perhaps even a piaffe pirouette as a demonstration of the highest degree of collection and perfect balance.

Piaffe contributes considerably to bringing the hind legs more under the center of gravity and to the arching of the horse's back. Even horses with sway backs can benefit from the gymnastic value thereof. The topline remains flexible and the horse can learn to build up his problem zones in-hand without the weight of the rider at first. Later, the rider can ask the help of an experienced trainer to lightly touch the horse with the whip from below to improve the ridden piaffe.

In a Grand Prix test, a good piaffe gives information about the willingness and degree of collection of a horse, and also reveals all kinds of shortcomings of the training very clearly. Therefore, it is marked with a coefficient of 2, which emphasizes its importance.

When horses are already in an advanced phase of training, the piaffe can also be used at the beginning of a training session to aid in the loosening-up phase and to help remove tension. This can also turn the freshness of the horse into controlled work where the horse still has enough power to perform the exercise well. It is important for the horse to do fewer but good quality steps, rather than to compromise the expression and overtire the horse by doing too many steps at once.

After some successful steps of piaffe, where maximum contraction and tension is required, it is absolutely necessary for the horse to stretch in complete calmness. This will prevent the muscles from stiffening. The horse gains confidence and performs the exercise powerfully and without stress.

12.2. Passage

Definition: *In the classical art of riding, the passage develops from the piaffe, with the horse lengthening the stance and the suspension phase in such a way that the impression of weightless, cadenced floating arises.*

This exercise originates, like the piaffe, from "showing-off" behavior of a stallion, who courts the mare of his choice in an elevated position to make her notice him. The back of the horse must be very active in this exercise, in order to bring the maximum spring energy of the hindquarters to the front. The classically developed passage guarantees this by allowing the piaffe to proceed forward, resulting in a so-called swinging back passage with high movement (fig.12..2.a). When the passage is achieved without sufficient activity in the back or only by touching the front legs with a whip, one gets a very accentuated lifting of the legs (fig12.2.b) which may look spectacular, but has no gymnastic value due to inadequate activity of the back. These horses look as if they are divided in two, have distinctly hollow backs and sometimes even drag the hindquarters, since the legs do not step under the center of gravity, but [in this poor manifestation] instead, stay behind the horse. These horses often get behind the bit as well, and thus loose the contact.

The transition from medium trot into passage and passage to medium trot is interesting for the muscular development of the hindquarters, for it will help develop a reciprocal transformation of the springy power into weight bearing power and vice versa. The result can be powerful hindquarters and a very balanced horse.

These transitions should only be performed a few steps at a time to improve the bending of the haunches and the development of forward thrust. Horses that have trained in this way will easily, and with little influence can sustain longer episodes of passage.

Fig 12.2.a The classical correct swinging from the back passage, developed from the piaffe, is recognized by a very active back and good activity from the hind legs. The rider can sit easily. The contact with the mouth is reduced to a minimum and the author waits for the forward impulse without interfering with the movement.

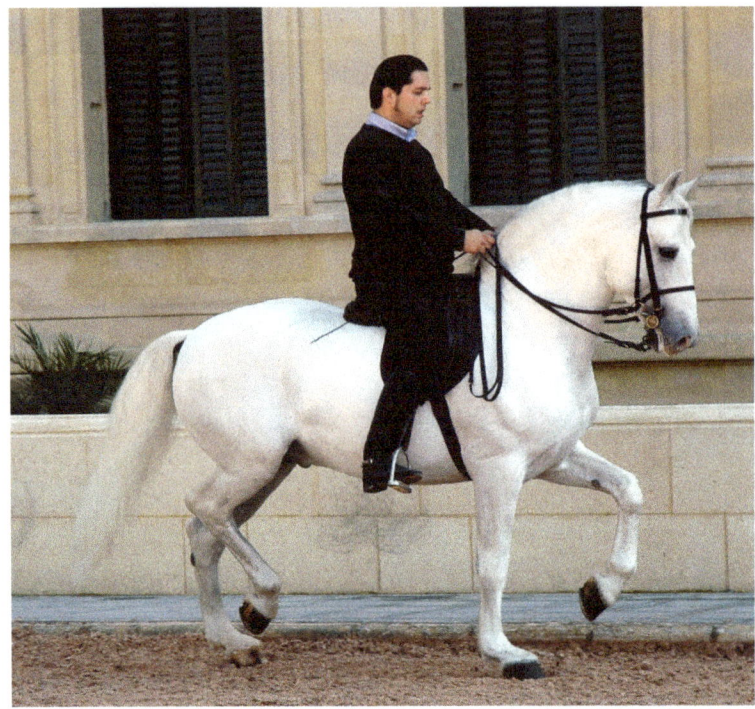

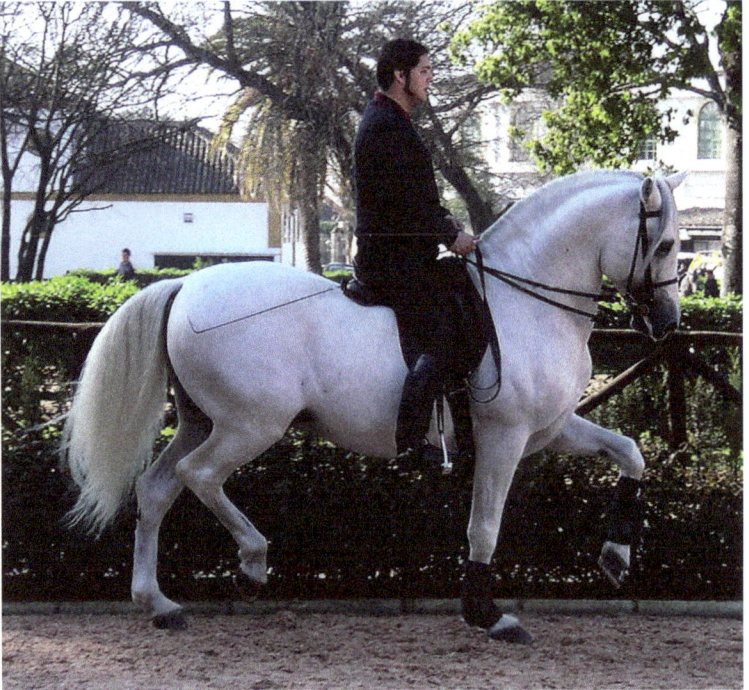

b. The accentuated lifting of the legs might look very spectacular, is often a shortcut of the classical way or lacking activity of the back or a hollow back.

Since passage and the transitions to piaffe and extension are very exhausting, the exercises must be well-planned in order not to forfeit brilliance and expression. Muscular tiring and the resulting overloading of the tendons and ligaments can be prevented in this way. When horse are not yet trained up to passage and piaffe, one can vary the tempo of the transitions between the working, medium and collected trot to increase the activity of the hindquarters. Sooner or later a few piaffe steps will appear through quick changes of tempo.

12.3 Canter pirouette

Definition: *The canter pirouette is also scored with a coefficient of 2 in the Grand Prix test and it represents the highest degree of collection in canter. In this exercise, the horse must jump 6-8 canter strides on the spot in a circle around the hindquarters. (fig.12.3)*

Here, strong bending of the haunches with very active hindquarters is required, so that the canter rhythm can be maintained while moving almost on the spot. Basic mistakes include fast turning around the hindquarters or the hindquarters not jumping in the pirouette. Horses often avoid sitting correctly in this exercise and tend to overload the knee joints and the tendons

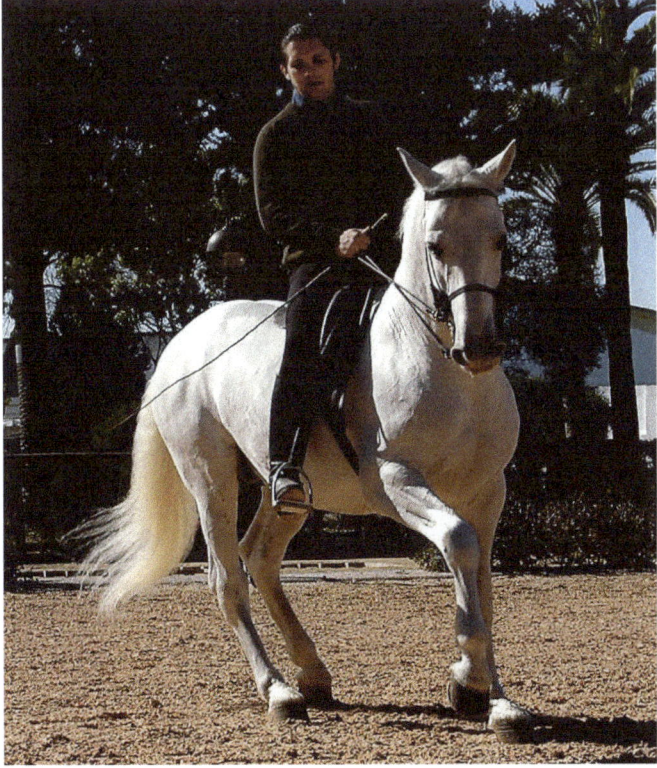

Fig.12.3.a The introduction to the canter pirouette occurs in a horse's haunches bent to the maximum in a very collected canter, where the three-beat canter must not be lost. The pirouette should only be done with weight aids and as with little influence from the hand as possible to avoid disturbing the horse's execution of the movement.

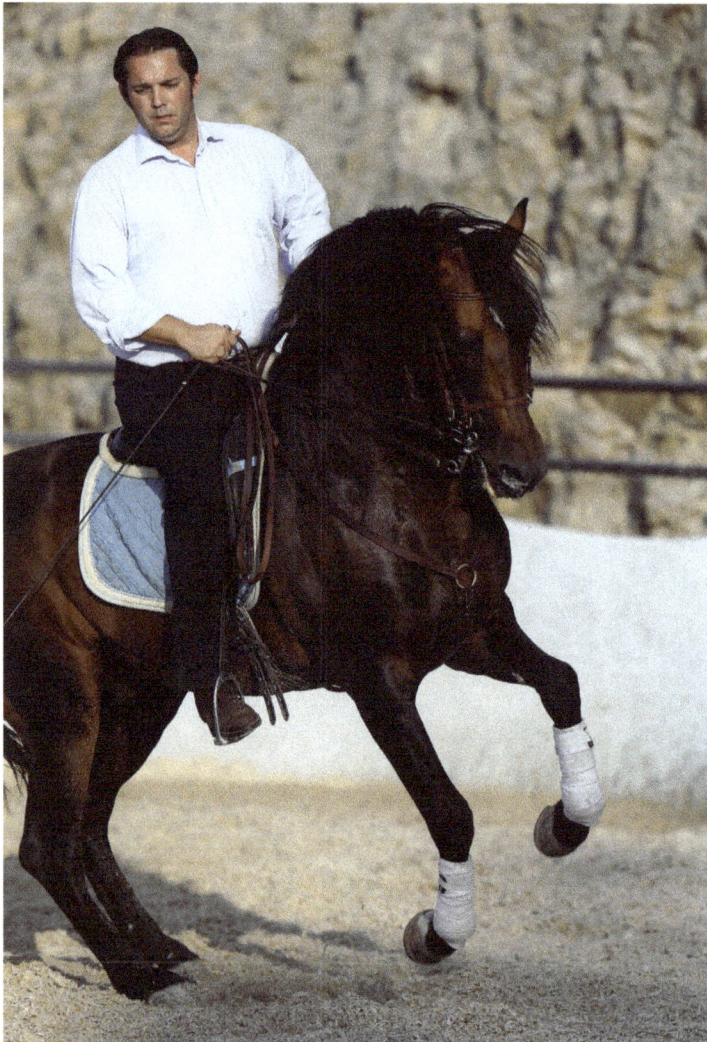

Fig. 12.3 b. Canter pirouette is the smallest turn on the horse's haunches; only possible if the horse is completely supple in his back and mobile in his haunches. Lateral bending and the position of the horse's neck and head must be perfectly placed according to the required level of collection. Note the small circle the horse is describing with his hindquarters and that the author's weight is born on the inside seat-bone.

and ligaments around it. The quick turn is a way of avoiding strenuous longitudinal rounding—and the gymnastic effect is thereby, lost.

Keeping the longitudinal roundness in this exercise makes it an even more difficult exercise, for the whole body must be completely worked in a gymnastic manner in order to perform it correctly.

To develop power in the hindquarters, a square pattern with a quarter pirouette on each corner can be practiced. The horses must be able to lengthen and shorten the canter strides until they can canter almost on the spot (the accordion-effect as preparation0. This exercise promotes willingness to be ridden and the development of the gluteal muscles and strengthens the abdominal muscles.

Once the horse is established in the canter pirouettes, he has enough power to start the flying change at every stride.

12.4. Flying changes

Definition: *A flying change is a unified change from right lead canter into left lead canter (or the other way round) during the canter's moment of suspension.*

The horse will "begin a new canter" in the moment of suspension, and the hindquarters will initiate the change of lead (fig.12.4.). Horses must be prepared in the canter to collect on a straight line, such that the uphill tendency of the canter can be developed and ultimately, guaranteed. The horse must be kept as straight as possible in the change, which requires a good feeling of balance and strength to carry weight. Swaying in the changes is a sign of insufficient strength and balance.

Horses that perform the change in two strides due to tension in the back, must, first of all, have their top-lines stretched and need to improve their basic canter. The accordion effect, where the canter strides are lengthened and shortened will be beneficial for stretching the topline while simultaneously improving the engagement of the hindquarters. This exercise will improve the control over the canter.

Horses that change late with the hindquarters can correct this problem by practicing the change from shoulder-in to renvers, so that the hindquarters have a shorter route to go. If the change is too short, it can be improved by changing to the outside, from canter to counter canter. This will make the canter

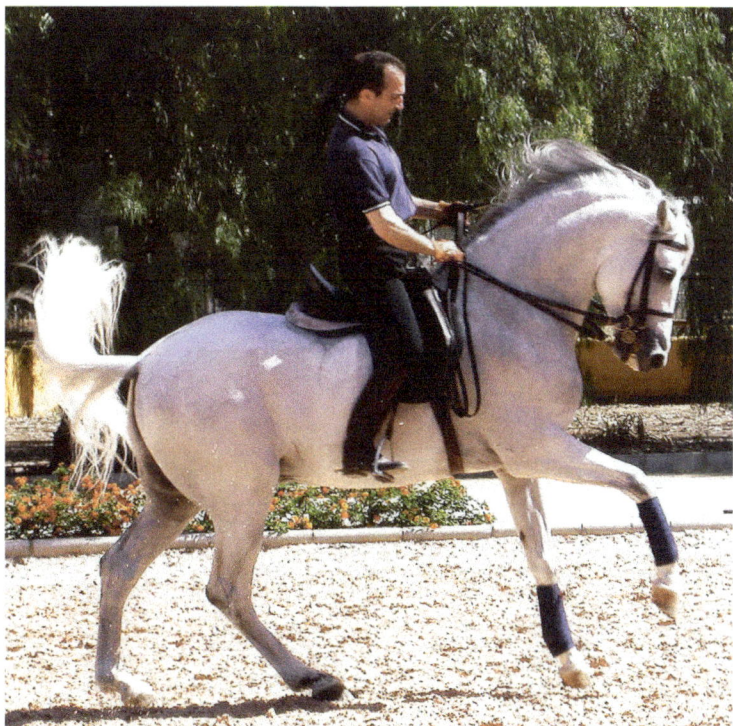

Fig 12.4 The one-time flying change is the crowning glory of flying changes and requires the highest collection and a high response rate from both sides. The rider, Alfonso Ruiz from the REAAE demonstrates this to perfection.

stride longer and will stretch the topline. For the opposite problem, of the change being too long, the change can be done from the outside to the inside.

When horses run after completing the flying change, they can immediately be calmed down by a transition into walk and a preliminary exercise such as canter-walk transitions with a change from canter to counter canter performed. This will improve the horse's rhythm and he should, in this way, develop more trust in the exercise. The change should, in all cases, be made with as little aids as possible, almost immobile, so that the quality of the change does not suffer due to unnecessary movement by the rider.

Tempi changes, up to one-time flying changes, improves the strength to carry weight, obedience, balance and willingness to be ridden and thus adds to the gymnastic effectiveness of the back and hindquarters.

12.5. Spanish walk—Paso Español

Another exercise that is valuable for shoulder freedom, but not classified as classical by the F.N., is the Spanish walk. Ethologically viewed, it originates from the fight between stallions, where it takes on the meaning of a request to play or fight.

Definition: In this exercise, the horse stretches his front legs slowly, alternately and almost horizontally to the front and slowly lowers them again. (Fig.12.5.a)

This exercise gives the horse the possibility to release tension and free the shoulder from strain. The triceps and trapezius muscle get stretched. The biceps brachii and the brachialis muscles become activated and the forehand is prepared for a higher knee action. A good combination is to ride shoulder-in followed by Spanish walk across the diagonal. This promotes the length of the steps and the action of the Spanish walk.

Horses that have too little action in the passage or extended trot can be improved with the help of this very valuable exercise.

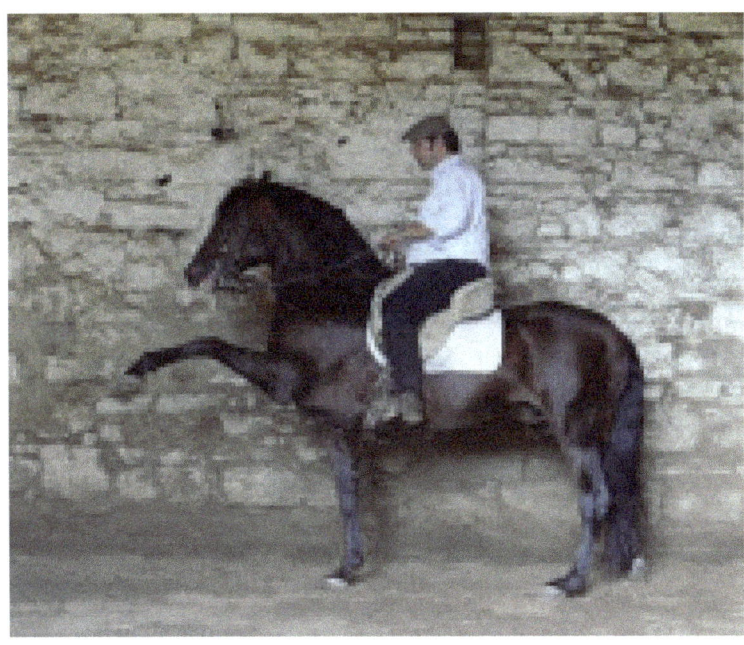

Fig 12.5.a. The Spanish walk promotes a degree of extension that is possible in the shoulders and can be used to reduce aggression in stallions. Here the exercise is expressively demonstrated by the author on his stallion.

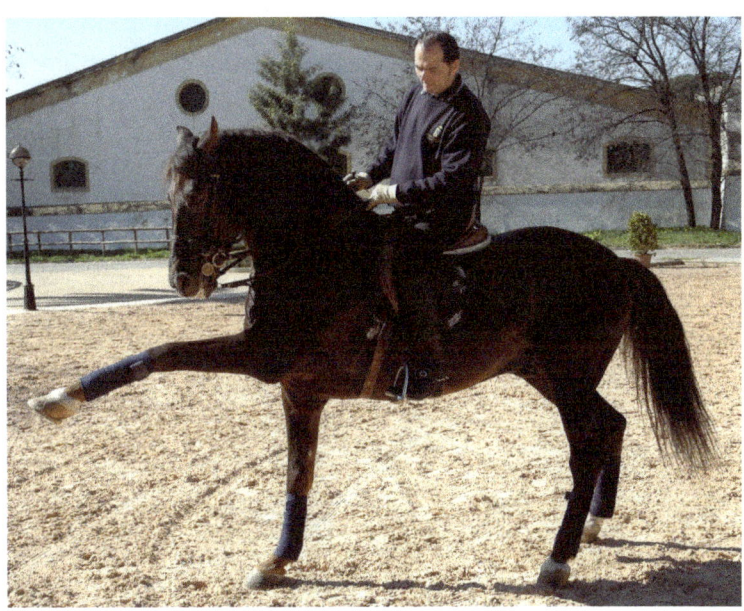

Fig 12.5.b. The jambette, or stretching of one leg only, serves, on the one hand as preparation for the Spanish walk and, on the other hand, to a great extent as a exercise to improve the muscles that lift the front leg up, such as the M. biceps brachii and the extensors. J.M. Sanchez Cobos demonstrates this on his stallion Impetigo.

13. Cavaletti work

Cavalettis were already used in the 19th century, by the Italian, Caprilli[12] —who was the inventor of the light seat—where he used it to do gymnastic exercises to develop the horse's back. Cavaletti work has its merits as long as it is not applied for too long and does not tire and overtax the horse.

The easiest way to improve the horse's proprioception is to work over slanting poles that are placed at irregular distances. This teaches the horse to consciously adapt his stride length to the poles on the ground. It is better to use low cavalettis in this context, as the danger of injury when the horse accidentally steps on it is much smaller.

The ideal length for cavaletti is 2.80m [9 feet], and the cross-support at the ends makes it possible to choose three different heights. In the rehabilitation phase it is better to start with the lowest so as not to overtax the muscles of the horse.

Initially, one should use one cavaletti for each quarter of the circle, and start to lunge the horse over them in the walk and later at the trot. This procedure is necessary for the horse to adapt to the new obstacles on the circle and so as not to jump over them in an uncontrolled manner and injure himself.

Thereafter, one can add up to four cavaletti in a trot distance of 1.30m [4'-4"]. This will allow the horse to complete at least two trot sequences with sufficient activity in the back. It is important that the horse only trots over these 5, or a maximum of ten times in the beginning to prevent fatigue.

Later on, one cavaletti can be put higher to make the horse contract his stomach muscles more and attain more articulation of the joints. Once again this exercise should not be done for too long and should only be used for certain, specific indications.

Canter distance can be 2.6-3meters [9-10 feet]. The horse then has to step well under his body through the in and out jump [using two cavalettis] and will thus round his back more. The psoas muscles and the hamstrings can thus be specifically trained. Canter work should only be added much later in rehabilitation work.

The benefits of cavaletti work both on the lunge and under the rider is in the ability to selectively address the stomach muscles, the flexors and the psoas muscle. These flexor muscles in the body of the horse must also be trained as their antagonists that stretch the spine like the M. longissimus

---

[12] Captain Federico Caprilli (8 April 1868 - 6 December 1907) was an Italian cavalry officer and equestrian who revolutionized the jumping seat. His position, now called the "forward seat," formed the modern-day technique used by all jumping riders today.

dorsi, for one, can quickly over-train one muscle type and the horse will then show deficiencies in the sequence of movements as a whole. In this context 1-2 cavalettis must be put at their highest for the horse to go over. Horses must be functionally fit and should round and arch their backs in the moment of suspension over the cavaletti. The supraspinous ligament will stretch, the spinous processes will open and the mobility of the back will be improved.

All of these exercises should be performed in a round pen or lungeing circle, where the horse can achieve a stretch in the outside back muscle through the visual boundary [of the wall of the round pen] on the outside.

Cavaletti work can be optimized with the use of a Pessoa training system or the double lunge line.

Completely unsuitable for cavaletti work are the rigid rein aids [side reins] normally used for lungeing, for they will hinder rather than help the stretching posture. They can also provoke the horse to push his back down when moving over the cavaletti instead of arching, which is the true intention of cavaletti work.

Robert Stodulka, D.V.M.

14. Mobilization exercises in-hand

14.1. Mobilization according to François Baucher[13]

The old French riding masters like François Baucher, General Decapentry and later, also James Fillis, already knew the special benefits of a horse that has been mobilized in-hand, that could become used to the movement of the bit in the mouth prior to being asked to take on the weight of the rider. The basic idea is to obtain a supple horse through the systematic treatment of an individual area in order to be able to work the horse without tension.

In the age of mechanization, the horse was also seen as a machine that had to function according to specific physical criteria. In this context, the first biomechanically minded approach was brought into the systematic training system. Through the numerous possibilities of physical explanations, there

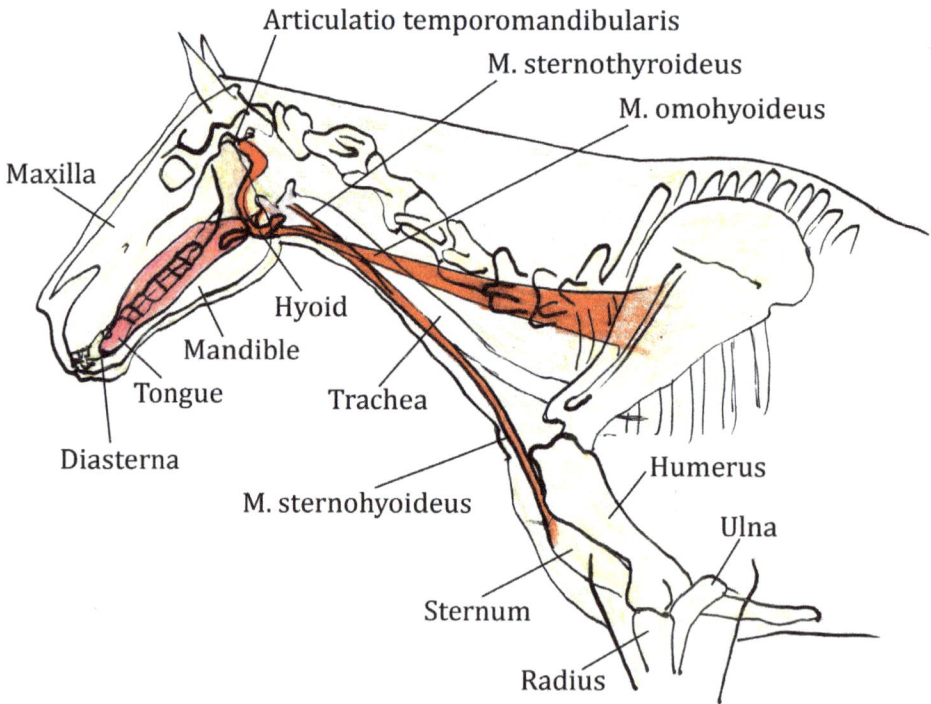

Fig. 14.1.a Biomechanical context of the hyoid bone, temporomandibler joint and shoulder.

---

13   François Baucher (1796–1873) was a French riding master whose methods are still debated by dressage enthusiasts today. His philosophy of training the horse changed dramatically over the course of his career and is often considered in two distinct phases or "manners."

are naturally many wrong paths that have been trodden, which have already been mentioned in the history of riding. It is only a horse, free of tension and with a relaxed jaw that can move in a relaxed manner under a rider.

This highly modern-minded approach from the 19th century has stood the test of time and is used in veterinary osteopathy. The most important insight was that the horse might have a physical problem (for example tension in muscles) that makes him unable to cooperate with the rider and not because of mere unwillingness.

One can compare the writings of the founder of osteopathy for horses, Dr. Dominique Giniaux[14] to the teachings of Baucher. However, one should not disregard that the best mobilization exercises in-hand are only as good as the rider with an independent seat that does not disturb the horse in his movement. The mobilization exercises in-hand at the halt are similar to the osteopathic mobilization techniques and therefore do not fall short in their impact when applied correctly.

From a physiological or biomechanical point of view, it is only possible to have a relaxed horse when he can relax the hyoid muscles, the M. sternocleidomastoideus, M. sternohyoideus and M. omohyoideus, leading to a calm chewing of the bit with foam forming. The parotid gland starts to produce saliva because the ducts in the mouth are properly open, which increases the sensitivity of the tongue.

This parasympathetic reflex will also relax the muscles of the tongue as well as the M. masseter, which, in turn, influences the temporomandibler joint in its mobility. It is for this reason that a relaxed mandible and temporomandibler joint is the foundation of any further influence from the rider. If any tension occurs in the horse's body, the first place where it will be noticed is in the contact with the hand of the rider. This is manifested by horses looking for support in the hand or simply leaning on the bit.

When the jaw becomes tight, tension will also go to the Musculus-rectus-capitus group, which, in turn, will also cause the poll and neck muscles to resist the influence of the rider. This muscular kinetic reaction can be carried through right up to the lumbar part of the M. longissimus dorsi; it becomes impossible to sit the horse, the horse refuses to bend longitudinally

---

14   Dr. Dominique Giniaux began his career as an allopathic veterinarian in 1968 and treated horses in the "classical" manner until 1981. Although very adept at this established knowledge, he later turned to "holistic" medicines, like acupuncture and osteopathy, which he studied first on humans. Dr. Giniaux was first in the world to practice structural osteopathy with the equine. His fame soon spread when he was called to lecture in the United States for the International Veterinary Acupuncture Society. Author of *Equine Osteopathy: What the horses have told me*, Xenophon Press 2014 and *Healing Hands: a treatise on first-aid equine acupressure, 2nd edition*, Xenophon Press 2014]

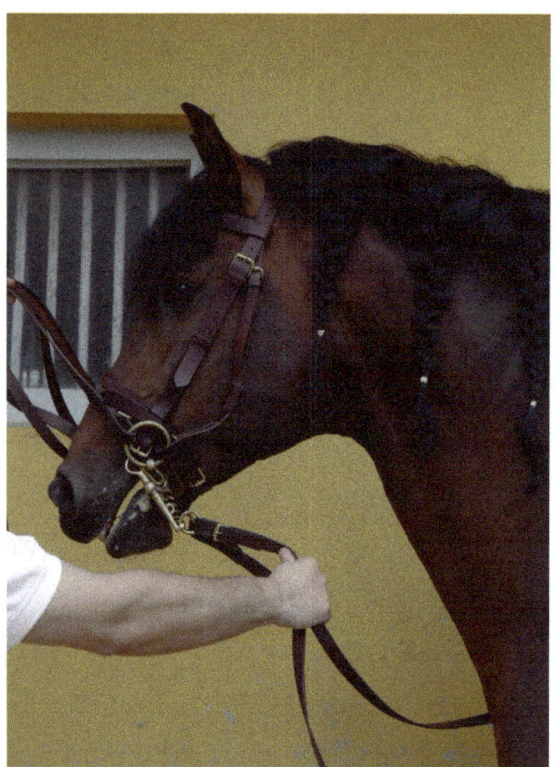

*14.1
b. Relaxing the mandible according to Baucher. The influence of the snaffle to the front and the curb to the back causes an unblocking of the temporomandibler joint and relaxation of the mandible and it's muscles, initiating a chewing on the bit. As soon as this is achieved, the impulse must be yielded to immediately.*

and is ultimately not capable of collection. In this stage [of tension], character changes and complaints about the willingness of the horse can often be found (rearing, pulling etc). Systematic exercises to loosen the horse, starting with the jaw (Fig. 14.1.b), can prevent such chain reactions and release tensions that do not have organic origins.

When mobilizing a horse in-hand, it should wear a bridle with or without a nose-band. One of the most common mistakes is to buckle the nose-band too tight, in order to gain more control over the horse, which is usually unsuccessful. Horses need to be able to chew on the bit to relax, and they need to breathe in the process. A constricting nose-band can lead to obstruction of the airways, depending on the kind of nose-band used and on how tight or loose it is buckled. When the horse is especially sensitive, this can become an intolerable stress and many horses become very bothered by the contact and start to fight against the rider's hand.

Stand in front of the horse, take the rings of the bit with both hands, turn the mouthpiece for a time towards oneself until the horse starts a slight chewing movement by opening his mouth (fig.14.2.a). It is only possible to relax the jaw and the muscles of the hyoid bone in this position, with the mouth slightly open.

Once the horse understands this mechanism, one starts to turn the head slowly first to the left and then to the right, all the while making sure

Fig 14.2.
a. By stimulating the chewing of the bit the mouth opens, thus relaxing the jaw joint and the M. masseter and allowing the temporo-mandibler joint to be mobilised.

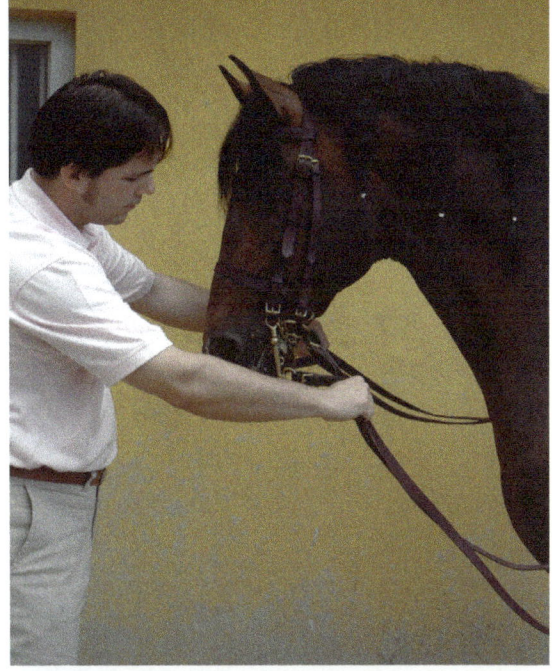

b. Sideways turning of the head to stretch the M. splenius on the opposite side. Notice that the ears should always be at the same height. The poll should never be tilted!

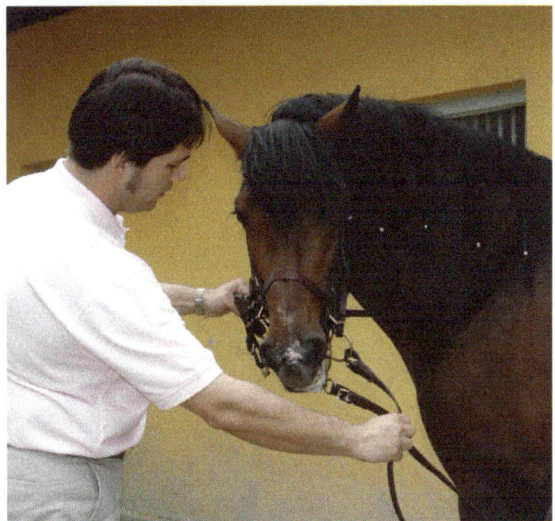

that the head stays straight (not tilted) (fig.14.2.b) and the horse should continue chewing the bit. The neck muscles on the opposite side will thereby be stretched (M. brachiocephalicus, M. splenius, M. scalenus) and will be able to relax. The horse also learns to accept and understand the bending influence of the rider's hand. The horse should not evade the bend by moving the hindquarters. This sideways evasion prevents the horse from stretching and yielding the outside muscles which are exactly the ones needed to relax in order to promote chewing of the bit.

Beginning with this exercise in the halt, rotation, extension and flexion of the stretched neck vertebrae can also be triggered to mobilize the spine in

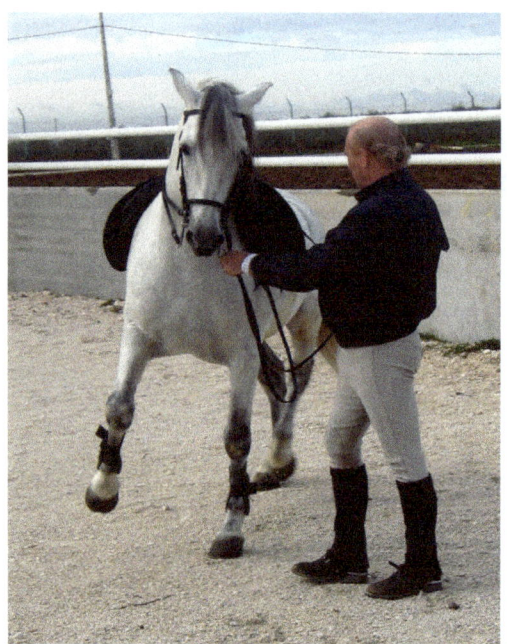 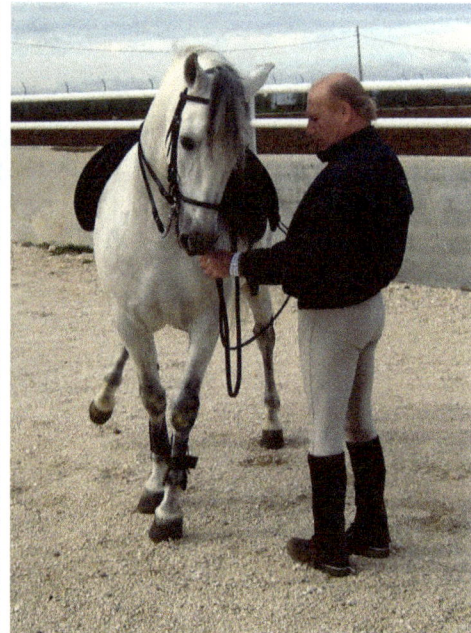

Fig 14.3. a. & b. Through the slow crossing according to Baucher it is possible to specifically loosen the forehand or neck, as shown in the photo, in order to eliminate tension. The well-known Spanish bullfighter, Antonio Ignacio Vargas demonstrates this exercise on one of his stallions. Note the way the reins are held.

an axial plane too. After successful latero-flexion, a forward and down stretch should finally be carried out to stretch the supraspinous ligament.

Once the exercises in the halt have been successfully carried out, one can commence with turns on the forehand and haunches as well as crossing the legs and shoulder-in in-hand. (fig.14.3 and 14.4)

For this purpose, the outside rein is taken over the "*axthieb*" (light indent in the neck in front of the wither) in the right hand, which also carries the whip. The left hand takes the left rein near the bit, so it is possible for the trainer to keep good control over the outside shoulder while, at the same time, maintaining the position of the horse's head to the inside. These exercise can be seen as the prerequisite for the ridden half-halts and riding in "position." The horse must never be locked into position by the use of auxiliary reins, and can thus rediscover his movement possibilities at all times. It is for this reason that this manner of mobilization works well on horses that have been "previously been damaged by lungeing aids," for [in this method] they are not constricted and can gain confidence in the trainer.

At first, one starts with generous sideways steps to the right on a large circle. The horse should not just stay fixed on one spot since the trainer walks with him. The crossing of the legs is achieved by lightly tapping the horse with

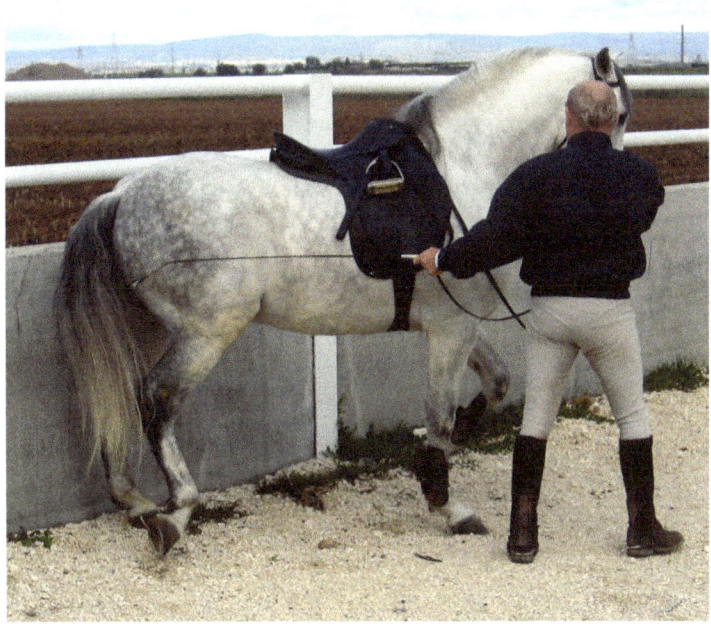

Fig 14.4. The shoulder-in, in-hand is an excellent way to teach the horse this valuable exercise without the weight of a rider, making it easier to perform it under the rider later. Note the sideways driving whip and the influence of the outside rein in the hand of the trainer.

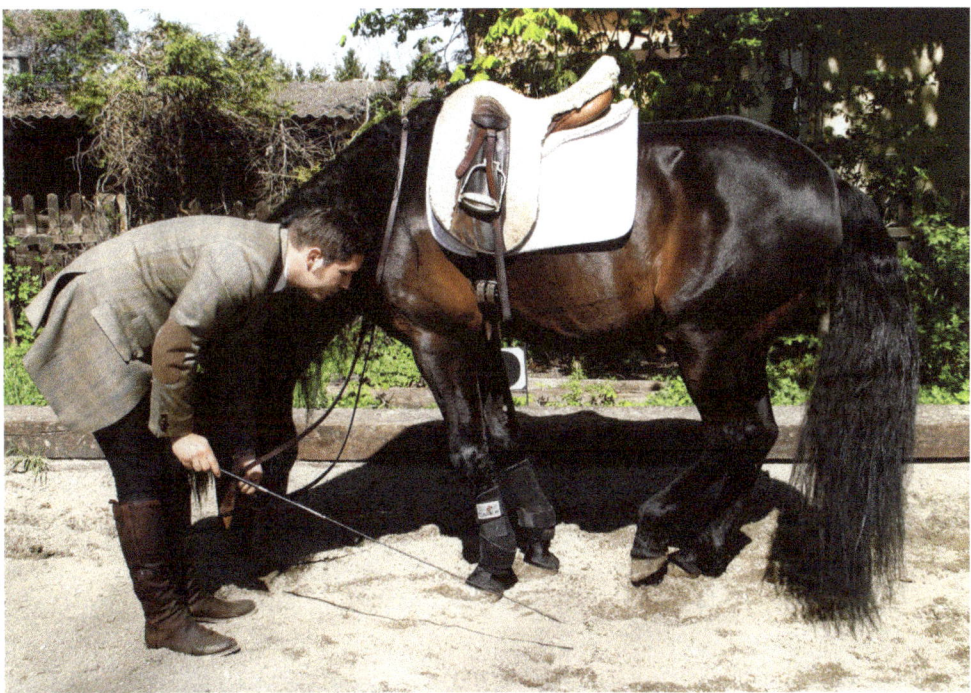

Fig 14.5. An almost forgotten exercise from Baucher, "goat on the peak." Through the hind legs that approach the forehand, the topline can be stretched well, especially in the rectangular shaped horses. Here is the author with the 22 year old English thoroughbred stallion, Nerine. The left front leg could have been slightly more to the back.

the whip at the height of his knee [or hock]. When the size of the circle is reduced, the result is a turn on the forehand against the direction of the movement.

The triceps and hamstrings can be stretched really well with this exercise. A the same time, the start of the longitudinal bend will cause the inside Musculus-obliquus-externus-abdominis and Musculuc-obliquus-internus-abdominis to contract while the outside M. iliocostalis gets stretched.

When the trainer moves somewhat slower in the direction of the head of the horse while crossing the legs, a turn on the haunches can easily be provoked, and this will strengthen the gluteal muscles and cause a stretch on the ipsilateral [same] side, i.e. the side of the trainer.

All of these exercises should be repeated in a mirror-like fashion on both reins to prevent over-training of one side.

Another useful exercise is the "goat on the peak," invented by Baucher. (Fig. 14.5) In this exercise the hind legs approach the front in such a way that the topline is strongly arched and the neck is stretched forward in the long and low position. This can train an optimal balance and can help horses that have problems commencing the piaffe. This is also an isometric exercise for the stomach and back muscles and really promotes balance.

When these exercises are done every day before training, the warm-up phase in walk can be put to good use without overtaxing the joints and, at the same time, obtain profit from the suppleness they give.

14.2. Physiotherapeutic mobilization techniques to improve maneuverability

Every muscular effect is based upon an interplay between contraction and relaxation and each muscle can only work in the context of its opponent (agonist-antagonist[15]).

Based on this principle, it often happens that inadequate use of different groups of muscles will cause neglect of the opposing partner, shortening it. Thus the possibilities of movement are thus restricted. Muscle shortening will, on the one hand, cause elongation of the tendons, which imparts more tension on the tendons, making them more prone to injury.

It is for this reason that specific mobilization techniques are of great use to lengthen and to re-establish mobility. When mobilization techniques are to be applied, it is advisable for the horse to be warmed up beforehand,

---

15 A drug which exhibits some properties of an agonist (a substance that fully activates the neuronal receptor that it attaches to) and some properties of an antagonist (a substance that attaches to a receptor but does not activate it or if it displaces an agonist at that receptor it seemingly deactivates it thereby reversing the effect of the agonist).

since cold muscles will be more prone to injury.

By the same logic, each mobilization should be carried out slowly, cautiously and only as long as the horse will tolerate the stretch in a psychologically relaxed manner.

Every stretch should only be done up to the point where the horse offers a slight resistance to the therapist and should be held in this position for ten seconds. This guarantees the optimum stretch and mobilization effect—stretching of the fibers so that tears will thus be avoided.

All abrupt, rough and erratic movements should be avoided, as they can injure the horse and break the trust for future treatments.

The basic requirement for any therapeutic intervention is the horse's complete willingness to participate and his complete psychological relaxation, which, in turn, will have, through the parasympathetic system, a reflex effect on all of the muscles in the body that will make it easier to work on these muscles. A higher tone in the muscles of the body makes it more difficult to do a proper mobilization and carries a higher risk of injury for both the horse and the veterinarian. The specific mobilization techniques for specific regions will be discussed in the following sections.

14.2.1. Neck

When mobilizing the neck, one should be especially cautious, for these vertebrae may be the most agile, but are also the most susceptible when it comes to injury.

Fast, unsympathetic mobilization can block vertebrae, pinch a nerve and, even worse, cause fissures or fractures of the neck vertebrae.

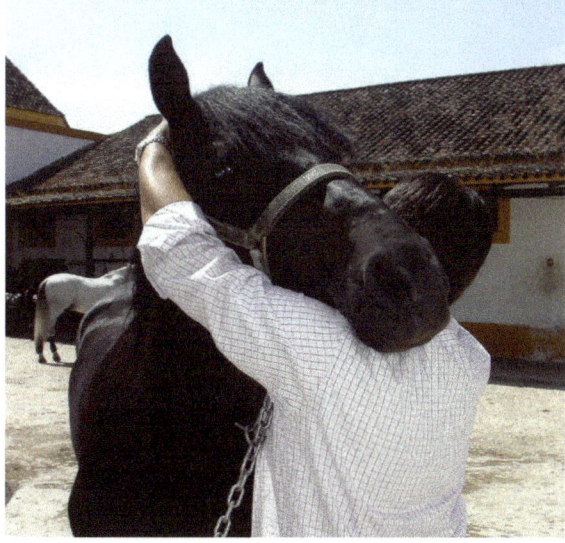

Fig. 14.6.
By circling the atlas with both hands and slowly sideways bending of the neck, performed by therapist, one can achieve a relaxation of the muscles in the area of the poll.

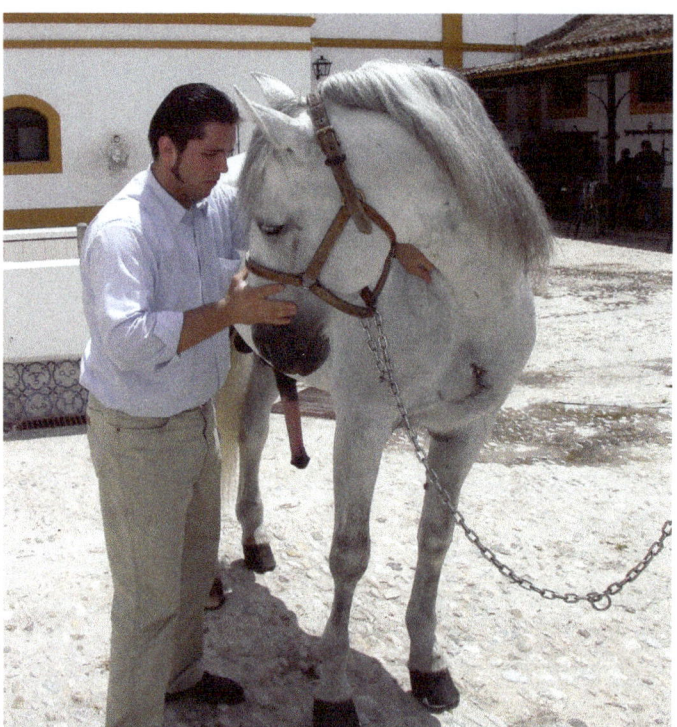

Fig. 14.7. By supporting sections of the neck with the hand closet to the body and bending the neck sideways one can mobilise the neck vertebrae. Abrupt movements should be omitted in order to avoid damage to the neck vertebrae. The author demonstrates maximum sideways bending on the stallion Distinguido.

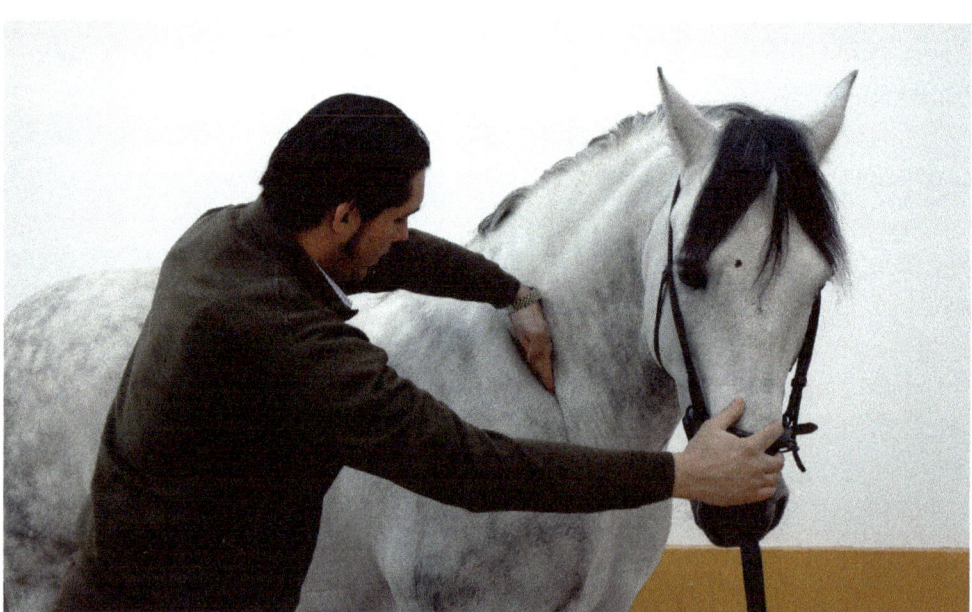

Fig. 14.8. With the parascapular technique, tension in the serratus and neck muscle area can be released easily. Careful reaching behind the scapula will stimulate the nervous structures like the brachial plexus and the ganglium stellatum, and the horse will arrive at a deeper state of relaxation.

The Science and Art of Riding in Lightness

In Practice: *In the carrot stretch, where a carrot is held on the pelvis and the horse stretches for it with a rapid and even neck movement without turning the hindquarters away from therapist, one mobilizes the opposite neck muscles. It is also a good test for the neck muscles. When the carrot is held between the front legs, one provokes an arching of the back and an opening of the occipital joint.*

When one stands in front of the horse, and encircles the lower jaw with both hands, one can achieve an over stretching of the atlanto-occpital joint, mobilizing it at the same time, while stretching the M. sternocleidomastoideus and M. braciocephalicus.(fig.14.6)

For manual mobilization of single sections of the neck, one grasps the bridge of the nose with the hand furthest from the body of the horse, move the nose towards oneself whilst lightly holding against the neck with the other hand, keep the head in this position for a few seconds to stretch the neck muscles on the opposite side (fig.14.7). Tension in the neck area can be influenced with the para-scapular technique (fig.14.8).

14.2.2. Front legs

To mobilize the front legs, stand in front of the horse, to be held by a helper; take the front leg at the fetlock and stretch it straight ahead until a light resistance is felt, keep it in this position for a few seconds and repeat several

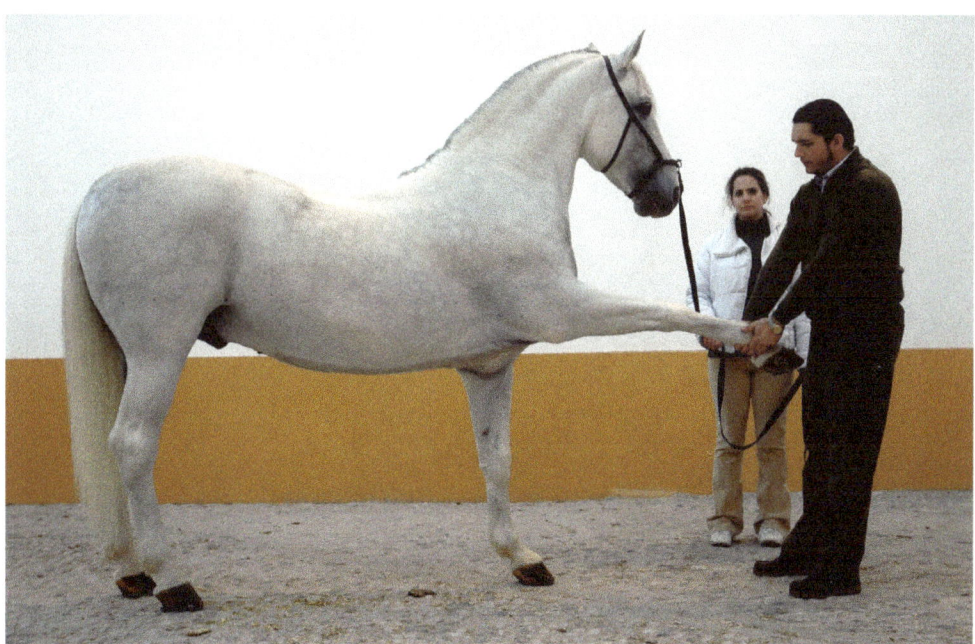

Fig. 14.9.a. Through the extension of the front leg, the tricep group and the M. lattisimus dorsi will be stretched, which can increase the range of movement.

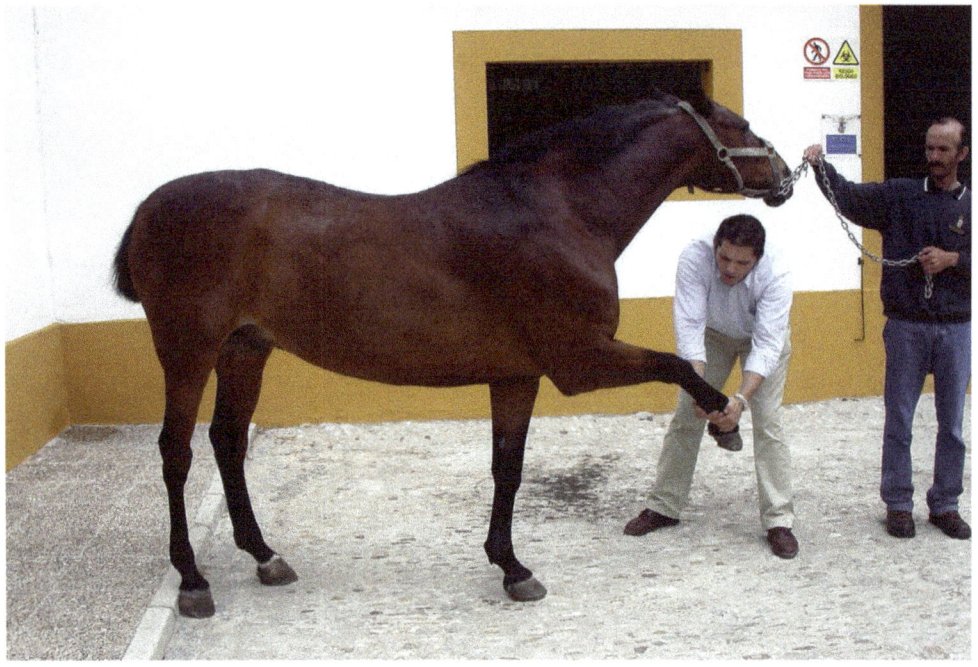

b. The pull in the direction of adduction will increase the stretch on the shoulder and upper arm muscles.

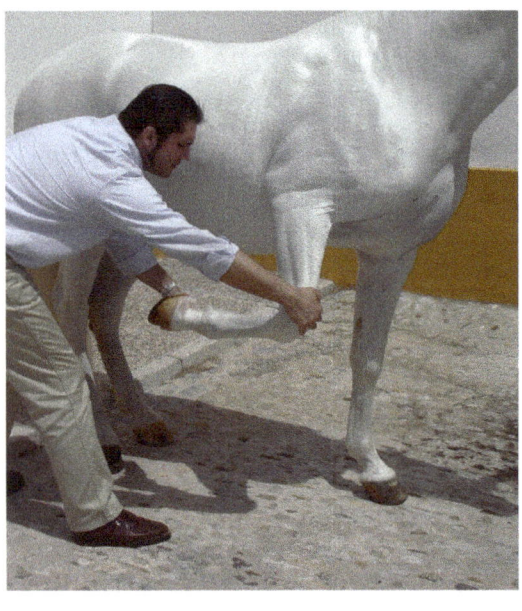

Fig. 14.10. Pulling the leg to the back can achieve a good stretch in the M. brachiocephalicus and the shoulder joint.

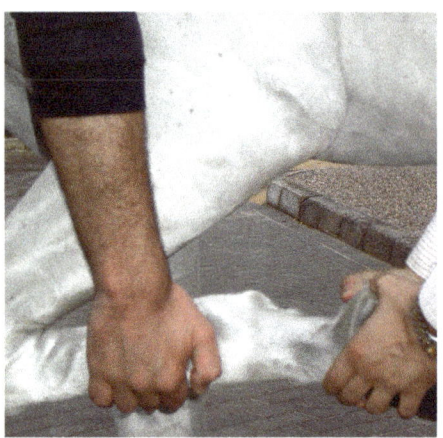

Fig. 14.11. Mobilization of the fetlock with light rotation and traction.

times (fig.14.9.a).

By stretching the leg straight to the front, the M. trapezius, M. deltoideus, M. triceps, M. pectoralis, M. lattisimus dorsi and all flexors are stretched. When the stretched leg is taken over the mid-line in a light adduction, an increased stretch of the outside shoulder and upper arm muscles is achieved. (Fig. 14.9.b).

In abduction the serratus and pectoral muscles are stretched. When the lifted leg is move caudally in half a circle, a stretch of the M. brachiocephalicus, the extensors and M. biceps brachii is achieved. (Fig. 14.10).

When the leg is moved backwards, therapist can also mobilize the leg in a cranio medial direction to stretch the M. trapezius, M. rhomboideus and M. lattisimus dorsi. By supporting the bent front leg on his upper leg, therapist can provoke a specific mobilization of the pectoral muscles when his free hand can grip medially under the elbow.

The last mobilization technique for the front legs would be the hoof joint mobilization, where the horse is either asked to stand on a 30 degree slanted surface, or the stretch can be administered manually (fig.14.11). The horse is asked to stand on an increasing slant, up to 30 degrees, and in the beginning only the wither has to be pushed down to reach this stretch in the deep digital flexor.

14.2.3. Hind legs

Along the same lines as the mobilization of the front legs, one can also

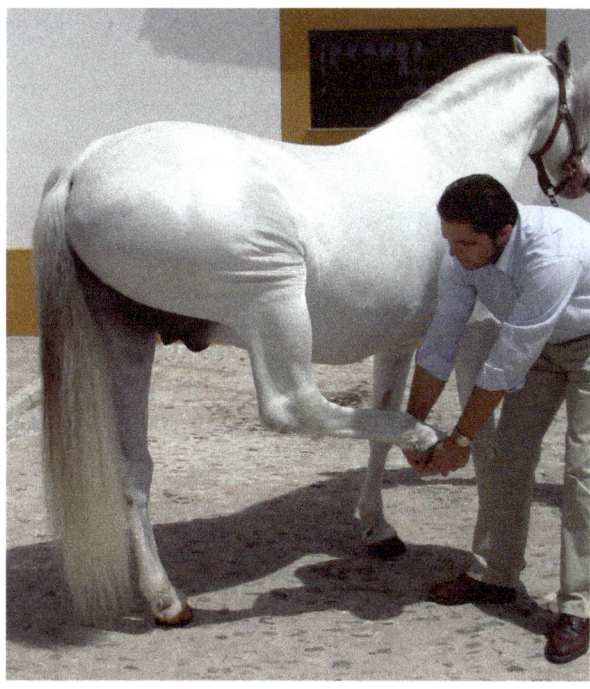

Fig. 14.12. Taking the leg forwards will stretch the M. biceps femorii, M. semi-membranosi and M. semi-tendinosi and improves the ability to step under the center of gravity.

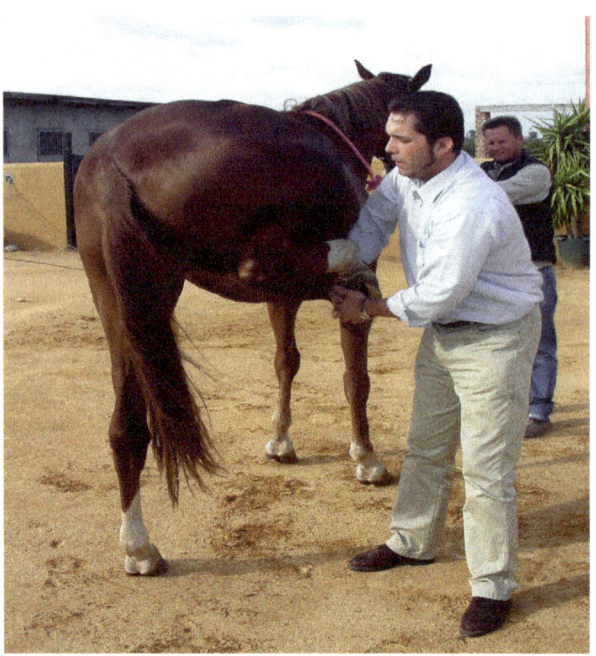

Fig 14.13. Abduction of the hind leg with slight rotation of the pelvis makes it possible to mobilise the sacroiliac joint and the lumbar vertebrae in a gentle way.

carry out mobilization of the hind legs. First, one stands next to the horse's thorax facing backwards, pick the hind leg up at the fetlock and move the leg forward to stretch the M. semi-membranous and M. biceps femoris (fig.14.12).

When the leg is now bent at the hock and moved away from the horse in abduction, the adductors of the hip joint can be mobilized (fig.14.13). In order to improve the crossing of the legs in the lateral work, then therapist

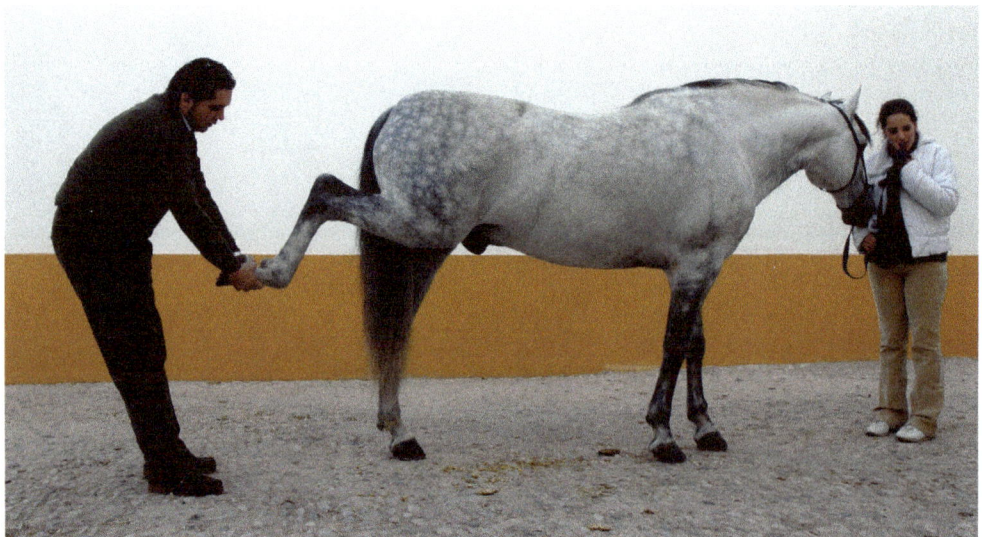

Fig. 14.14. Stretching the leg straight to the back will improve the elasticity of the lumbar area, for the M. longissimus dorsi as well as the psoas group can be addressed. The M. tensor fascia latae can also be stretched in this way.

can bring the leg from the opposite side over the median line in adduction to stretch the above mentioned muscles.

When the therapist stands behind the horse and stretches the hind leg straight back, he can stretch the M. quadriceps femoris and all its components. (Fig. 14.14) At the same time, the hips and knee joint will be mobilized. When therapist stands in the farrier position next to the horse and pushes down on the calcaneus, he can mobilize the hock, M. gastrocnemius and the Achilles tendon. Mobilization of the hoof joint follows in the same manner as in the front legs.

14.2.4. The back and sacroiliac joint

Mobilization of the back also includes the significant testing for mobility exercises. Execution of the lateral flexion is shown in fig.14.15.

To lift the topline, therapist stands at shoulder level, facing the horse, and tries with ever increasing pressure in the Regio sternalis to achieve a lifting of the back (fig.14.16). This movement will increase the distance between the vertebrae and the long back muscles and the independent postural muscles will be stretched. When used regularly this can improved the activity of the back. The horse is thus prepared for the arching of the back under the rider.

Hollowing the back can be achieved by triggering the extension reflex

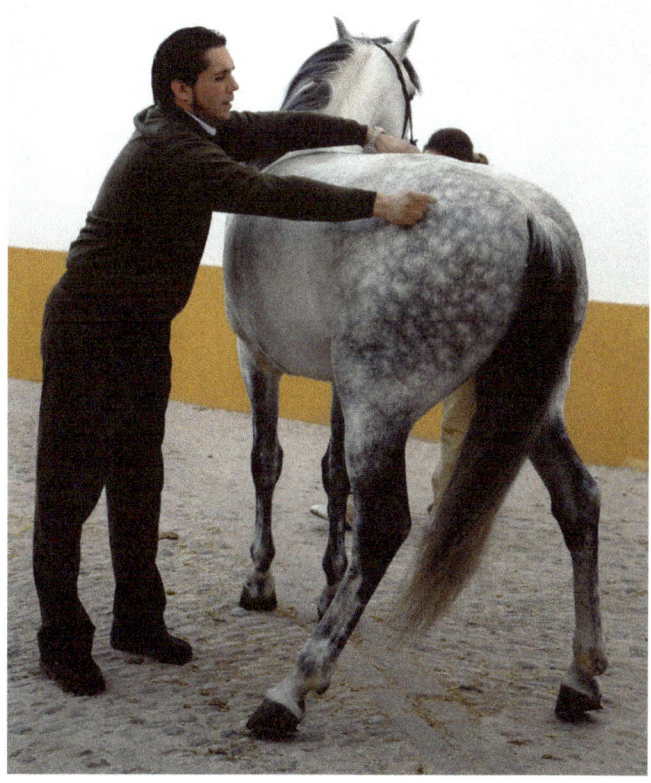

Fig. 14.15. Lateral flexion can be achieved when a reflex point is triggered near the hip joint while holding against the saddle area with the other hand.

when therapist briefly pushes down in the saddle area with both hands. (fig.14.17) This will mobilize the thoracic and loin vertebrae downwards and must then immediately be provoked in the upward direction by the previous technique. This interplay follows the rules of the agonist-antagonist game.

A cat-like arching of the back and flexion of the sacroiliac joint can be achieved when therapist stands behind the horse, and applies pressure about a hands breadth from the spine of the horse, on both sides. The first mentioned muscles will be mobilized in this way. Many horses prefer this to the lifting of the back in the region of the sternum. (fig.14.18)

An extension or flexion of the sacroiliac joint can be achieved because of the existence of two reflex points on both sides, almost a hands breadth in the area of the third lumbar vertebra. This will cause a specific mobility of this very important anatomical structure. (fig.14.19).

In order to improve the mobility to the side, the therapist stands beside the hip of the horse, facing forward and places the hand furthest from

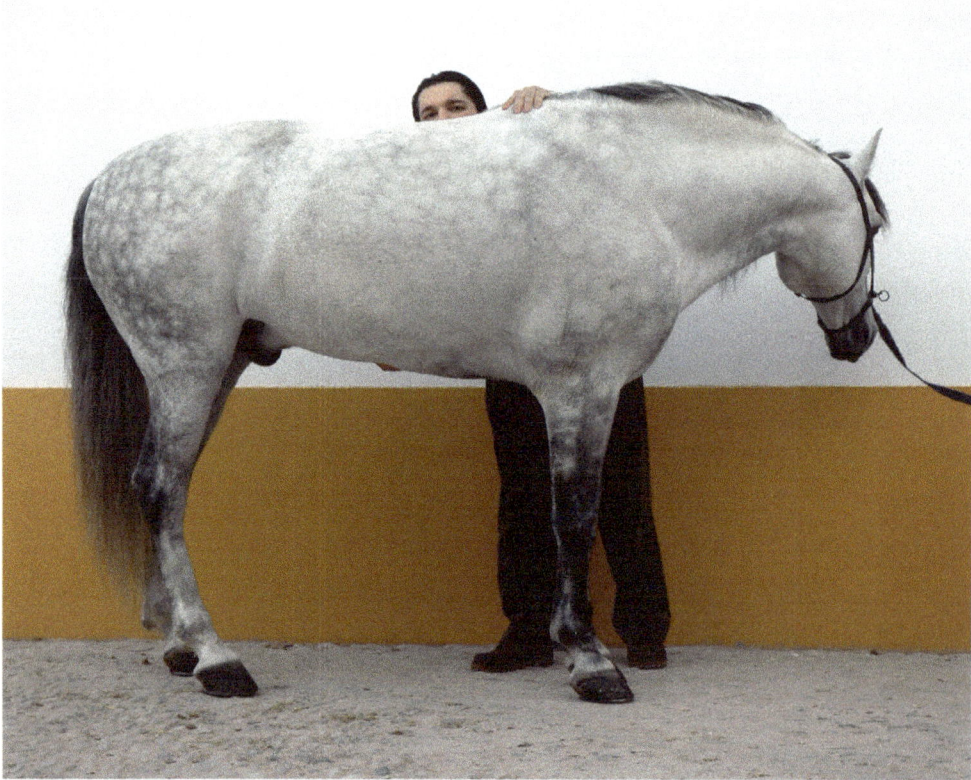

Fig. 14.16 Therapist stands near the shoulder, facing backwards and tries to achieve an arching of the back by softly putting pressure behind the xiphoid. The horse should lower his head for optimal stretch of the supraspinous ligament.

Fig. 14.17. Even pressure in the saddle area can achieve lordosis, and when used with the arching of the back technique can improve the mobility of the back tremendously.

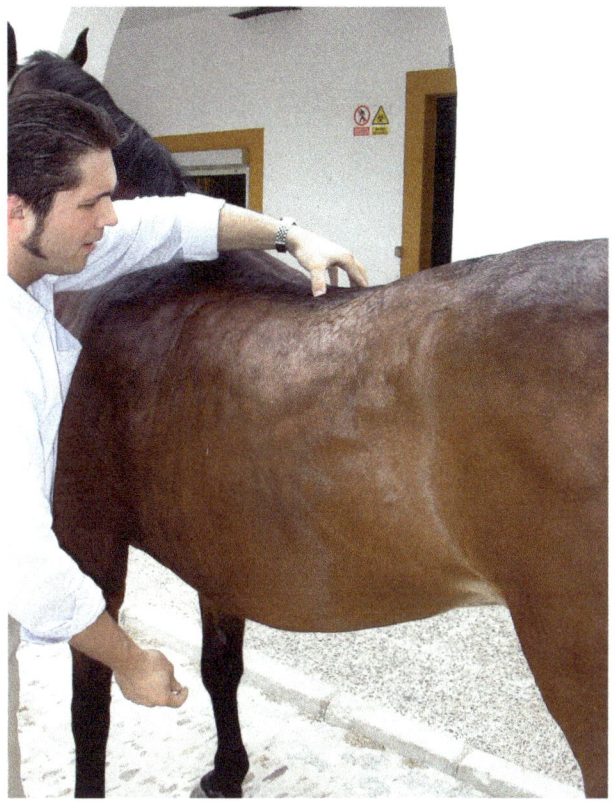

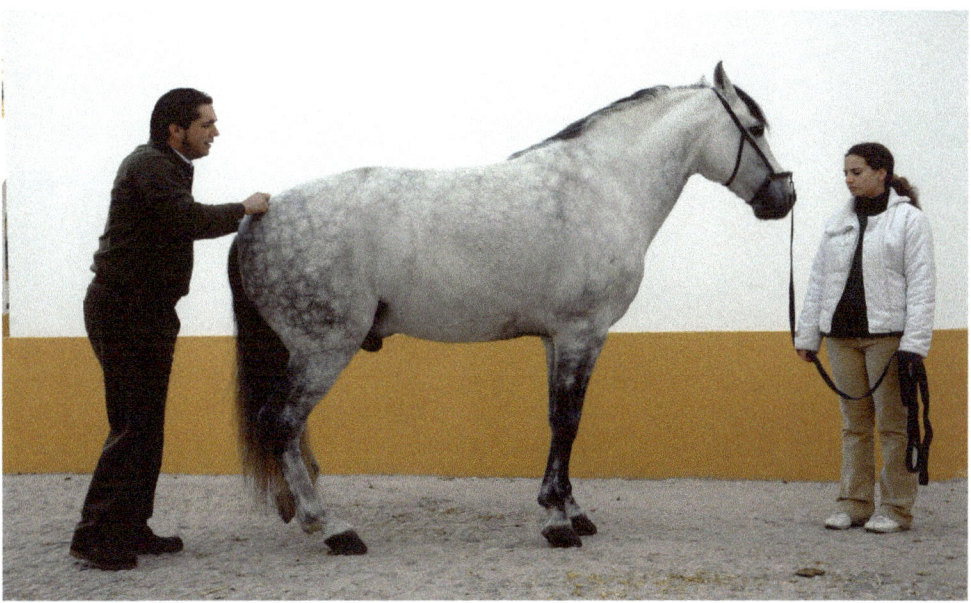

Fig. 14.18. Therapist stands behind the horse, and with increasing pressure, one hand from the spine and starting just in front of the sacroiliac joint and ending in the same height as the hip joint, tries to achieve an arching of the back. Through this technique, a suitable relaxation of the long back muscles is promoted and arching of the back is encouraged.

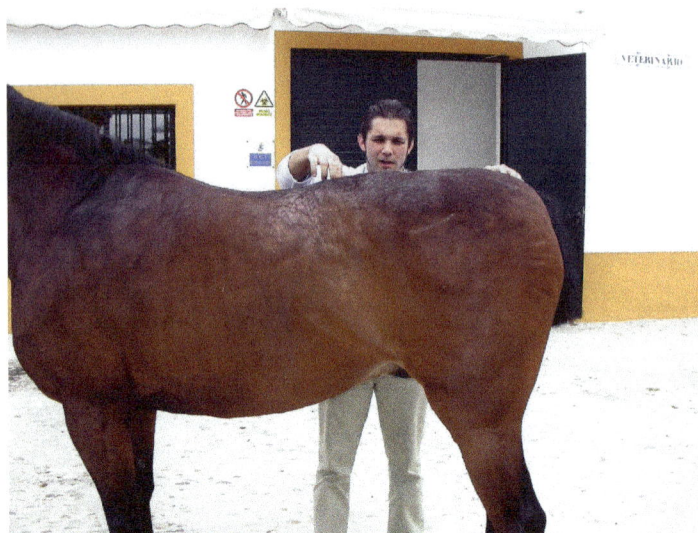

Fig.14.19.
a. About one hands breadth in front of the sacro-ileac joint one will find the reflex point that produces an extension of the sacro-ileac joint.

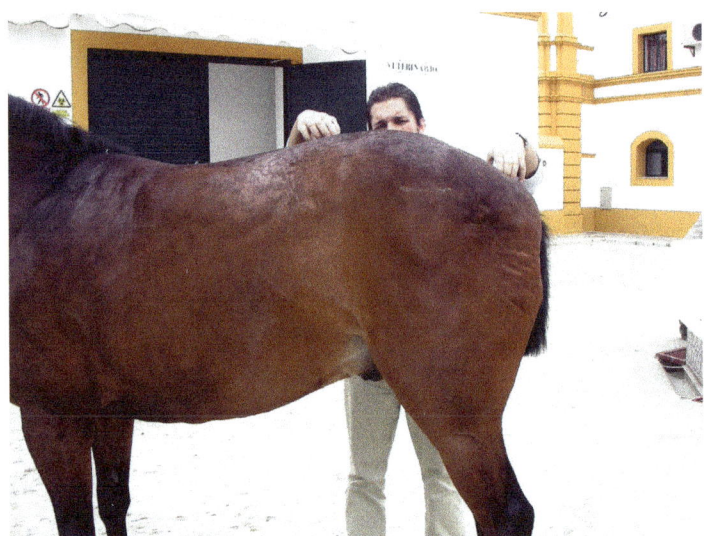

b. On the caudal side of the Sacrum lies the reflex point that produces flexion of the sacra-ileac joint. An interplay between this and extension can achieve highly effective movement.

the body where the legs of the rider will be. The other hand puts pressure over the hip and causes arching of the thorax with simultaneous rotation in the loin area. This will improve the ability for longitudinal bend.

In daily grooming, one can always integrate the carrot stretch, where the horse must fetch a carrot in the area of the pelvic bone, or the cat-like arch where the reflex points next to the sacroiliac joint are pressed, thus loosening the loin area easily.

14.3. Spanish work in-hand

In general, the Iberian work in-hand is different because no training aids are used, only the double bridle or lungeing cavesson with lead is used. A second person is not needed as the trainer has the reins over the withers

*Fig. 14.20.
a. Targeted tapping of the cannon bone can increase stepping under the body as well as the action. This is demonstrated in perfection by one of the riders of the REAAE in preparation for airs above the ground.*

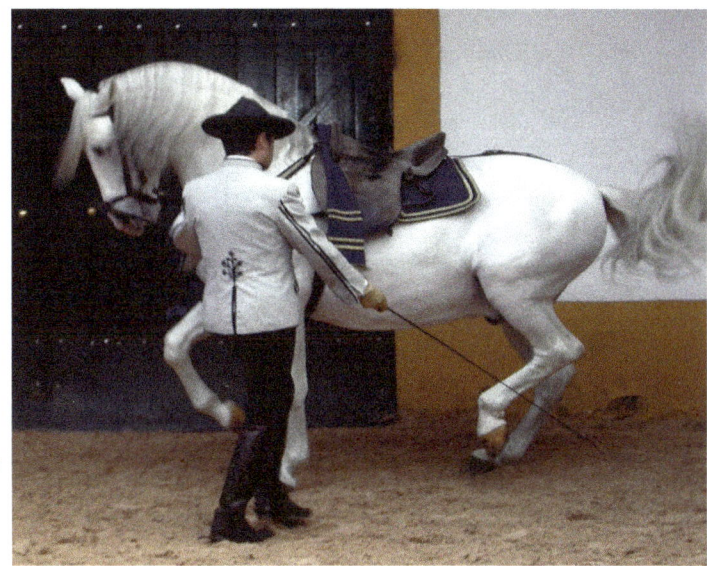

and in his hand closest to the horse's head, and the whip in the other hand. (Fig. 14.20) Through voice aids and body language the trainer can influence the horse in a decelerating manner near the head and in a driving manner near the croup. Many possibilities for intervening can arise, that bring with it a playful and creative lightness.

The hand controlled position of the head allows the trainer to yield quickly to the respective needs of the horse in terms of head position and also allows a lowering of the head without first undoing some reins.

In the hindquarters there are different areas that can influence the activity and action due to the reflex points. Tapping on top of the croup can cause a lowering thereof and increase the frequency of the steps. (fig.14.21) When one taps in the area of the hip or knee, stronger bending of the joints can be the achieved which will result in higher action of the hindquarters. Tapping the back of the hocks and the cannon bones can increase the

*b.
Holding the reins for work in-hand by the Spanish method.*

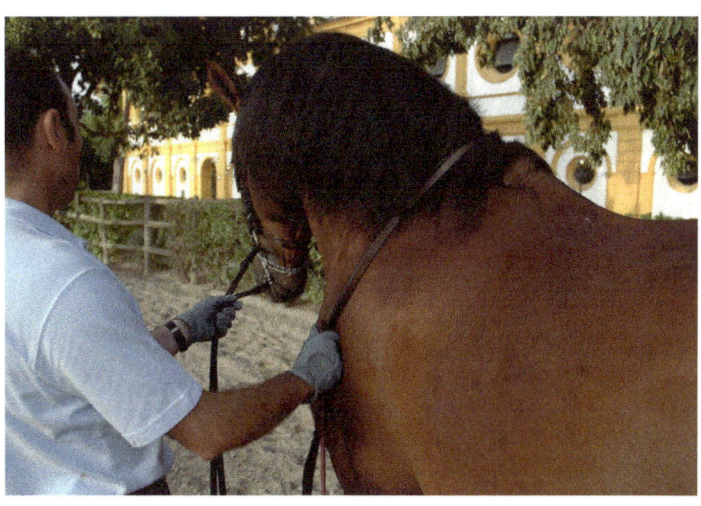

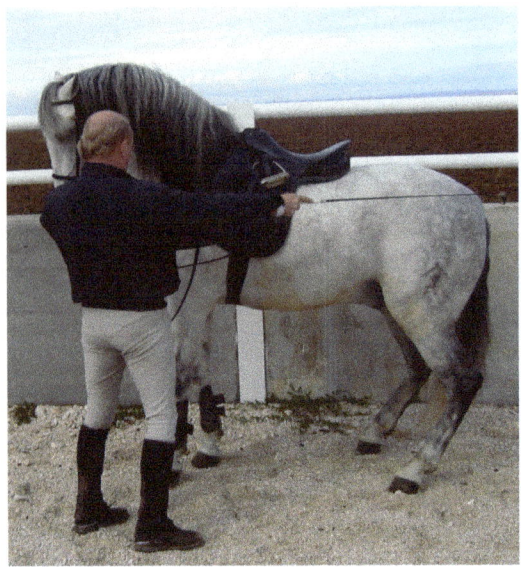 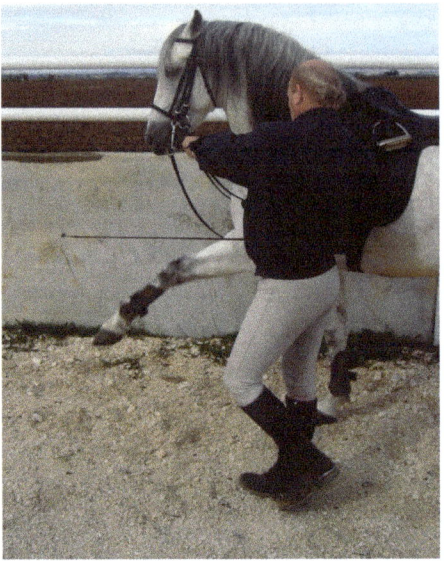

Fig. 14.21.
Lowering of the croup is achieved through the contraction of the psoas and abdominal muscles.

Fig. 14.22.
Holding the whip in front of the horse or tapping on the breast can provoke extension of the front legs, whereby the Spanish walk can be developed.

stepping frequency and convince the hind legs to step more under the center of gravity, whereby more collection can be achieved. In the same way more stepping under the body as well as higher action can be achieved by beneath the abdomen. Tapping on the shoulder joint can cause a stretching of the leg, which will clearly improve the action. (fig.14.22) When the "axthieb" is tapped, the stepping frequency and action of the front leg can be improved.

14.4. Work in-hand according to the school of Vienna

Work in-hand according to the Spanish Riding School in Vienna requires a lungeing cavesson, side reins, lead rein, plus an extra lead rein on the outside ring of the cavesson, the so-called jumping lead. (Fig.14.23a) This system requires a knowledgeable helper on the lead rein that stops the horse from running forward and keeps him straight. The experienced trainer on the jumping rein leads the horse, with the rein over the withers to help keep the horse straight, to the middle of the school while tapping the various areas with the whip. This method is ideal to teach horses the airs above the ground, capriole, courbettes and levade, but requires a skilled trainer and an experienced team who can support the horse accordingly.

15. Long reins

A special training method is the work on the long reins. This method represents the completion of collected work in a fully trained horse, as the horse should perform all the lessons learned from the saddle with only the long reins, voice and whip from the trainer who walks behind him. (fig.15.1) Due to decreased possibility for intervening with the horse, the horse must be finely trained, and have no tendency to kick, for that could lead to dangerous injuries for the trainer.

The riderless, or weightless work of the horse in collection, can improve the activity of the back and assist in re-muscling in the rehabilitation phase, especially with older horses. Even horses with leg problems, that cannot be ridden, can find a type of activity with this work, without having the feeling that they are forgotten.

Work on long reins is a specialized field which requires the trainer to have much empathy and expertise in order to encourage the horse properly.

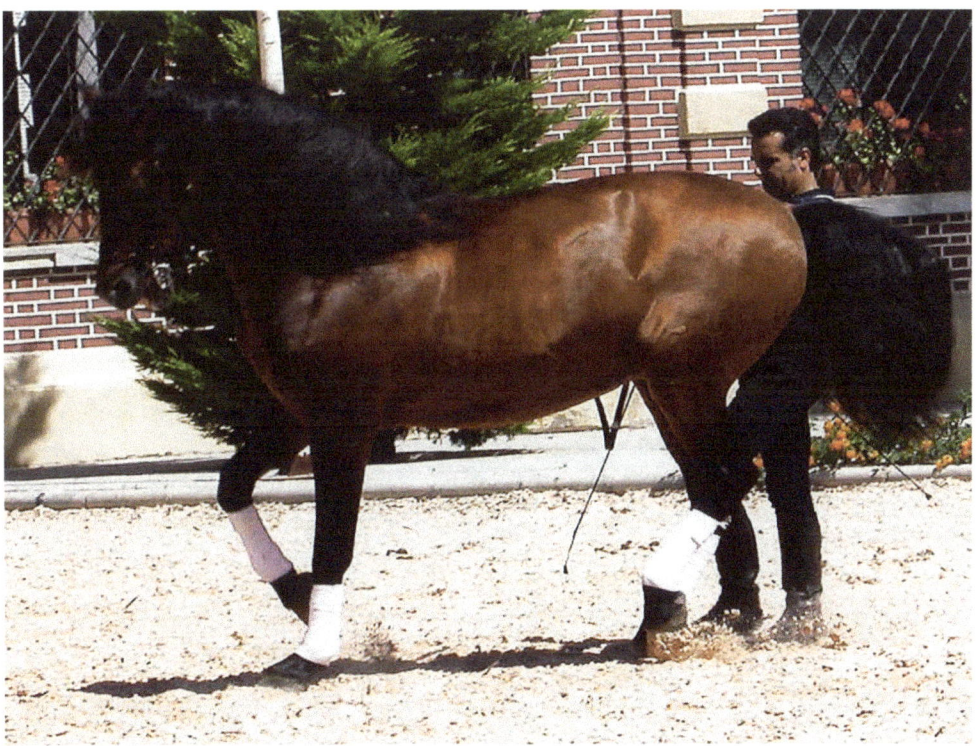

Fig. 15.1.
Work on long reins, canter pirouette to the left, here demonstrated by Manuel Ruiz, chief rider of the REAAE, with his stallion Judio.

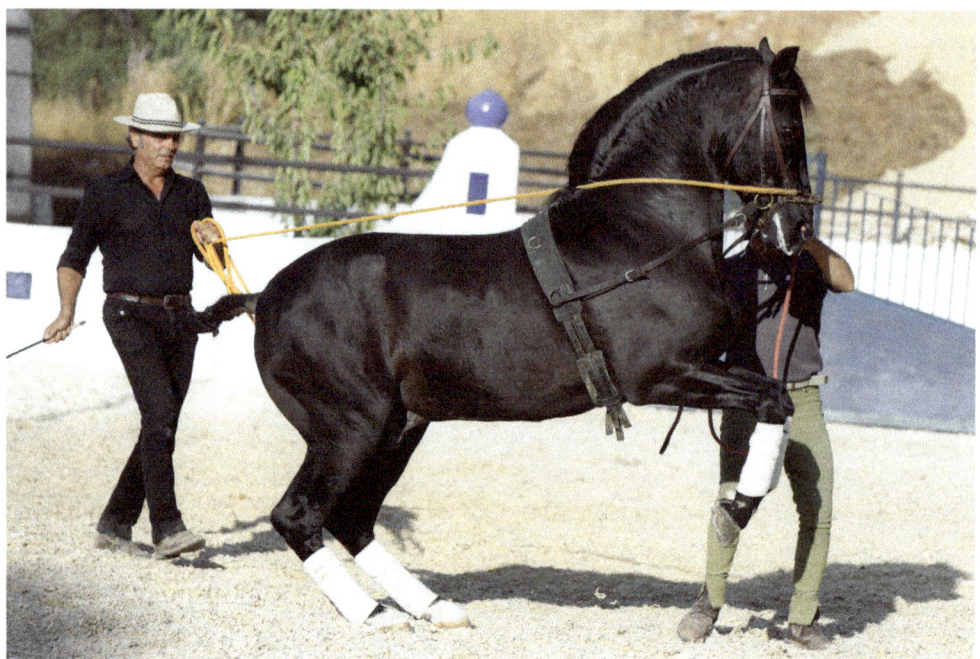

Fig. 14.23 a. Miguel Barrionuevo preparing his horse for the Capriole by collecting him in a perfect terre a terre. The terre a terre is a two beat canter-like movement which enables the horse to turn to either side without changing lead; it also strenghtens the hindquarters.

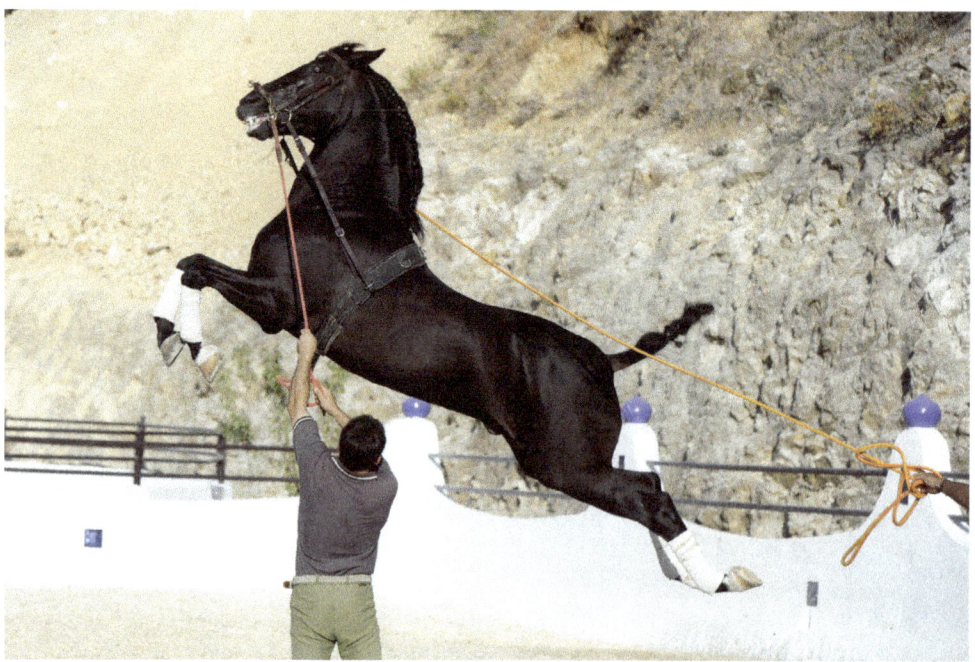

Fig. 14.23 b. Capriole—note the excellent upward position of this air above the ground, and the equally extended hind legs.

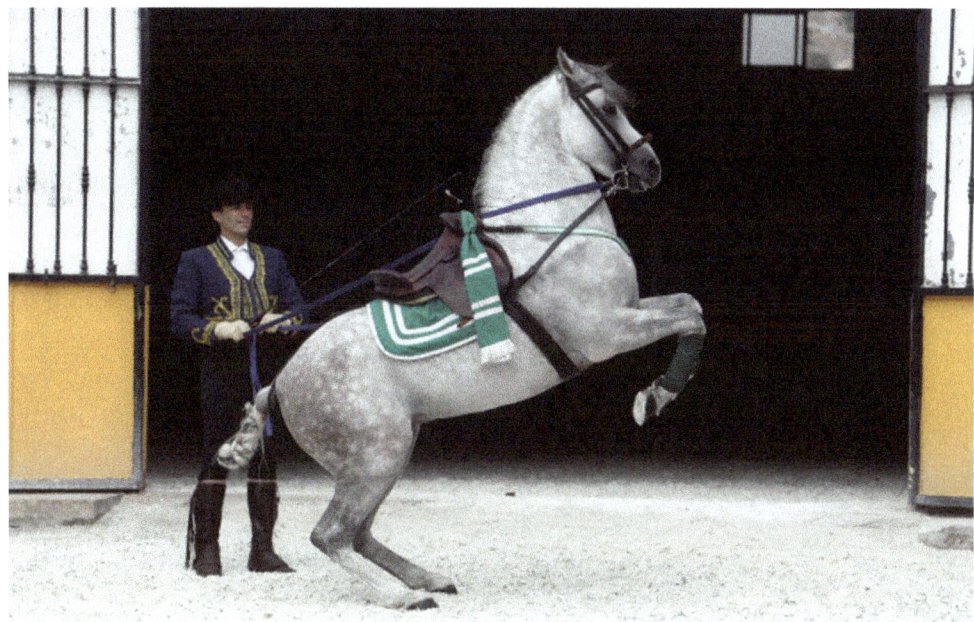

Fig. 14.24 a. Carlos Gonzalez prepairing the classical courbette, which is a more elevated terre a terre *achieved by gaining more ground under the body. The change between the up und down of the legs makes this a very special, beautiful, high school air. The jumps on the hindquarters which the Spanish riding school of Vienna performs is an invention of the 19th century and has nothing to do with the classical courbette that was described by The Duke of Newcastle and de la Guérinière.*

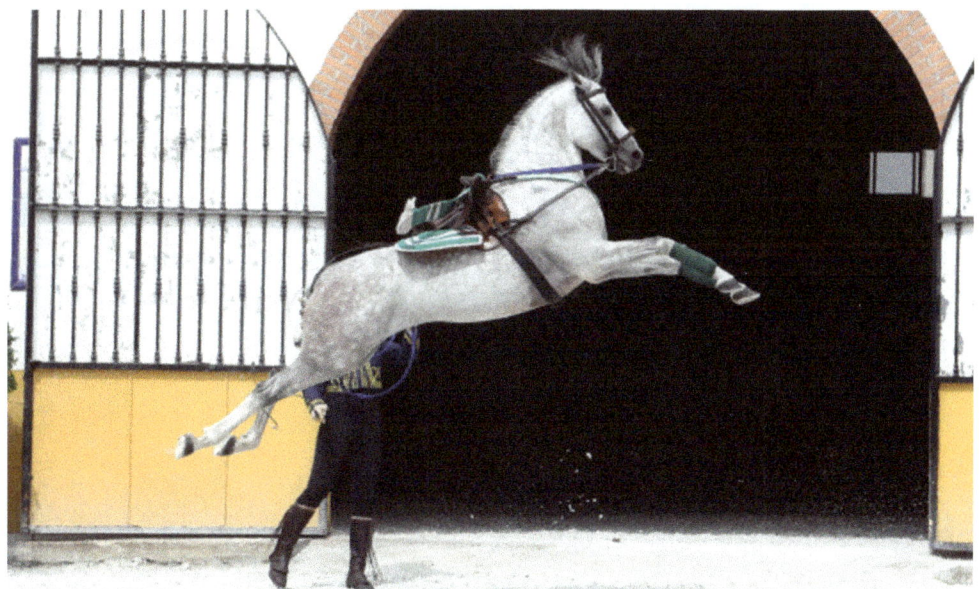

Fig. 14.24 b. The capriole is the crowning jewel of the airs above the ground—here realized by the spanish master, Carlos Gonzales in a very spectacular way.

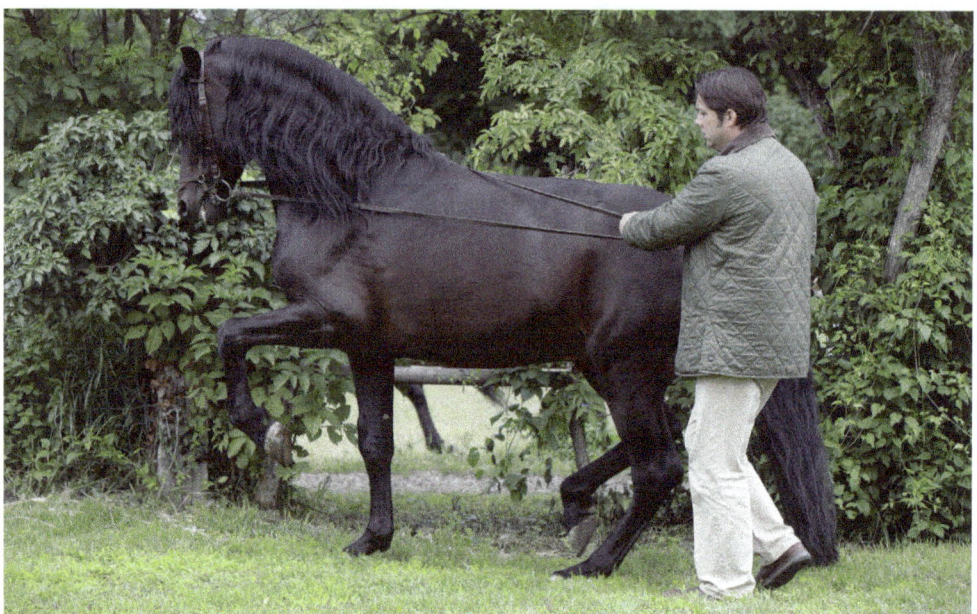

Fig. 15.2. a. Piaffe in-hand is the most important high school movement because it concentrates all the forces in the horse's middle. Please note the very good lowering of the haunches and the arched loins. A good rassembler in the piaffe is the basis for all other airs above the ground.

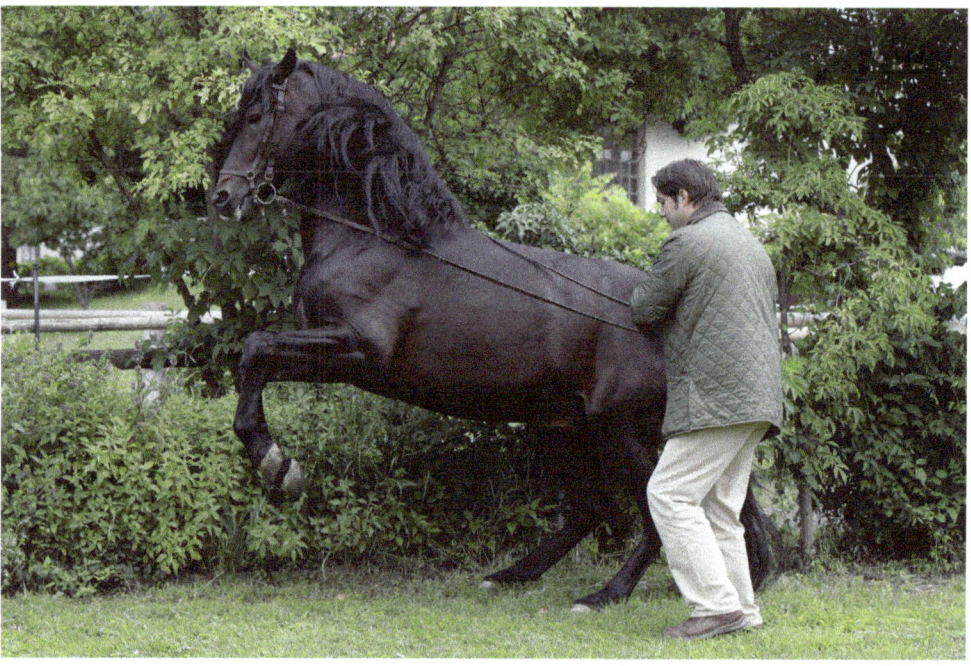

Fig. 15.2. b. Levade—not every horse is able to maintain this position (an angle between 30 and 35 degrees) on his haunches. The most important thing is the slow elevation of the forehand which ideally, should be folded at the carpal [knee] joint.

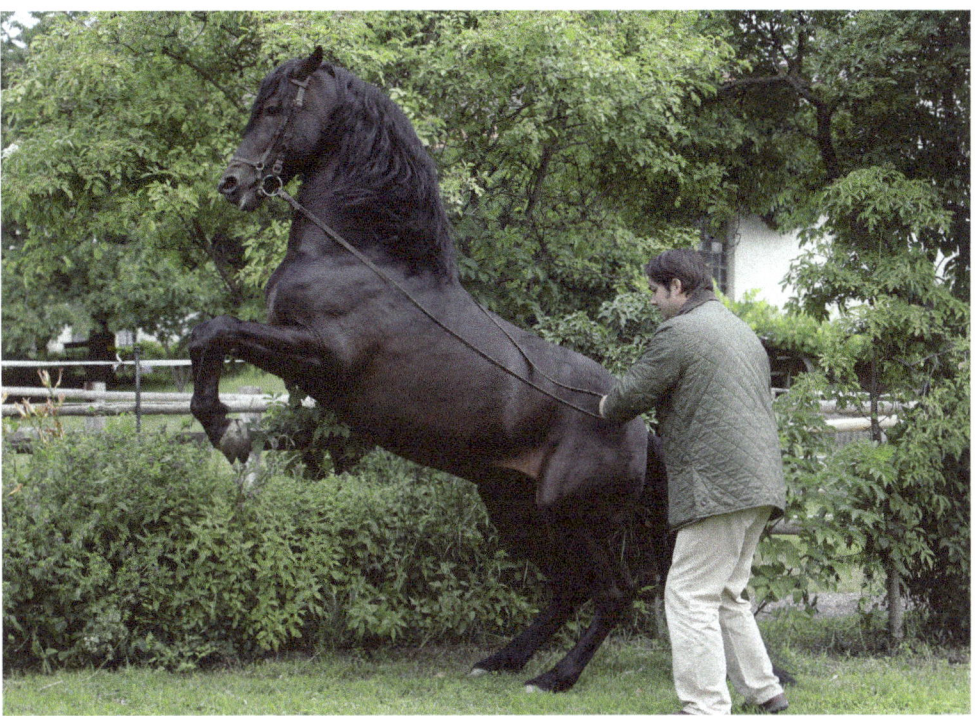

Fig. 15.2. c. The pesade is an air above the ground which has a higher degree of elevation of the forehand and can be developed from the piaffe and levade. It also schools the feeling of balance and strengthens the loins. It is very important to end every training session of airs above the ground with a good piaffe because the horse should not learn to use the airs as a way of defending himself to avoid too much work. [The horse should not finish his "airs" lesson with the air itself, lest he learn to use the air as an evation to other work—always finish with piaffe.]

PART III: CORRECTION OF PROBLEMS AND SPECIAL PHYSIOTHERAPY

16. Course of examination

As described in the previous Chapters, any kind of training that does not follow biomechanical rules can be detrimental to the health of the horse. Recognizing tension or lesions is therefore, the first, and simultaneously very important step to introducing a suitable form of rehabilitation.

The physiotherapeutic course of examination is an additive for further study in classical veterinary work, and orthopedic and neurological examination of the patient, in which the orthopedically relevant areas will be further discussed. First of all, tension, blockages and restriction of movement should be explored with the so-called "motion-palpation-analysis" (MPA), so as to initiate a corresponding therapy.

In contrast to the classical orthopedic course of examination, the physiotherapeutic examination is especially useful in analyzing and diagnosing restrictions of movement of myogenic origin. For this reason, it is very important to have a sound knowledge of the biomechanical context and the anatomical basis in myology, in order to make a diagnosis in this system.

In the case of lameness, the horse must be examined orthopedically by an experienced veterinarian with flexion tests, palpation of the hoof with hoof testers, and diagnostic anesthesia to localize precisely the origin of his lameness. If necessary, the examination must be extended to include x-rays, ultrasound, thermography CT, and/or MRI to get a sure diagnosis and to determine whether the case can actually be treated with physiotherapy. As a rule, the examination is composed of three parts.

16.1. Case history

In the first place, the information of the medical history should be documented, where the name, age, breed, sex, color, purpose and level of training must be noted. This is beneficial from a forensic view, for the veterinary duty of care is complied with according to the mandatory recording law.

Keeping an examination protocol gives the certainty that everything is systematically and properly covered and nothing overlooked. It also makes it easier for the veterinarian to detect changes in findings and to compare them, so that possible progress, stagnation or setbacks are easier to recognize.

The most time consuming, but important part of the examination, is to collect information for the case history. One is often called by an owner that says his horse is lame, has never been lame and has not had any problems. In these cases detailed questioning of the problem of the alleged healthy horse is important and knowledge of riding and driving is necessary to understand the problem. When there is a trainer, he should also be questioned about the training and subjective assessment of the problem. The order of the questions should at least shed light on the following:
- When did the horse begin having problems?
- What are the problems?
- Was there an accident, fall or injury before the change of pattern?
- When was the last time the horse had his teeth done?
- When was the last time the horse was shod? Were there any problems (rebellion when giving the foot)?
- What saddle and bridle is used? How the owner saddles and bridles his horse should be immediately assessed with the horse.
- Riding discipline (Western, English, Baroque etc)
- How does the training normally proceed (warm-up, cool down, length of time)?
- What is the stage of training?
- How are the exercises performed?
- When was the last show/competition and when is the next one?
- How is the horse lunged, and more specifically with what equipment and how long?
- Does the horse get medication, muscle building products, dietary supplements etc?
- Does the horse have permanent orthopedic problems(tendinitis, spavin etc)?
- Has the horse been treated previously and with which therapy? What was the diagnosis?
- Is the horse still being treated, do two or more vets or therapists treat the horse, is there a doping possibility etc?

16.2. Examination at rest and in movement

Ideally the horse should first be observed in his stable, how he moves and behaves. Is he friendly and interested in his environment, is he grumpy with his groom or does he turn away, does he threaten with ears pinned back and biting or is he withdrawn and shy? Are the walls dirty, do they have marks where he kicked, are there chewed wooden components or trenches in the floor? All of these give valuable hints to the horse's well-being in his personal space and reveal possible problems or reactions the horse might have while being examined.

16.2.1. At rest

The correct physical examination of a horse includes a properly placed horse, that, in contrast to the conformation assessment should stand squarely.

Definition: *A horse standing "square" will stand on a rectangular shape, all legs evenly loaded and calm.*

Nervous and fidgeting horses make the examination and the findings difficult to interpret.

The place for the examination should be bright, without a draft, have a non-slip surface and be far enough from the normal stable chaos to create a calm atmosphere. The horse should be set up squarely on a flat surface for the physical examination, so the legs do not create an inaccurate impression of asymmetry. The therapist moves slowly in a safe distance(2m) around the horse, to get an overall impression of the patient, to better assess atrophy, relieving posture and asymmetry. In this phase of the examination, a calm environment is advantageous so the horse can stand quietly and not dance around nervously and give the wrong impression of the problem (for example showing off by a stallion).

16.2.2. Presenting the horse in-hand

The horse should either be wearing a snaffle bridle or a lungeing cavesson for the physical examination in movement. The person leading the horse goes on the left of the horse.

The lighter cavesson like the ones used in Portugal or Spain, should take preference over the more padded ones, for the horses can be handled better and with more safety. The lead rein must be attached to the middle ring; this guarantees an even action on the bridge of the nose. The lead rein should not be longer than 1.50m, for too much rein in the hand is uncomfortable. If the horse becomes disobedient, one should aways correct the horse with a downwards movement of the lead rein to restore basic obedience.

When the horse is presented with a bridle, the reins should not be on the neck. The right hand should take both reins about a hand's width under the bit, with the left rein between the thumb and index finger and the right rein between the index finger and the middle finger. In this way one can specifically act on the bars of the horse's mouth and thus maneuver him better.

The end of the rein, at the buckle, is held in the left hand. This will allow the person to have the rein in his hands if, by accident, he falls while presenting the horse.

If a whip is carried, it should be at least 1.30m long to get the horse to trot. This should be held in the left hand, with the lash to the back, and parallel to the horse. Thereby a fast and precise action is possible. A whip should never be carried upright or pointed at the horse's head.

A combination of the cavesson and bridle is recommended when a problem horse (rearing, pulling, etc) is presented, for the bridle can keep the horse straight to a point and the cavesson can affect the horse in a way that will stop too much forward movement due to the influence on the bridge of the nose. In this case, the left hand takes the lead rein of the cavesson and the left rein of the bridle while the right hand takes the right rein of the bridle over the withers to achieve a straighter line with the use of half-halts. The lead rein and left rein of the bridle is separated in the left hand to influence the horse on the left bit and cavesson independently.

The horse should be presented without saddle, bandages, blanket. One should also find a flat, straight surface so the horse does not adopt unwanted misalignments.

Assessment of the horse starts in the halt and then the walk, such that the horse should be led away from therapist on at least a 20m track and then straight back to therapist again. It is important that the person leading the horse not keep the rein too short so that it does not disturb the movement of the neck, making the assessment more difficult or even impossible.

The presentation should be calm, but brisk and even. Turns or changes of direction should always be made so the handler is on the outside of the horse, and travels on the bigger circle. This way the inside shoulder of the horse is more visible to the therapist.

Trot should occur in a similar way in which great value should be put on an even and calm rhythm so as to best assess the swing of the pelvis and any rotation in the lumbar spinal cord. Flashy trots or horses that jump around make the assessment impossible and increases the risk of injury.

In general, one assesses the first ground contact of the hooves when the horse moves away from and towards the therapist, any relieving posture, load relief and lameness. This should always be done on both hard and soft surfaces, since many illnesses show themselves better on one terrain more than on another.

Horses with arthritis will, for example, go worse on hard surfaces while a horse with patellar ligament lesions will go worse on a soft surface. Improvement or deterioration of a disorder in the movement can also provide valuable hints on the course of the prognosis of the problems. Inspection on a circle and small turns without the use of lungeing aids can further help with conclusions of lameness and constrictions in the movement.

When movement disorders only appear in particular exercises (extensions, half-pass, flying change, etc) or in intended uses (riding, lungeing, jumping, etc), these areas should be analyzed together with the owner or rider of the horse. Horses often move without problems during the inspection in-hand and only show the real problem once they are ridden.

Rein-back at the end of the inspection is not only for obedience, but horses with back or pelvic problems can show immense defensive reactions, such as rearing, which can be an important diagnostic reference to the problems.

16.2.3. Presenting the horse on the lunge

When the inspection in-hand has been done, the horse should be moved free on the lungeing circle, first in walk, the trot and canter as well. Shortening the lunge line can provoke increased loading of the hind legs and influence the longitudinal bend and positioning of the horse.

The horse should wear brush boots or bandages and possibly overreach boots and a lungeing cavesson without any rein aids. The lunge line should be at least 12m long and the lunge whip must have a long enough lash to reach the horse exactly on the right spot.

Ideally the horse should be worked in a lungeing circle or round pen of at least 20m in diameter. If one only has a riding arena available, one should move around every so often, provoking the circle-straight-circle sequence and thus assess the irregularities of the gait in a better manner. Likewise, many changes of gait, decreasing and increasing the diameter of the circle should be asked to evaluate the pattern of a gait and the activity of the spinal cord.

The surface should have enough grip and not be too deep (not more than 8cm=3 inches).

Horses should move freely in the lungeing cavesson, and one should, every so often, try to abandon the contact to see how the position and longitudinal bend of the horse changes.

16.2.4. Presenting the horse under saddle

When the horse has specific movement disorders in only specific patterns of movements or tasks, he must be ridden in his usual environment, with his usual saddle and bridle, with or without extra aids in order to see the problems.

It is often visible when a horse is ridden that many problems are due to incorrect influence of the rider or shortcomings in the training that should, in the first place, be corrected in a very diplomatic way, for even the best intentions can be inadequate and the blame put on the therapy.

In this presentation, one often sees incorrectly fitted saddles and bridles (too-tight nose-bands, wrong size bits, narrow saddles etc) that can frequently be the cause of all the resistances of the horse. It is for this reason that the assessment of the equipment used is meaningful.

16.3. Movement-palpation analysis

The use of a halter and lead line is advisable for this inspection, as the therapist can injure himself when he gets caught in the leather or buckles of a bridle when the horse makes any defensive movements. What is more, the mobility of the neck and jaw can be better performed with a halter.

Before actually starting with the examination, the horse with halter and lead, not tied, should be spoken to in a friendly way, patted and caressed. Through this the horse will learn to accept the therapist and surrender to touches in unpopular areas such as the stomach.

This examination must be done in a calm environment, for a hectic stable aisle will lead to incorrect results due to the inherent tension that accompanies this restlessness.

In practice: *Different breeds react differently to pressure. For example, one can find a thin-skinned English Thoroughbred reacting with extreme defensive movements when just slightly touched, whereas an Island pony will not even look back when much stronger pressure is applied.*

16.3.1. Head and neck

Once contact with the horse has been established, one stands on the side of the horse and palpates gently along both the Christa facilis to test the M. masseter for any tension. The last portion will be to palpate the temporomandibler joint for any trigger points (see Chapter 18.6) and to check the mobility. (fig.16.1) To do that, take the mandible and maxila and try to achieve a sideways movement, similar to that of chewing. Likewise an opening and closing of the mouth should be provoked. In these two examinations any restriction in the range of motion is sought.

Next, one palpates the atlanto-occpital junction, for any asymmetric appearance and sensitivity to pressure. One palpates distally along the neck vertebra and tries to feel for muscular tension (M. splenius, M. rectus capitus) in the form of a higher muscle tone (trigger points). (fig.16.2) In order to arrive at a clear conclusion, one must have a lot of experience in the

Fig. 16.1.
a. Examining the temporo-mandibler joint for trigger points

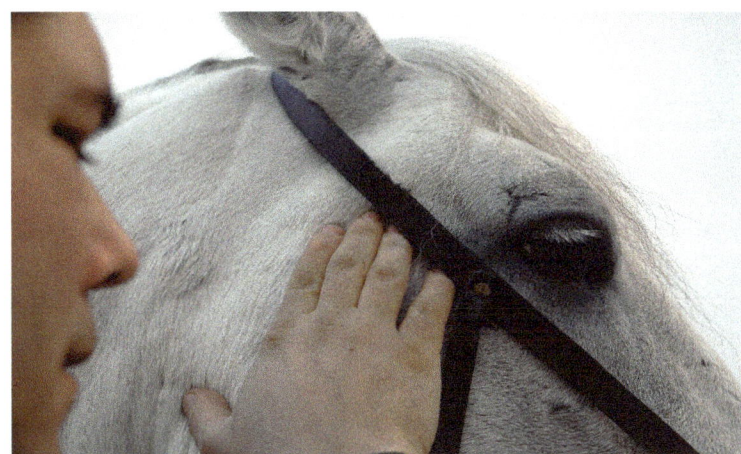

palpation technique. From the occiput, one palpates ventrocaudodistal all the muscle groups of M. trapezius, Pars cranialis, M. brachiocephalicus and M. sternocleidomastoideus and tries to also find reaction to trigger points.

After this, mobility tests are done on both sides, where the hand furthest takes the bridge of the nose and with the other hand holding against, segment after segment is touched, while the other hand pulls the head of the horse toward the body of therapist (see fig.14.8).

> **Note:** *It is very important not to do any rough movements or movements against the will of the horse. An inexperienced hand can cause irreparable damage to the neck vertebrae.*

b. Mobilization of the jaw.

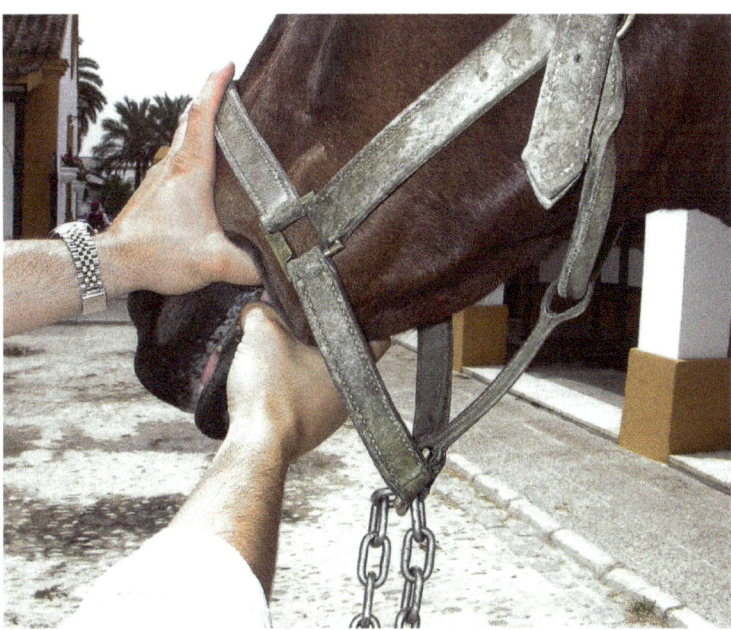

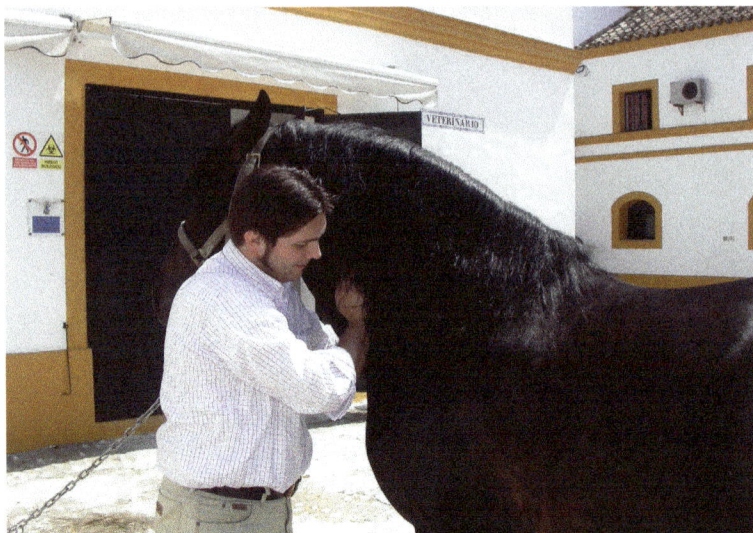

Fig. 16.2. Palpation of the neck vertebrae must always be bilateral for comparison.

Easier, but much less specific, is the carrot test, where the horse must follow a carrot as far as possible in the direction of the hip and only perform a rotation movement in the last third of the neck vertebrae.

16.3.2 Forehand

In the shoulder, one carefully palpates the cranial and caudal sections of the M. trapezius, and slowly over the M. supraspinatus and M. infraspinatus to the triceps muscles, where one palpates superficially at first, and then gradually goes deeper. Here the position of the two shoulder and elbow joints are compared, the tenderness tested and trigger points are sought. Deeper palpation of the triceps can occasionally lead to heavy defensive reactions, for there are often painful tensions in this area.

The bursa of the bicep tendon is of great interest in the shoulder. One palpates along the extensors and flexors to the tendon and tests it for increased thickness and painfulness to pressure.

Subsequent to that, shoulder and elbow mobility is tested. One carefully stretches the front leg forward and up and moves it slightly in the adduction and abduction planes to explore painful reactions and movement restrictions. Then the shoulder is pulled in a half-bent position, caudally to put tension on the tendon of the biceps and test it. (See fig.14.10 and 14.11)

The bent legs then get tested for movement restrictions in the Os carpi accessorium (fig.16.3) as well as adduction and abduction of the carpus.

The fetlock is carefully bent and the sesamoid bones are tested for their tendency to slide and the restriction of movement to the side is also assessed. In this case, a helper can hold the cannon bone, making it easier

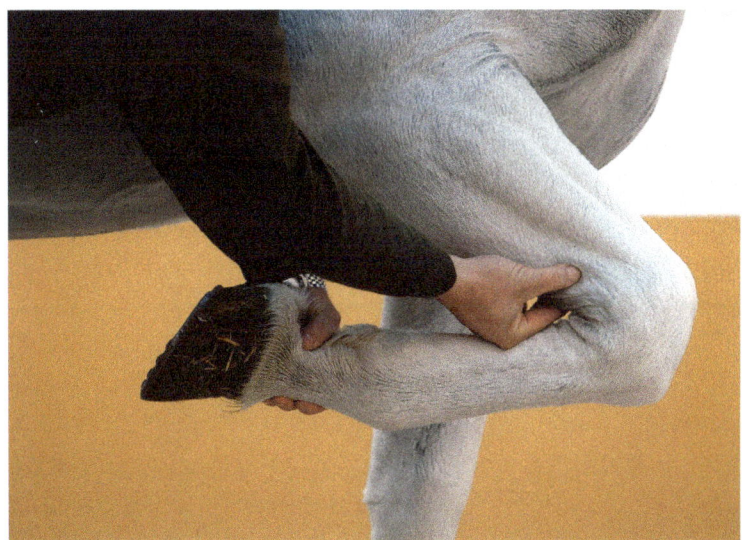

Fig. 16.3. Palpation of the Os carpi accessorium. Here it is tested for restriction of movement. It should be done on both legs for comparison.

for therapist to lightly rotate the fetlock joint with both hands, and to feel the possible blockages in the joint. The tendons must also be checked at this opportunity, first with a superficial palpation and then a deeper palpation and the check ligament must be assessed for tenderness.

After comparing the two front legs, the withers and the vertebrae should be checked for any swelling, unevenness and blockages. At first, one palpates with the fingertips along the spine up to the sacroiliac joint.

Thereafter, one palpates along the trapezius muscle across the M. lattisimus dorsi to the M. longissimus dorsi and the M. iliocostalis. These are inspected for tension and trigger points.

16.3.3 Hindquarters

The sacroiliac joint must be examined for asymmetric points of the bone structures. Thereafter one palpates along the croup muscles between the M. semi-tendinosus and M. semi-membranosus to find tense spots.

In the area of the croup the N. ischiadicus should also be examined. When one-sided sensitivity to pressure is found, one can possibly speak of neuritis of the N. ischiadicus which is often accompanied by asymmetry of the sacral tuberosities and the croup muscles.

The hip joint can only be tested indirectly for trigger points around the joints, with an ab- or adduction movement. Painful reactions and short blocking of the movement are possible indicators of a lesion in this area.

The knee must be examined for instability of the patellar ligaments. In doing so, therapist pulls the horse to his side while examining the patella for the tendency to slide with the other hand. When the ligaments are unstable, the patella will be too loose. The knee must then be bent in such a way that the therapist stands next to the horse and the leg is positioned similar as with the farrier facing backwards. In this position one can apply pressure on the calcaneus and thus test the Achilles tendon.

The mobility of the hock can be tested in the bent leg as follows: the bent hock is moved in an ad- and abduction movement from the cannon bone, more and less under the belly of the horse. The fetlock joint is examined in the same manner as the front legs.

16.3.4. Vertebrae

Once the horse is used to being manipulated, the movement possibilities of the thoracic and lumbar vertebrae can be examined. For this, one stands caudally, looking towards the head of the horse, puts the hand on the height of the seat bone opposite, and by pulling and pushing causes a rocking movement.

In this process the hand stays on the parts that are examined and checks them for movement restrictions. This procedure also requires a lot of practice and feeling.

Subsequently one stands closer to the shoulders and attempts to achieve an arching of the back through light pressure on the breast bone (see fig.14.16) At the same time one can palpate the pectoral and abdominal muscles. Caution should be exercised with mares and thoroughbred horses, as they often paw with their front legs when they feel harassed.

After this mobility test, a light pressure in the saddle area should provoke a hollowing of the back (see fig.14.17.) When this is possible, one can, segment by segment, try to get rid of all the restrictions in the movement.

In conclusion, one stands behind the horse and with both hands provokes an arching of the back by pressure on both sides about a hand's width from the sacroiliac joint. (See Fig.14.18) The vertebrae of the tail is the end of the spinal cord and by bending and rotating, it can be tested for any problems.

16.4. Thermography

Definition: *Thermography is an imaging procedure to view superficial temperature distribution. Thermography measures infrared waves, radiated by every living being, and converts them into a color heat pattern. This imaging procedure can give important information on inflamed or under-supplied areas.*

Seeing that the body surface is about 5 degrees cooler than the inside body temperature, the difference is clearly displayed with thermography. A difference of 2 degrees when comparing sides is significant. By comparing sides the regions with a higher temperature are shown in a different color scheme, making it possible to come to a conclusion regarding pathological matters in these regions. In some pathological cases a reduction in circulation can be a problem caused by edema.

In the course of healing and monitoring complimentary therapies, the use of thermography can be an advantage for documenting the progress of healing and improvement in the circulation after successful therapy.

Raised temperature differences resulting from overloading in training can manifest up to two weeks prior to a clinical lameness, making this system especially useful in recognizing early tendinitis. A corresponding change in the training can be made after a thermographic examination which can often prevent lameness.

Note: *Thermography does not replace advanced imaging such as sonography or x-rays. It is only capable of narrowing down diagnostically relevant areas.*

To avoid distortion of the surface temperature, it is important to stable the horses at least two hours before an examination without any exposure to the sun. Stable bandages and rugs should also be removed as they will otherwise give an incorrect positive result. (fig.16.4)

When horses are lunged or ridden before the examination, one can often see the impressions of the lungeing surcingle or saddle for several hours after, making a correct interpretation more difficult. Even grooming the horse before an examination can make a difference.

In winter, when the hair is longer, the interpretation of the heat

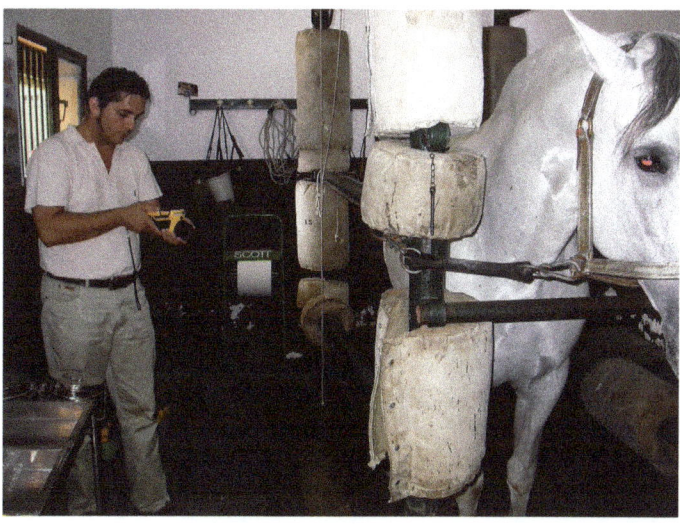

Fig. 16.4.
A thermogaphy examination must always take place in an environment that is free from sunshine and drafts. This horse is in the examination stand at the REAAE.

Robert Stodulka, D.V.M.

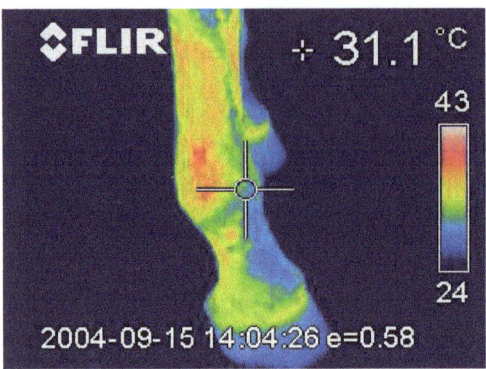
a. Arthritis of the fetlock

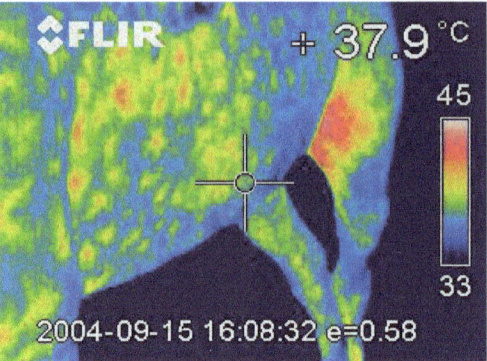
b. Desmitis of the middle patellar ligament

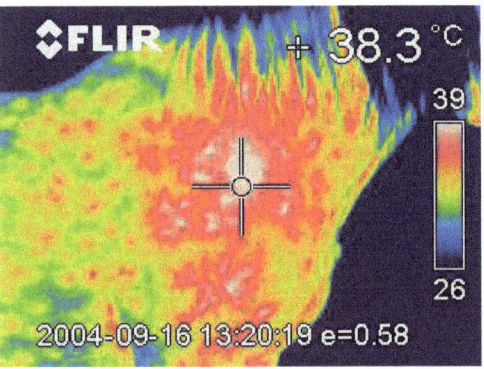
c. Tear of the M. supraspinatusligament

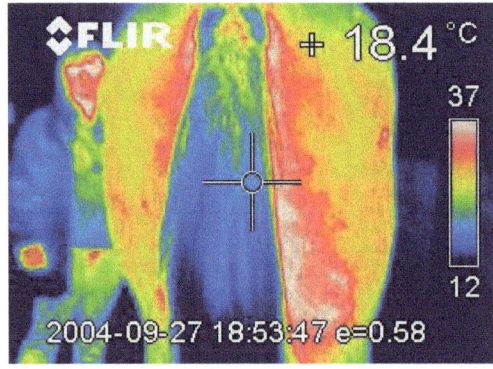
d. Tear of the M. semimembranosus

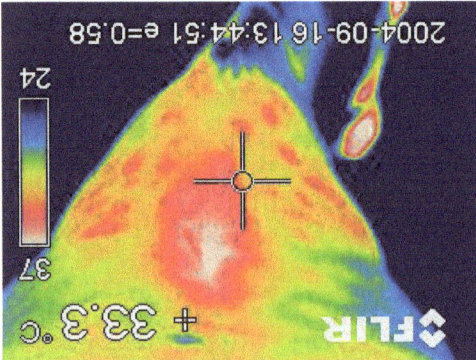
e. Kissing spines

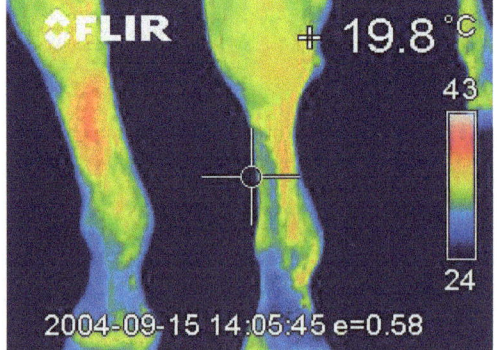
f. acute periostitis(front right medial)

Fig. 16.5. Illustration of different lesions with the help of thermography. (all findings obtained were verified with sonography and x-rays)

pattern can often be more complicated. Hairless areas, whorls, scars or brand marks all appear warmer in a thermogram and must therefore be especially considered so as not to interpret results incorrectly.

Sweating horses or an environment with a high humidity will also falsify a thermogram, making the tool difficult to use.

Furthermore, application of cool gels and liniment must be omitted two days before an examination. Showering and airing the stable before an examination should be avoided and the administering of anti-inflammatory medication should be avoided for that may cause a general cooling of the legs which does not allow for any kind of reliable interpretation of thermogram.

In Practice: *In the ideal case, one has a dark room without any draft with an inside room temperature of 20 degrees, where the horse can become acclimatised for 2-3 hours. Practically speaking this is almost never possible, and one should adapt to the circumstances, but it should at least be without a draft and direct sunshine, for horses can "warm-up" or "cool down" relatively quickly.*

Muscle injury, joint disorders and decreased blood flow through obstructions (laminitis) can be shown well if the therapist has accurate anatomical knowledge and experience with thermography. (fig.16.5) To avoid an incorrect diagnosis, it is recommended to compare both sides of the body so the individual differences can be better outlined.

As mentioned before, a temperature difference of 1-2 degrees is significant. This statement stems often only from academic interests as the examination cannot be made standard in everyday practice.

Note: *In the first place the comparison of both sides is decisive for the outcome, whether further imaging procedures are to be done or not.*

In this context, it should be mentioned that an accurate knowledge of the blood vessels is necessary for there is always a temperature increase in subcutaneous vessels which is purely physiological. It is for this reason that a diagnosis for the hock is made difficult for the beginner due to the location of the saphenous vein.

As a zone to calibrate, the coronet is seen as the hottest part of the horse's body. The machine must therefore be calibrated from scratch every time for a new patient in order to get a clear heat pattern that is easy to interpret. Automatic calibration is not suitable for horses as the horse emits a lot of infrared radiation due to his body surface and the sweat from the glands can also give a faulty reading.

Apart from its diagnostic use, thermography can be used as demonstration for the owner when used to justify treatment to the skeptical owner. It is especially useful to show the owner that the horse, although no longer lame, should not yet be burdened with competition, which can be of great help to prevent further tendon damage. Unbalanced feet or incorrect loading and overloading can be well documented due to the changing thermographic patterns and can provide valuable information for further action and management of the daily training.

The only disadvantage of this system is the high purchase price although it can be justified due to its versatile fields of application.

17. Movement Therapy: Rehabilitation and Training.

In the world of rehabilitation, movement therapy plays an important part. Not least because the horse is a movement and flight animal that is programed to move, but also, it significantly contributes to his spiritual welfare, and helps in the healing phase, improving the handling of the horse tremendously.

In movement therapy, all aspects of **"Riding in Lightness"** can and should be involved in order to rehabilitate the horse. According to the required outline, the horse can be worked with a rider or without a rider (lunge, walker, treadmill, work in-hand, mobilization).

> **Definition:** *Rehabilitation training includes all the measures taken after the acute phase, after the first three post-traumatic days, to bring the horse back to his original state of movement as fast as possible. In rehabilitation training, apart from physiotherapy, various movement programs are used to improve the mobility, injury and illness of the restricted patient.*

In this context, great importance should be given to the indications for therapy, for it makes a considerable difference whether the horse is rehabilitated after a surgically repaired fracture, a tendon problem, or back pain.

> **Note:** *As the most important criterion is the earliest possible, controlled recovery of the range of motion. (ROM)*

Range of motion is the physiological movement radius of a joint. Osteopathic lesions will have a reversible restriction on this and will provoke functional restrictions for example shortening of the stride, and the result may be anything from a relieving posture to atrophy and muscle shortening. If this is left without treatment, it can delicately impede the normal regeneration period. The reintroduction of the horse as an athlete will be delayed.

> **Note:** *It is important in all rehabilitation measures that a controlled, slow and directed movement is carried out, so that it does not lead to more damage when the horse gets into unpredictable panic situations.*

How rehabilitation programs can be applied to specific indications will be dealt with separately in Chapter 19.

17.1. The difference compared to normal training.

The major difference and limiting factor between general training programs and rehabilitation training programs is the poor state of health of the horse. Many horses are subjected to a rehabilitation program after orthopedic surgery and are only able to work in a limited way because of insufficient carrying capacity.

Habituating the damaged parts to a recovering physiological movement can only be done one step at a time in a modified adaptation phase. This plan must be both matched to the problem and specific to the indication.

Leading the horse in-hand over different terrain will improve proprioception of the posture and the positioning reflex.

Working the horse at the walk 12cm deep gravel will act as massage for the coronet and promotes the circulation of blood through the hoof which, in turn, will stimulate the pump action of the digital cushion. These sessions should last no longer than 10-15 minutes.

Alternating between hard, soft, and gravel surfaces will promote the horse's attention, proprioception and the purposeful lifting and planting of the feet.

Often, horses lose their ability to place their feet, due to very damaged nervous structures (radial lameness). In these cases, an assisted passive demonstration of how to use the legs, initiated by therapist is indicated. This can be done by the use of a cloth or the lunge line being wrapped around the leg. Every forward step of the leg must be supported by a soft pull on the cloth, whereby the muscle can be passively activated and can thus be reprogrammed in the memory of the nervous system, supported by massage.

Cavaletti and poles on the ground are also helpful for the recovery of the proprioception and for developing of the abdominal muscles.

Lungeing, the work in-hand and mobilization exercises should be granted a wider application in rehabilitation, for these therapies play a key role next to therapeutic riding.

Training sessions should be kept to a few intensive minutes. In most cases the movement therapies will be supported by manual therapies.

17.2. Lunge work

17.2.1. Correcting of badly trained horses

Definition: *A badly trained horse is a horse that has learned to effectively oppose his rider due to faulty training methods, which can lead to dangerous situations for both horse and rider.*

Rearing, nappiness, bucking etc are often signs of incorrect training where physical pain and psychological over-taxing were inflicted upon the horse. Depending on the horse's temperament, he will either fall into one of the above mentioned patterns or internalize the conflicts and become restless.

Due to non-compliance or faulty execution of the individual points of the scale of training, we need to correct the horse's training and consider him as if he were a green horse, yet one that has learned (incorrectly) to oppose the rider with his mass.

> **Note:** *Punishment and harsh handling are fundamentally wrong for correction, because the problems can become worse due to the addition of fear of punishment. Calm but consistent handling is necessary to solve these problems.*

All acts of insubordination that are caused by orthopedic and osteopathic reasons should be restored accordingly, before the horse enters a rehabilitation program.

Auto-equilibration is also of great importance in these corrupted horses for many horses have never learned to confidently stretch or accept the contact.

There is a popular recommendation that: Most "horses with back problems" should be corrected with the use of auxiliary training aids to make it easier for the rider to prevent the horse from pulling and to help him 'go on the bit.' This train of thought is basically incorrect when one looks at the training scale. The neck is the most important method of balancing for the horse in order to bring himself into equilibrium and move in rhythm, relaxed and in correct contact with the bit. However, when the horse has learned to fear the training aids, it is urgently necessary to coax the horse back into inner ease to reach physical relaxation. This process of building trust takes much longer than breaking the trust. The horse must learn to move calmly around the trainer in a stress-free manner, without training aids, so he can find his own rhythm.

In principle, various steps of the work for green horses must be repeated, for most "problem horses" lack basic training. The old claim, retraining is more difficult than new training, is true.

The goal of work on the lunge is to achieve a correctly stretched posture and to lengthen the supraspinous ligament and the long back muscles in a rhythmic gait, full of impulsion with maximum relaxation. Only after this is achieved, can one think of working the horse under saddle in the same manner. At this stage, we are at step 3-4 of the training scale.

Many horses associate being ridden with over-taxing, pain and stress. It is exactly for this reason that they should be gradually progressed from easy to difficult and only introduced to movement possibilities after therapy has been successful. Of course this is achieved better without the weight of a rider. The

Nelson Pessoa training system modified by Dr. Stodulka, is an excellent tool in the rehabilitation phase. When it is used correctly, it supports the activity of the hindquarters while simultaneously showing the horse the way to stretch forward and down. After 3-4 weeks, the activity of the back, rhythm, relaxation and contact improves so much that even the quality of the gaits can be dramatically improved. Horses quickly learn that framing of the hindquarters helps them to step more under their bodies, which promotes the arching of the topline. At the same time, the deep adjustment is ideal for stretching the supraspinous ligament which has a positive influence on balance and the rhythm.

Once the horse has learned to move fluently in all three gaits, one can support the work by introducing 3-4 cavaletti (see Chapter 13). In the beginning, a low cavaletti should be placed at the 12, 3, 6 and 9 "o'clock" positions on the circle to aid the horse when he still shows faults in rhythm. Once the horse accepts the cavaletti, one can set up trot cavaletti with a distance of 1.30m [4'-3"] for a big horse. [Correspondingly, the distance can be reduced for shorter-striding horses].

Setting up 3-4 cavaletti at a lower height will make it possible to intentionally lengthen the moment of suspension as well as the stance phase, making the topline arch more and, at the same time, lower the neck. The horse should trot over the cavaletti in a calm and rhythmic manner. Higher cavaletti in canter distance of 3.20 m [10'-6"] will especially promote the hindquarters to come under the body through several in-and-out jumps over small hurdles. This also strengthens the loins but should only be started once the horse is confirmed in the trot cavaletti work.

Cavaletti work is very strenuous due to accentuated stepping, stretching of the topline and contraction of the abdominal muscles, and should therefore not be repeated more than 10 times in each direction. Trotting over too-high cavaletti should be completely discouraged, since the horse is only tempted to lift his legs without arching the back, easily producing "a leg-mover." Only sensible use of training aids has gymnastic value.

It is also important to use solid and stable cavaletti and not poles that can roll on the ground so the work does not become dangerous for the horse. When horses step on poles on the ground, the distances change and they can get serious injuries and pulled ligaments from the rolling poles. It is therefore important to work with proper equipment.

17.2.2. The rehab patient on the lunge

There are some important basic details to be considered when recuperating and rehabilitating a horse on the lunge: Is this an orthopedic patient that has to be rehabilitated after conservative or surgical care for his lameness, or is it an orthopedically healthy horse that is a "back patient"?

In the first case, we have to decide whether circular movement is meaningful or not on the basis of the indications.

Surgically treated fracture patients drop out of this scheme, for the danger of overloading the reinforced limb is just too great. In the same way, bruised tendons and ligaments should not be worked on the lunge, unless they are sedated and can be controlled at the walk only.

> **Note:** *In this context it should be mentioned that the main gait of orthopedic rehabilitation patients is the walk, since this gait has the smallest centrifugal shearing force.*

Lungeing is also only advised after two to three weeks of leading in-hand on straight lines, to allow the inflammation to subside after the horse has completed conservative lameness therapy using anti-inflammatory and intra-articular injections. Thereafter, the horse should be worked principally in trot with training aids and lungeing cavesson to get rid of tension.

It is recommended to lunge a horse in an arena where one can constantly change the position and move on straight lines, thus decreasing the additional centrifugal and shearing forces in the damaged joints. This will motivate the horse and minimize the circular movement.

As mentioned before, the main goal for "back patients" is twofold: the rebuilding of atrophied muscles of the back and restoring the full spectrum of movement of the horse. Reaching the often-mentioned stretched posture therefore remains the most important criterion, such that the topline can be stretched and loosened. Training over cavaletti, gymnastic jumping and similar exercises can all improve the horse's activity of the back and the strength to carry weight. Horses that are already further in their training can be worked on the double lunge by an experienced trainer to improve the activity of the hindquarters.

Horses with neurological fail through exogenic trauma; for example, impact injuries or falls, can gain better proprioception when 2-3 poles are put down in irregular distances to improve coordinated use of the feet. Naturally these obstacle runs should be carried out at the walk. Different depth and texture (sand, gravel, asphalt) footing can also obtain improved proprioception for it promotes the depth sensibility of the foot.

In some rehabilitation centers, one finds lungeing circles with a light slope to the outside, whereby a different loading possibility on the outside pair of legs can be obtained to improve the concentration and balance of the horse. Posture and position reflexes can be promoted in this way; the horses move more calmly and rhythmically due to the slope, thus reducing the centrifugal and shearing forces.

The use of weighted boots can help to strengthen parts of a muscle and help to attain muscle symmetry. In order not to overtax the joints and the ligaments, these horses should be worked at the walk only for the weights can lead to a stronger centrifugal force at other gaits. When the weighted boots are then removed, the horse becomes more free in his movements due to specific muscle development. This means when weighted boots are sensibly used, they can actually improve the action of a gait. Nevertheless their danger regarding overloading when used in faster gaits should be remembered.

17.3. Use of training aids and their importance in rehabilitation and training

In orthopedic physiotherapy, the use of training aids, that can lead a horse in an easy and understandable manner to the stretched position, is of great value.

> **Note:** *Every kind of gadget that fixes the horse's head in one position is unsuitable for rehabilitation and should be rejected.*

This includes over-check reins, martingales and, to a lesser degree side reins, although side reins can be very useful in the collected work in-hand for a short time.

As follows from the above, for rehabilitation measures: the use of suitable training aids that can aid in reaching an unhindered forward and down stretched position that prepares a horse to be used as a riding horse, is necessary and meaningful.

However, when choosing training aids, individual limitations of conformation for each horse should be considered. Changing over to a new system requires time for adaption and this time should likewise be alloted to the horse.

In the author's daily practice of rehabilitation, the modified Pessoa system is almost exclusively used (see Chapter 9.3). This system allows for the possibility for adjustment to a lower or higher position of the horse's head, making it possible to work different muscles between stretching and tensing with one system.

When a horse is lunged with this system, he learns within 2-3 weeks to find his own rhythm, improve their back activity and to keep their own rhythm in the gaits. The canter is often tremendously improved as the harness softly animates the haunches to step under more.

Running side reins can also be used to reach the stretched position, but due to the lack of possibility for collection, they offer less in the way of rehabilitation training.

"*Halsverlängerer*[16]" and chambon should not be used in the rehabilitation phase, for too much pressure is put on the poll which could provoke a defensive reaction in sensitive horses.

Side reins usually prevent the horse from stretching forward and down for they frame the horse at a specific limit. This promotes a down and backwards position of the head and the necessary stretch for the topline can never be achieved. This can be desirable for a short period of time when working in-hand or beginning piaffe, but only has limited usefulness in a therapeutic lungeing program. Nevertheless, should side reins be used, they should be only of leather, with no rubber rings or rubber inserts, so the horse cannot lean on them.

The chambon[17] and the Gogue[18] generate too much pressure on the poll, and abandon the horse in the decisive moment of yielding. The horse is left on his own without further contact possibilities. Since rehabilitation training is a preparation for being ridden with a light contact to the mouth of the horse, these systems seem to be of little use. Furthermore, horses with back problems often have greater sensitivity to pressure on the poll.

The rubber "*halsverlängerer*" provokes leaning or bearing on the rubber elements, that can later only serve as an insufficient contact, for horses lean on this and go more on the forehand. In addition, it generates pressure on the poll where many horses with back problems already are sensitive.

---

16   *Halsverlängerer* are elastic draw reins, which are run down from the saddle girth between the front legs through the bit rings behind the ears over the headpiece.

17   The chambon is a strap that runs forward from the bottom of the girth or surcingle, and forks. The forks continue to a ring on either side of the bridle or halter, at the base of the crown piece. Running through those rings, the forks follow the cheek pieces to the bit. They may attach to the bit or pass through the bit rings and attach to themselves below the horse's neck.

18   The Gogue is a leather piece with cords attached. These cords fork at the horse's chest and each run through one of the bit rings. The cord then follows the cheek piece of the bridle up to a ring or pulley at the side of the browband, before going back down to snap to the leather piece near the chest. The leather extends so that it can attach to the girth.

Robert Stodulka, D.V.M.

18. Complimentary Physiotherapeutic Methods at a Glance

Definition: *Physiotherapy is a form of therapy that takes advantage of all physical foundations and variables, whereby a healing impulse is given.*

In this context, variables such as warmth, cold, pressure, current, light (laser), sound waves and magnetic fields are to be mentioned, and can be used according to specific indications.

In the following article, the most common methods of physiotherapy and rehabilitation medicine, including pain treatment, will be briefly presented. In the process, the medicinal care of the rehabilitation patient is intentionally not discussed, for it is about the physical therapies and only the ones that are seen as practical are discussed. Conventional pain therapy can and should be used in rehabilitation medicine and has corresponding value. Movement therapy is discussed in Chapter 17, mobilization techniques in Chapter 14.

18.1. Manual therapies

Definition: *Manual therapies, (derives from Latin "manus" meaning hand) are all therapeutic measures done with the hands of therapist. This includes massage, stretching, mobilization, acupuncture, lymph drainage, and in a broader sense, also osteopathy and chiropractic.*

Through these more or less structural techniques, depending on the procedure, muscle bundles will be mobilized on the one hand, subsequently ensuring an improved range of motion, and on the other hand, vasodilation caused by the massage will supply the affected area with increased blood and oxygen. The relaxation effect from these therapies takes place via the autonomic nervous system through the parasympathetic system, that makes itself noticeable through deep relaxation and satisfied chewing.

18.1.1. Stretching and mobilization

Definition: *Stretching and mobilization are both active and passive techniques that can improve the mobility of individual body—and joint sections.*

Stretching and mobilization have as their main aim, via the Golgi tendon organs, to stimulate the muscle spindles and thus reach an improved function through the lengthening of the designated muscle parts.

In contrast to osteopathic and chiropractic techniques, that can at first glance seem similar, stretching and mobilization are not used as a correction for osteopathic lesions, but only to improve the likelihood of mobility through systematic stretching. This will for example resolve the stickiness that is formed with tendon injuries.

Mobilization can and should be practiced before riding in order to promote the horse's joy of movement. (See Chapter 14)

In practice: *Stretching and mobilization are always progressively carried out in such a way that the affected leg is stretched to the point where a light resistance is felt. At this point the stretch is held for 10 seconds and the leg is replaced.*

This will cause a synergistic interplay between tension and relaxation, whereby the best effect regarding increased range of motion can be achieved. This will prevent muscle tears and lessen the danger of injury for both the horse and the rider. Abrupt attempts to stretch however, can be very painful for the horse and lead to massive protest reactions.

18.1.2. Osteopathy and chiropractic

Osteopathy is a holistic procedure, founded by A. T. Still[19], which theorizes that every disease must be preceded by fundamental structural changes of the axial skeleton. Correction of these structural changes with the use of osteopathy allows the body to mobilize the inherent powers of healing. Restoration of the functional health of the axial skeleton is of fundamental importance.

Definition: *An osteopathic lesion is a reversible, functional movement restriction, that is not found in the pathophysiologocal space in the joint.*

Subluxations with destruction of neighboring structures cannot be influenced through osteopathic techniques.

Normally longer levers with low speed thrust is used in osteopathy, which is one of the differences to chiropractic, which works with short levers and high speed thrusts. The direction of the manipulation in osteopathic treatment goes into the blockage—similar to the release of a handbrake—which is not painful.

---

19 Andrew Taylor Still, MD, (August 6, 1828 – December 12, 1917) was the founder of osteopathy and osteopathic medicine. He was also a physician and surgeon, author, inventor and Kansas state legislator. He was one of the founders of Baker University, the oldest four-year college in the state of Kansas, and was the founder of the American School of Osteopathy (now A.T. Still University), the world's first osteopathic medical school, in Kirksville, Missouri.

A special form of osteopathy is craniosacral therapy, which stimulates the cerebrospinal liquid through the meninges, by the influence of the seams of the skull, and carries out corrections to the axial skeleton by means of deep relaxation.

This method developed from the teachings of the American, chiropractor Daniel Palmer[20], who saw changes in the spinal cord as disease-causing and wanted to influence them. As said before, chiropractic differs from osteopathy regarding the direction of manipulation. In chiropractic the levers used are clearly shorter than in osteopathy. Chiropractic adjustments, unlike osteopathy, can be painful.

18.1.3. Massage

Massage is one of the oldest forms of therapy that has its origins in the therapeutic use of hands. In linguistic history, the word comes from the Arabian "mass" which means touch. The origin of this therapy is said to be from the Orient.

Definition: *Massage has the following goals in animal physiotherapy: increased circulation, improved metabolism, faster removal of waste products, improvement of performance and mobility, increasing the subjective well-being, and a secondary analgesic effect (relaxing of trigger points, releasing tension etc).*

The therapeutic effect of massage is the relaxation of the lymphatic and vascular systems. Improved circulation can furthermore provoke an adjustment of the muscle tone.

Furthermore, the improved supply of nutrients to the tissues can cause a tightening of the connective tissue and a reduction of pain sensation through the "gate-control-mechanism." Subsequently, psychogenic relaxation can be achieved.

By the same token, massage can loosen scar tissue and adhesions. Apart from classical massage, lymphatic drainage and connective tissue massage expand the therapeutic spectrum.

Note: *All massage techniques must be adapted to every individual horse with regard to tolerance to pressure and duration.*

A massage carried out on an unwilling horse not only causes a bad atmosphere for the next treatment, but really does not help as the horse cannot reach a state of physical relaxation.

---

20 Daniel D. Palmer, the founder of chiropractic

Indications for classical massage are:
- myogelosis
- tendinopathy
- tension, muscle hardening
- trigger points
- flaccid paralysis
- muscle atrophy
- post-traumatic and post-operative orthopedic states
- osteoarthritis and arthritis

Absolute contra-indications are all inflammatory processes of the skin, thromboplebitis, lymphangitis, any general disease with fever, poor well-being, tumors, fresh fractures and a danger of embolism.

Classical massage uses different hand techniques such as mechanical pressure, traction, vibrations and displacements of the skin and the connective, neural and vascular tissue beneath it. A secondary improvement in the mobility of different joints can be achieved. In principle, one distinguishes two types:
- All deep techniques, like effleurage, deep petrissage, strong tapotement[21] and the frictions have a toning effect.
- All superficial, soft tapotement and vibration act in a relaxing way

Effleurage (stroking)

Definition: *Effleurage is a technique which covers a bigger area (flat hand, ball of the thumb, knuckles only in deep effleurage) and is applied superficially to gain the trust and consent of the horse. It is also used in the palpation examination.*

Through a relaxing effect, increased circulation is achieved in the treated areas of the body. The massage should also be ended with effleurage. Deep effleurage will influence the connective tissues and muscles, improving the circulation and in turn, speeding up the removal of waste products from the body.

---

21 Tapotement is a specific technique used in Swedish massage. It is a rhythmic percussion, most frequently administered with the edge of the hand, a cupped hand or the tips of the fingers. There are five types of tapotement including Beating (closed fist lightly hitting area), Slapping (use of fingers to gently slap), Hacking (use the edge of hand on pinky finger side), Tapping (use just fingertips) and Cupping (make your hand look like a cup and gently tap area). It is primarily used to "wake up" the nervous system and also as a stimulating stroke and can release lymphatic build up in the back and gently tap the shoulder of the client. The name of the stroke is taken from the French word "Tapoter", meaning to tap or to drum.

Petrissage (kneading)

> **Definition:** *The main effect of petrissage is the lifting of the skin from the connective tissue underneath it and the loosening and the stimulation of blood flow. The tissue is taken crosswise or diagonally to the run of the muscle fiber, lifted and moved, in this manner achieving an effective loosening of adhesions.*

Adhesions below the surface of the skin should be broken up and lymph drainage stimulated, thereby having a positive effect on muscle tone.

The C-grip can be well-used on the neck and hamstring muscles. In the process, the subsequent layers of the tissue mass will be lifted little by little and mobilized in the direction of the lymphatic flow.

Due to the size of horses, one mainly uses double handed petrissage or the C-grip.

Friction

This is a very deep technique and therefore highly stimulating. One distinguishes between moving technique, sliding technique, gelotripsy [local kneading massage of myogeloses] and transverse friction.

In the moving technique, the hands work deep into the muscles, achieving a strong stretching of the tissues, a stronger metabolic activity and improvement of elasticity of the muscles.

In the sliding technique, the knuckles or joints of the hands are first superficially used, then certain points are treated in a circular movement, and these areas are stretched and lifted.

Localized treatment of myogeloses is done with gelotripsy. The therapist uses the finger tips or elbow and works towards the trigger point or myogelose (muscle knots) in a circular movement, in order to achieve a release. This can be a very painful procedure, so the therapist should be sensitive to the magnitude of the horse's response.

Transverse friction, as used in all tendinopathies, is a special form of friction. The area is moved crosswise to the fibers with two fingers. The already tense tendon area will be stimulated by the Golgi tendon organ[22] to relax through a reflex action.

---

22 Present in all vertebrates, the Golgi tendon organ, named after Camillo Golgi, is a sensory organ of depth perception. It is a kind of nerve plexus, which is used to measure and control muscle tension. It is located at the junction between muscle and tendon and is responsible along with the muscle spindles for the proprioception of the muscles.

Vibration

Definition: *Vibration is a muscle relaxing technique that can be used by reason of its relaxing effect, also while mobilization and traction techniques are being applied. They can be used locally with the finger tips or the palm of the hand.*

Shaking the legs can have an enormous relaxing influence on the muscles of the legs. A vibration massage on the front legs relaxes the triceps muscles. Vibration massage can be applied manually or with the use of vibration machines or ultrasound apparatuses.

Tapotement[23] (Schüttelungen)

Definition: *Tapotement is a strong circulation promoting and tone stimulating technique, performed with the edge of the hand.*

A more rigid carpal joint [of the practitioner] can strengthen the tapping movement and a light cushioning can soften the effect. Tapotement can also be executed with a cupped hand, which is less precise, but the patient can tolerate it better. The taps can be used in a large area such as the back, upper arm and hamstring area of the horse. Care should be taken with sensitive horses, for many of them find tapotement an irritating, unpleasant harassment and can react to this sudden exposure by kicking orbiting to show their discomfort.

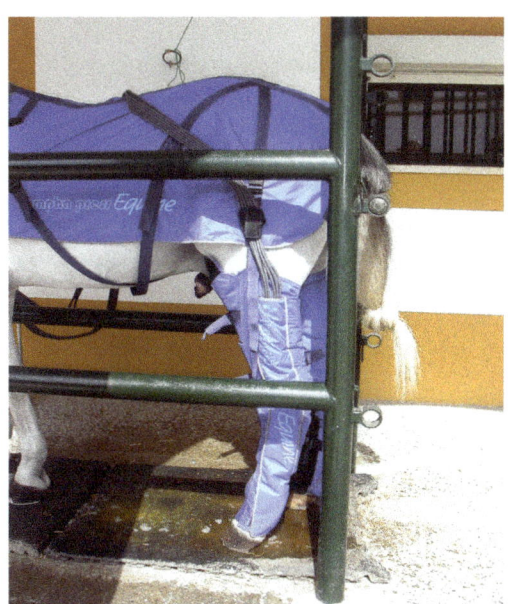

Fig. 18.1. Mechanical lymph drainage

---

23   Massage in which the body is tapped rhythmically with the fingers or with short rapid movements of the sides of the hand.

Lymph drainage

> **Definition:** *Lymph drainage represents a special form of massage, which promotes the removal of interstitial fluid via the lymphatic system.*

The lymphatic drainage works through increased lymphatic transport, thus activating the parasympathetic nervous system and the stimulation of the local and systemic immune system. In lymphatic drainage, one uses different techniques such as pumping circles, cupping and wringing.

> **Note:** *The direction of the massage is to follow the flow of venous blood toward the main lymphatic duets. This can cause problems when directed in the wrong direction. The field of application includes all kinds of edema and all post-traumatic and post-operative swellings.*

Acute and chronic inflammation, thrombosis, circulatory decompensation and all tumorous illnesses are contra-indication.

Apart from manual lymphatic drainage, one also uses compression machines that rhythmically massage the legs from the bottom to the top. A crush pen is necessary for this as it could become expensive if a horse accidentally breaks a machine due to some defensive movement. (fig.18.1)

It is actually irrelevant which method one uses, but the last mentioned is more expensive to purchase. However, it is important that the big lymph nodes are opened and activated, so the lymph can actually be drained.

Connective tissue massage

In connective tissue massage one performs a tangential traction force on the subcutaneous connective tissue to eliminate local swelling. Depending on the area, it can be skin, subcutaneous tissue and fascia involved. This occurs as a consequence of the "vicerocutaneous" reflex, as is often heard in neural therapy, where the mutual influence of the organs on the body segments, and vice versa, lead to poor condition of the corresponding area of skin. This is felt as swelling or thickening of the subcutaneous tissues.

These nodules are painful. In small animals they can be easily felt, in horses they are usually less apparent. This technique is mentioned for completeness.

18.2. Device therapies

In device therapies one finds all the machines that are seen by the layman as "physiotherapy." Apart from the soft laser and magnetic therapy devices, one should look at TENS (transcutaneous electrical nerve stimulation), therapeutic ultrasound and iontophoresis.

18.2.1. TENS

Definition: *TENS stands for transcutaneous electrical nerve stimulation.*

Horses experience pain as muscles start to tense up while information from the brain or spinal cord is transferred into action by a relevant stimulus.

In TENS, an electrical current that blocks the transmission of pain to the brain is sent and in return is processed by the central nervous system.

Through this process, an analgesic and vasodilatory response is provoked at the appropriate location. TENS is also very effective in paralysis caused by muscle atrophy (sweeny[24]). The effect also produces rapid reduction of swelling. Investigations have proved that daily use for 14-28 days can improve capillary circulation between 50 and 100%.

In Practice: *TENS devices for use on horses should always have 2 exits and be easy to use because horses are highly sensitive to electrical current and show defense reactions easily.*

The device must have electrodes that are easy to stick on the horse, for the hair makes an air pocket that makes connection difficult. (fig.18.2) In good machines, one can adjust the intensity, frequency and wavelength, all of which are important for an efficient TENS therapy. Before attaching the electrodes, the machine must be switched off.

Note: *A good analgesic effect can be reached with a frequency of 2 with a wavelength between 230 and 250. For a relaxation effect, frequencies between 20 and 80 with a wavelength of 50 is sufficient.*

When a stronger stimulation is needed, one should slowly increase the intensity until a tolerable measure is found.

With a little practice, one can quickly find the reactive zones and the horses enjoy the rhythmic tensing and relaxing of the muscles, which improves circulation to the tissue.

Definition: *E1 and E2 are the pair of electrodes that should be attached paramedically on the site to be treated.*

---

24 Sweeny: atrophy of the shoulder muscles in horses.

When the two electrodes are attached in a longitudinal direction relative to each other, there will be no rhythmic contraction. It will then only be possible to keep the analgesic effect of the impulse.

Tips for the treatment of pain or tension in the back or simply for a better warm-up effect are the following:

1. Pain in the thoacolumbar area, gluteal area, sacroiliac joint. The E1 attached one hand lateral to the end of T18. E2 at the side of the tuber sacral.
2. Pain in the loin and sacrum area. E1 placed one hand lateral to and between L3 and L4. E2 lateral at the third sacral vertebrae.
3. Pain in the gluteal area, irritation of the ischias. E1 placed laterally near L5. E2 on the pelvic bone.
4. Pain in the sacroiliac area. E1 placed directly in front of the wings of the ileum. E2 in the area of the second or third sacral vertebra.

In all of these combinations, one should look for a light rocking motion of the area. All easily accessible muscles can be treated as long as the electrodes do no slip for anatomical reasons.

18.2.2. Soft laser

Soft laser is one of the most useful machines available in physiotherapy today, for it has an excellent bio-active effect on damaged tissue through combined light beams of different wave lengths.

Through the effective principle of laser, one can initiate a process of regeneration, stimulating mitochondria, endoplastic reticula and all cellular organs with light rays increasing metabolism. Soft laser can also be used in wound healing disorders, treating trigger points and in laser acupuncture.

Indication for soft laser therapy is supporting the healing process in tendon damage, ligaments and synovial joints. Even if the effect decreases as it gets deeper, it is still more efficient than most topical liniments. It promotes circulation in the back and difficult to reach areas such as the inside of the legs and the "arm pits," whereby it increases removal of waste products and at the same time has an analgesic effect.

In practice: *For horses, a laser with at least 50mWatt is needed, as weaker machines need a longer time per treatment and horses are not able to stay quiet for so long.*

18.2.3. Magnetic field therapy

The principle is similar to that of the soft laser, as it also influences the metabolism. Instead of light, it uses magnetic field waves. Based on the fact that all cells have their own energy of 4-6Hz, they can be influenced by other magnetic waves.

Note: *An analgesic effect is achieved at a frequency of 2Hz and a stimulating effect between 8 and 12Hz. Acute processes are influenced at a lower potential of 2Hz; chronic illness at higher frequencies (8-12Hz).*

Magnetic blankets for the back and neck and boots for the treatment of the legs are available. (fig.18.4) In this context it should be pointed out that only pulsating magnetic devices are scientifically proven as having a therapeutic effect.

Boots or blankets with magnetic inlays, although not harmful, do not add anything essential to the healing process—analogous to the early treatment of podotrochlosis where two magnets were applied on the hoof to improve circulation.

In practice: *During use, the horse should be secured, since many cables can often be a bother and the horse could cause damage to the machine.*

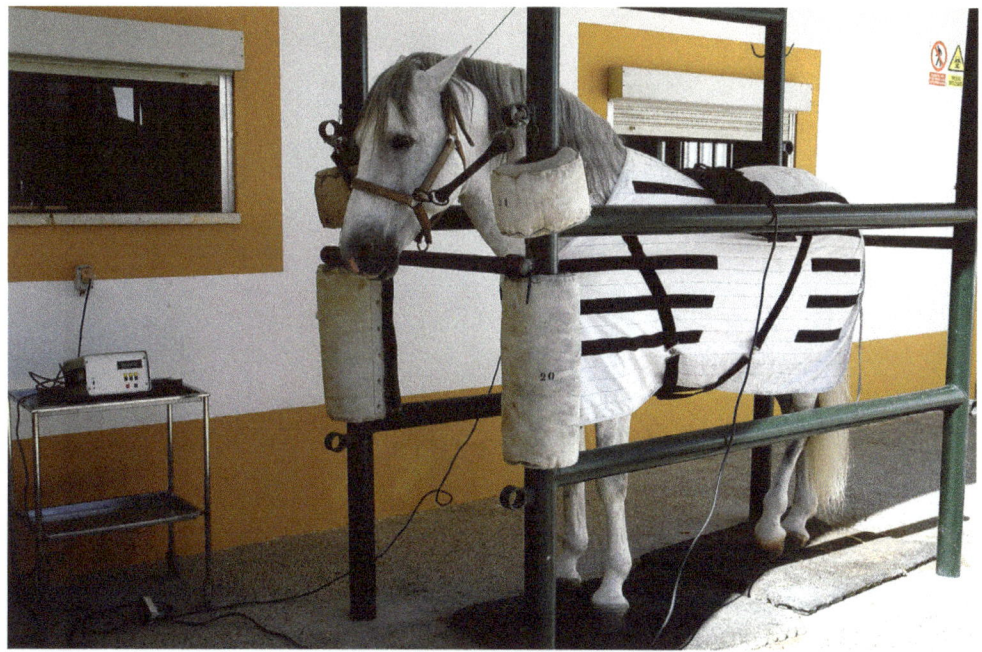

Fig. 18.4. Application of Magnetic field therapy on the back

Since there are so many different machines on the market, one should always read the instructions, because therapeutic recommendations are not the same for every machine.

18.2.4. Therapeutic ultrasound

Ultrasound waves are not absorbed by the skin and can therefore penetrate deeper. The low water content of collagen fibers causes the ultrasound waves to be quickly absorbed. In this therapy, short sound waves in three different frequencies are used, correlating with different depths of penetration. In human medicine, the penetration depth is assigned to the following frequencies:

- 7cm : 0,75MHz
- 4cm : 1,00MHz
- 3cm : 3,00MHz

In Anglican countries, the use of ultrasound for healing of muscle, tendon and ligament injuries is recommended at 0,5-1,5watt/cm for treatment.

Through the bio-active effect, the mechanically produced oscillations turn into vibrations and a rise in temperature in a 5cm radius of the treated area, and painful periostal reactions can occasionally be triggered.

The area to be treated must be shaved, de-greased and be lubricated with a contact gel. A good coupling is very important and this is often difficult in horses. There are 2 application techniques:

- Direct technique
- Immersion technique

In the direct technique, the sound head is directly coupled with the treatment area. The area must be shaved and lubricated with gel.

With the immersion technique, water is used as the medium of transport, thus diminishing the thermal effect. The sound head is held 1-2cm parallel to the area. This technique is only suitable for the distal extremities due to practical reasons.

Literature from human medicine demonstrates enhanced ossification within the first two weeks after a fracture. This could not be scientifically proven in equine medicine.

While ultrasound produces very effective therapeutic effects in small animal practice, the author believes that it has little use for horses. Apart from inadequate coupling despite shaving the area on a horse's leg for the treatment of tendinitis, the depth of penetration is too superficial. The results of ultrasound examinations differ only marginally from untreated horses.

18.2.5. Iontophoresis

Definition: *With Iontophoresis, one takes advantage of different electrical charges to administer medication delivering them between anode and cathode. With this method one can achieve good and deep penetration.*

Indications for Iontophoresis are all painful, inflamed processes; for example tendinitis, and arthritis. Open wounds are contra-indicated.

A good depth of penetration can achieve absorption, analgesia and vasodilation, depending on the medication used.

- Denoix is recommended for the treatment of distortions and tendon illnesses with an application of 2% Calcium chloride solution on the cathode(+).
- 1% potassium iodide solution in treatment of edema on the anode (-).
- 2% sodium salicylic acid on the anode (-) in painful inflammation; such as tendinitis, arthritis.

The treatment area is not shaved to the skin, for this can cause micro injuries and have a negative influence on electrical charges and even provoke burns. With extremely hairy horses, (winter coat) the leg can be partially shaved for better contact.

A moistened sponge-like protective cover with electrodes is placed on the moist skin, with the cathode on the painful area and the anode exactly on the opposite side. Both electrodes are then attached with a stable bandage to avoid loss of contact. When a larger surface (muscle) is to be treated, the electrodes should be no further apart than 5cm to avoid effective loss of effect.

Note: *The duration of the treatment should not be more than 30 minutes to avoid skin irritation. The intensity, depending on the horse, should be between 10 and 25mA.*

18.3. Cold treatment (cryotherapy)

This simple, inexpensive and effective treatment is one of the fundamental pillars of physiotherapy for horses. This is also the oldest therapeutic and regeneration measure known to horse people.

> **Definition:** *The effective principle of cold treatment is the vaso-constriction after 4-6 minutes, followed by an increased circulation-flood (heat rush) thus recruiting deeper lying structures.*

This cycle is repeated in 15 to 30 minute intervals. This means that the meaningful duration of cold treatment is limited. A few minutes several times a day is sufficient to get this physiological process going.

Apart from using cooling boots from the freezer, the easiest cold treatment is the use of ice, and due to thermal irritation of the nerve endings, it will cause vaso-constriction, reduce swelling and decrease the sensation of pain.

Ice can be applied locally on hematomas, muscle injuries, tendinitis and other joint problems. After the application of ice, it is then important to dry the skin, thus arriving at a massage effect for the area.

Hosing the legs of the horse after training and drying them off with a massage, will insufficiently improve the circulation of the distal part of the legs. The use of cooling aids will be more effective.

A very important thing to remember when direct or indirect cold treatment is used: protect the skin of the horse. One can get serious tissue damage due to excessive cooling effect. It is for this reason one finds boots with cooling elements that are inserted for they do not come in direct contact with the skin.

Cold treatment is only effective within 24-72 hours after trauma. Ideal would be a combination of cold treatment with external pressure; for example compression bandages or manual pressure.

Through hastened containment of swelling, post-traumatic or post-operative course of healing will be considerably shorter.

The cooling effect can—also through the vasodilatory reflex—relax muscular tension, for tension often causes pain due to inadequate circulation in the area. An analgesic effect also arises due to the "circuit of delay" induced by the cold irritation.

18.4. Heat therapy

The advantage of heat treatment is in the regeneration of chronic processes, increasing circulation and the metabolic activity.

Thus an increased oxygen supply will lead to "flushing out" of inflammatory mediators and waste products.

Arthritic processes often improve through heat treatment (radiation, warm water, wraps etc), and a reduction of pain is reached through the irritation of the heat receptors. Hence the heat treatment is effective for short term pain reduction.

Besides radiation (solarium), warm towels or heated pads, one can also use blood circulation stimulating ointments.

In order to reach an optimal effect, the areas need to be warmed up at least 5°C. When warming is more than 12°C, horses experience a painful sensation and they try to escape this pain. The skin temperature of a horse is approximately 33°C, therefore the heat treatment must be higher than this value. It may not, however, be higher than 50°C. Ideally it should be 43-50°C, or it can lead to serious structural defects.

The duration of the application should be between 10 and 20 minutes. When the duration arrives at 30 minutes, overheating of the area is provoked.

In Practice: *After heat treatment, mobilization techniques are performed really well, for the horse accepts them much better.*

The warm-up phase of the horse before training cannot be replaced by this routine of heat treatment. It is frequently assumed that the saddled horse under the solarium can be taken into high performance on the spot because his back has already been warmed up. This is not true and can damage the movement apparatus and all the muscles of the horse.

Relaxation of the muscles occurs only one hour after heat treatment due to increased circulation. At the same time, a recovery phase starts. It is for this reason that a one hour rest period is sensible after a session under the solarium.

Hydrosun therapy has a special position in heat treatment, where strongly filtered UV rays can penetrate deeply into the musculature and provoke relaxation. This is also done with mud-packing on the back muscles. Similar to the Chinese "vinegar-fire" back treatment, is considered invigorating.

Subsequently, remember that after every heat treatment on the back the horse should be returned to his stable with a blanket. If this is not done, the convection of the heat is lost, and the horse cools off rapidly, and the danger of getting a cold is high.

18.5. Acupuncture

Acupuncture is a wonderful supplement in the rehabilitation phase, but due to its complexity, is too much for this book, except for a small outline.

For successful application, it is absolutely necessary to acquire the appropriate basic knowledge of Chinese diagnostics and therapy, as anything less will not allow the therapist to fully exploit its possibilities. Western medicine and eastern therapies are only compatible when the veterinarian can manage to find his way around the eastern diagnostic scheme.

> **Definition:** *Acupuncture is about certain sites that have a diameter of more than 2cm and have both a decreased skin resistance and can be detected histologically. These areas are characterized by an aggregation of vascular and nerve bundles.*

Through the study of these areas, the energetic system of the horse can be influenced and a self-healing or regenerating processes can be initiated.

> **Definition:** *The meridian system can be seen as the energy streets in the body, and the acupuncture points as the stop signs and traffic lights.*

It is therefore also possible to influence the meridians by the stimulation of a point through which the Qi energy flows in this energy path. When Qi is accumulated in one area, it is called inflammation in western medicine. It is therefore important, according to our way of thinking, to get the inflammation to subside, which, in traditional Chinese medicine would be for the Qi to leave the area.

Due to the formation of the original neural tube into the nervous system in the development of vertebrates, organ systems can be influenced by their corresponding spinal nerves and vice versa. Over the viscerocutaneous reflex, acupuncture treatment areas can be built that can be instructive on the energetic and pathological situation of the organ. In the same way it is possible to stimulate these organs through a point that is far away from the actual structure.

The SHU points of the bladder meridian, found in the saddle area are the approval points on the energetic situation in the organ so named. Here it becomes obvious that a well-fit saddle not only has an impact on the back mechanics, but also on the organic systems via acupressure.

After successful acupuncture the original pain should be gone. This can be seen as successful therapy. Through the strong influence on the parasympathetic system, a deep relaxation is reached where the horse starts to chew and yawn. This content expression on the horse's face means he is completely relaxed.

Therefore it is important to leave the horse in peace after acupuncture and to do the treatment in a calm, stress-free area, so they can relax.

In Traditional Clinical Medicine [TCM], a pathological situation is seen as an imbalance of YIN and YANG, and depending on what predominates, a picture of the clinical illness can be seen.

Acute suspensory ligament inflammation is seen as a YANG state, and should be treated differently from a weak cough in the morning, which would be a YIN state. In one case, energy should be drained and in the other case energy should be reintroduced. Feeding energy can be with Chinese herbs or via burning Moxa over the corresponding acupuncture points, while draining energy can be done via micro-bleeding on the ting point on the coronet.

Acupuncture has been proven very effective as prevention, therapy, and control in chronic illnesses and in the strained back of the sport horse. The SHU points, found in the saddle area, provide important hints as to the energetic situation of a horse, and overloading symptoms can be recognized early in the corresponding joints.

Acupuncture can also produce an analgesic effect due to the release of endorphins. It also promotes oxygen transport through the relaxation of muscles and thus influences the regeneration process in a positive manner.

Critics always object that every horse in sport will get problems sooner or later. But one should ask why a horse moves well when a hock is x-rayed and two weeks later is lame on that same hock. A horse can obviously manage his problems for a while.

Through regular acupuncture, one makes it possible, in most cases, for the individual to move in harmony with his problems and thus stay powerful and vital. The psychological component of well-being should never be underestimated. Only motivated and relaxed horses stay healthy and powerful in old age.

18.5.1. Combined acupuncture and mobilization therapy

In this combined therapy, the advantages of acupuncture and mobilization therapy are used in an appropriate way.

With the use of acupuncture, where one has the analgesic effect and a strong relaxing effect, mobilization techniques can be more effective. (See Chapter 14) Furthermore, as sport veterinarian, one is safe from the danger of doping, for that cannot happen in this method, an important point for sport horses.

Serious tension and blockages in some body parts can frequently be mobilized only in an inadequate manner or with painful stretching. It is for this reason, not to jeopardize the success of therapy and to avoid further blockages and tensions, that the relaxing neuro-vegetative effect of acupuncture is used, thus influencing the integral posture and reflexes of the body.

Needling painful Ah-Shi points (local painful points in the area, similar to trigger points) can give significant short-term results with respect to pre-competition care.

This would include injecting small quantities of homeopathic remedies, vitamins and the individual's own blood into acupuncture points. Long-term therapy success is more likely than if only one type of therapy is used.

When the therapist is trained in classical acupuncture, it is recommended to use less painful remote points; for example on the legs, to get a longer-lasting response. In order to avoid a "do-it-yourself" sort of acupuncture process, there is intentionally no point combination mentioned here because each case should be diagnosed individually and must be treated as such. With the combination of stretch and mobilization techniques, one can reach a mobility-promoting effect very quickly, and horses can move better and without tension in competition.

Acupuncture is very suitable before a competition or race, as horses will be more loose and relaxed when they approach their high-performance discipline.

18.6. Neural therapy (trigger points)

Definition: *A Trigger point is a muscle hardening that results from muscular tension, that can react painfully when pressed (or even spontaneously) and can impair mobility.*

These reactive areas frequently develop from a relieving posture or an incorrect posture and lead to faulty and often uneconomical sequences of movement, and can make lameness worse.

Trigger points are often found near acupuncture points and are an essential component of diagnosis in physiotherapy. Their development is explained by Bergsman's musculo-kinetic chains: every relieving posture first brings a subconscious and later, an active contraction and increase of tone with it. Through the uneven loading of the legs, one gets a compensatory movement, which leads to overloading of other parts. The hardness of the muscle in a specific area causes energy and nutrient blockage in the tissue, making the removal of lactic acid poor, which will cause painful irritations at the end of the motor nerves. Further contraction and local malnutrition is the result.

This causes a vicious cycle, that should be treated with an appropriate pain therapy. Muscle relaxants, corticosteroids or non-steroid anti-inflammatory cannot solve trigger points, despite their potency. It is for this reason that neural therapy with mobilization techniques is of great importance in the rehabilitation of horses.

Trigger points are often found in the masseter, poll, neck and back muscles, sacroiliac joint, shoulder muscles and in the hamstrings. Due to the extensive possibilities of the existence of such points, it is important that they are found and treated via diagnostic palpation.

Local anesthetic is applied to the trigger points in neural therapy, in order to relax the surrounding muscles with the help of the viscerocutaneous reflex and to provide the patient with relief. In many cases, it is not possible to delete the "cell memory" from the nervous track without neural therapy, which helps break the vicious cycle of the pain spiral.

To perform an infiltration of the root of the nerve and plexus, one must have good anatomical knowledge of the areas and must work under sterile provisions (disinfection, shaving of hair) with disposable material (disposable gloves, needles, syringes) to avoid an existing danger of infection (deep abscess) of the treated area. A complete description of the appropriate techniques is beyond the scope of this book and should be researched in specialist literature.

Neural therapy is ideal in combination with mobilization techniques to ensure fast and effective success. Unfortunately all local anesthetic produces a positive drug screen which makes it unsuitable for competition preparation.

In Practice: *When a horse has been infiltrated in the back, it is better to lunge the horses a few days with the modified Pessoa system or running side reins in a long and low topline to keep the back round and improve upon the painless feeling with stretching and muscle activity in the back.*

19. Rehabilitation Measures for Specific Indications

As already mentioned at the outset, physiotherapy, using musculoskeletal instrumentation, should always be combined with a "post-treatment phase," involving a supportive workout regime. The key to success is choosing the right combination of training and physiotherapeutic measures, before and after competition—or in the rehabilitation phase with injured horses. However, these concepts should not be too programmed or dogmatic. One must always first evaluate the respective patient, and second, evaluate the possibilities with the owner with respect to feasibility and affordability.

19.1. Problems caused by the rider

When horses are inconspicuous from an osteopathic, internist and orthopedic point of view, one should, in any case, assess the horse and rider pair together to determine whether the disturbance of movement comes from too much hand influence or a not-so-independent seat of the rider.

19.1.1. Temporary loss of rhythm, bridle lameness, faulty gaits

Often, temporary loss of rhythm arises from lack of suppleness due to the absence of relaxation. Unyielding and inelastic hands act as additional hindrances. Unfeeling hands exacerbating the problem, especially when the rider mistakenly tries to support losses of rhythm with the reins.

In principle, most of these problems are avoidable when systematic training, according to the principles of the training scale, is applied. Problems can even be corrected, provided the rider has learned to direct the horse with an independently balanced and supple aiding system. There is no recipe for treatment of bad riding; the situation can only be improved when the training technique is well-developed.

Temporary loss of rhythm can often arise from riding forward too strongly; the horse begins to rush, the center of gravity moves forward so that the weight is on the forehand, the carrying power cannot be utilized, and the horse only runs after his center of gravity. The rider tries to compensate for the extra load on the forehand by pulling on the reins, which makes the horse even more resistant and the loss of rhythm becomes more evident.

Definition: *A 'pace' is a two-beat lateral movement with a moment of suspension; in some breeds it even replaces the trot. The left legs of the horse move in unison as do the right legs. (In contrast, the trot is a two-beat diagonal movement.)*

This faulty gait, the pace, can be seen in the walk as well as in the trot.

Note: *In gaited horses, where this gait is often congenital and belongs in their repertoire, the pace develops principally from too strong and an arhythmic influence of the hand.*

The horse fights back by going against the hand, pushing the lower neck forward (M. brachiocephalicus). He lowers the back and tenses the M. longissimus dorsi, M. trapezius and M. lattissimus dorsi. This leads to a fluctuating, often much shortened collected walk that has the following footfalls:

1. Left front and left hind
2. Hovering
3. Right front and right hind

Back problems can also express themselves in this way, especially when the horse becomes tired and therefore can no longer stay in rhythm; the rider moves from left to right, but the back does not move in an elastic way. Muscle hardening and sensitivity to pressure are the results and are often the reason for considerable contact difficulties and challenges to going 'on the bit.'

In the sport of dressage, the pace is seen as a crass fault in training and is evaluated as a sign of lack of suppleness to correct pacing, ride forward with impulsion, (returning to the first three stages of the training scale) along with a forward and down stretched posture. Shoulder-in on the circle can also improve the coordination of footfalls in the walk.

Definition: *Bridle lameness is a temporary loss of rhythm in the movement and only happens when the rider tries, inappropriately, to get the horse on the bit with the reins.*

These horses do not show any lameness when moving free and are also orthopedically sound.

Note: *Bridle lameness is often provoked through too-strong, unyielding hands, and a reflex chain of a tendency to pace can occur.*

When a horse is very sensitive in the bars of the mouth and has poor dentition and the pull of the reins on the bit hurts him, he may attempt to extract himself out of this constricting position by escaping through massive rhythmic irregularly. Points on the teeth can push painfully against the sensitive mucous membranes which causes a rhythmic raising of the head. When the saddle does not fit or the rider sits in a chair seat or leans too far back, it can influence the movement from the hindquarters to the back, such that the horse tries, with every step, to evade the punctual pressure by shortening the steps and hollows the back. The hollow back disappears when the horse moves on the lunge without a rider.

> **Definition:** *The disunited canter [a.k.a. cross-firing or cross canter] is a faulty canter, where the horse, for example, does left lead canter with his front legs and right canter with his hind legs.*

The disunited canter is a sign of lack of suppleness and loss of balance. Balance problems may not be as obvious in the trot due to the two beat nature of the gait. In canter, balance problems can occur on circular lines or in a corner and horses compensate for the loss of balance by changing lead with their back legs, in an attempt to restore the missing support. Horses that have a sacra-iliac joint blockage tend to strike off in a disunited canter, since the crooked position of the pelvis transfers the impulsion in a slanted manner onto the vertebrae and the horse thus tries to evade using the hindquarters. Apart from the osteopathic correction of an obviously blocked sacra-iliac joint, frequent change in tempo, transitions and stretching work on the circle with alternating shoulder-in with haunches-in can correct this problem. Frequent canter strike-offs from walk and counter-canter (fig.19.1) improves the activity of the hindquarters and increases the ability to collect.

> **Note:** *Temporary loss of rhythm is seen as a big fault in competition dressage and 99% of the time is caused by faulty influence from the rider.*

The most common is an inelastic, rigid hand that does not give the horse sufficient freedom for the movement in the three gaits during the execution of exercises. Continuous sawing with the reins and putting the horse behind the bit has a negative influence on the drive of the hindquarters, which are thus prevented from stepping forward and so tension develops in the loin area. Tension in the poll and pressure sensitivity of the M. splenius are often indications of a hard hand. Grinding of the teeth and emerging muscle outlines of the M. masseter are obvious signs of lack of relaxation and insufficient back activity. Faults from the hand and uneven rhythms are especially visible in transitions. A rider with an unbalanced seat cannot follow the movement of the horse's back, causing the rider to lose his balance, hold on to the reins [for balance] and then the harmony between horse and rider is lost. A [horse's] hollow back with the hindquarters out behind incapable

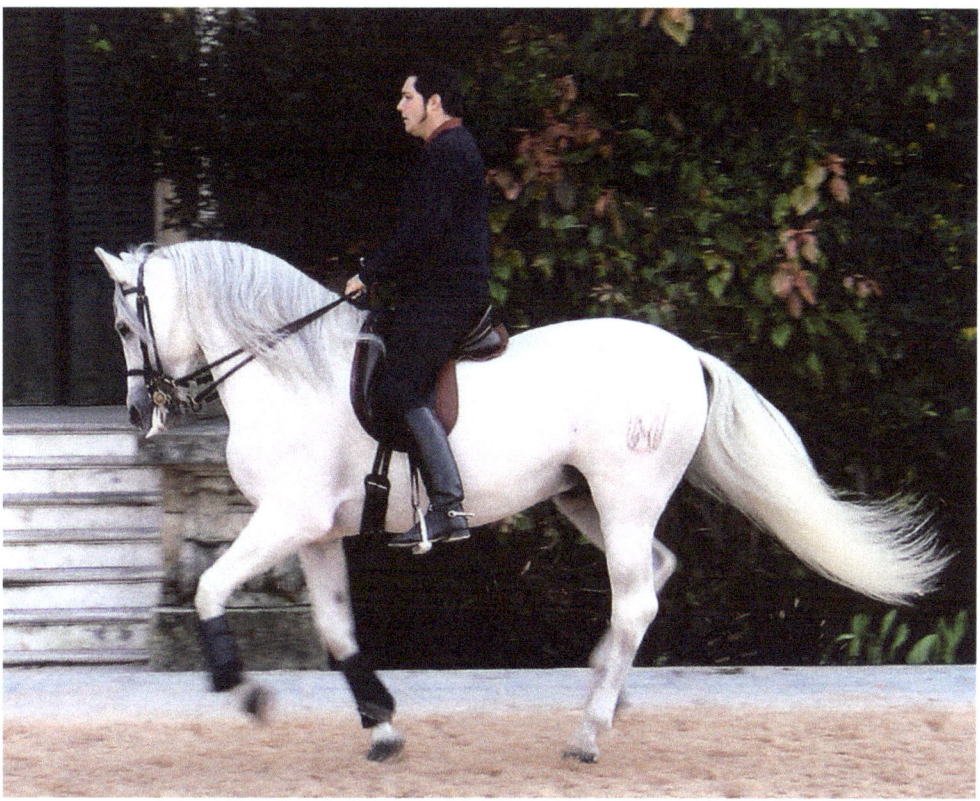

Fig. 19.1. Counter canter promotes straightness, ability to collect and the balance in canter. An established, well-balanced counter canter can clearly improve the canter and the flying change.

of carrying any weight results. When the rider pounds the horse's back with every extension, the horse will, through fear of pain, tense his longissimus and ileocostalis muscles to avoid the full blast of the rider's weight on the bony vertebrae. Consequently, loss of rhythm will arise when the horse leaves the corner on the diagonal. A crooked seat favors compensatory movements, especially when a lateral movement such as half-pass is requested. Loss of rhythm and nodding movements are then seen.

For all that, there are always horses that, due to orthopedic problems, tend to show a loss of rhythm, and they also show this without a rider; this should not be assigned to "loss of rhythm," but must be treated separately.

19.1.2. Over-bending and the "broken" neck

Definition: *A horse is over-bent when his forehead is too far behind the vertical and the nose is toward the chest. This leads to tension in the neck vertebrae and is caused by too strong an influence from the rider's hand.*

Depending on the position of elevation of the head and neck, the area in the jowl can become too narrow. The space between the throat and the Angulus mandiblee is so constricted that the horse can experience respiratory problems and tremendous difficulty extending the front legs. Through this strong shortening [of the neck] from a pulling hand, the horse "falls apart." The back hollows and the hindquarters cannot step under the center of gravity, for they are camped out. The croup becomes flat and a complete loss of impulsion occurs. Some horses are brought so far behind the vertical [of the forehead] with a horizontal neck emerging out of the withers that they can virtually bite themselves on the chest. This misunderstood deep position brings with it the effects of an incorrect stretched posture that has already been discussed. Both of these faults, caused by the hand, are common, and the artificially slowed forward impulsion results in the hind legs not being able to step under for weight bearing. This results in contact and mouth problems from being ridden incorrectly, because the missing support from the haunches must be found in the hand of the rider. In this incorrect position, it is biomechanically impossible for the horse to use his back or his body efficiently. He must increasingly work on the forehand and sooner or later gets physically damaged. (See fig.10.9.b)

Definition: *The broken neck is a head position where the third neck vertebra is the highest point of the horse instead of the poll. (See fig.2.3)*

The broken neck is much discussed, because the classical school requires the poll to be the highest point. In principle one must distinguish between two types of broken necks:

- One type results from an extremely developed neck, as is often the case with stallions and many Iberian horses. In these cases, it is important that the horse fulfills the criteria of correct relaxation and collection. When the horse is always able to assume a stretched posture, this deficiency is less serious, since the horse works correctly within the framework of his physical capabilities.
- The broken neck caused by too strong an influence of the hand, is characterized by the horse's nose being behind the vertical. The horse suffers immense loss of impulsion. The horse looks as if he has been pulled together and cannot stretch easily in a forward and down position, and huge errors in the basic training become evident.

Horses that are always "collected" by strong action from the hand will never be *truly* collected, since the appropriate basics, especially relaxation, is lacking. Without relaxation, true collection can never be achieved.

19.1.3. Problems with contact, the mouth and tongue

One of the most common problems for the physiotherapist is represented by contact difficulties and working on the bit. The horse refuses a correct position and bend, works against the hand, leans on the hand, stiff and insensitive in the mouth. When these horses are x-rayed, the outcome is mostly unremarkable and the teeth are also only marginally the reason for these problems.

When one reviews the first three points on the training scale, it becomes clear why these problems occur. Apart from osteopathic lesions caused by an accident and the tension that can then result in the neck muscles, rendering the influence from the rider almost impossible, it is in 90% of the cases an inactive and weak hind leg at the root. In combination with an unyielding hand of the rider, these problems increase. Lack of impulsion from the hindquarters will be further exacerbated by too strong of a hand. The hind legs do not take on any load and demand more from the hand, which is then used as a 5th leg in a vain attempt at keeping the balance.

Many transitions, voltes, turns-on-the-forehand, and especially shoulder-in on straight lines and on circles can help the horse learn how to use his hindquarters in a more coordinated manner. In the beginning, all exercises should be ridden in a calm and controlled walk and every small indication of yielding should be rewarded.

A tilt in the poll, where one ear is higher than the other, is often caused by unevenly pulling hands. A yielding hand carried at the same height should solve such a problem when used together with a driving leg aid. This is the only way to make the horse understand what is expected of him.

Tongue faults are almost exclusively attributed to too strong an influence of the hand or a bit that does not fit. Bits that are too large squash the bars of the mouth, while bits that are too small pinch. When the pressure on the tongue becomes intolerable, the horse will either let his tongue hang out of the mouth on one side, or put it over the bit, making him light in the hand for a short period, but he can no longer be controlled. When this happens, the horse must be stopped and the bit and nose-band re-adjusted. One should wait as long as it takes to have the tongue under a correctly fitted bit again.

Pressure on the bars of the mouth from double bridles is no rarity and should also be checked. When injuries occur due to the improper use of the double bridle, the method of training and the basic work must be questioned, for it can become an issue of animal welfare and protection.

> **Note:** *All "mouth difficulties" are caused by the rider and can only be improved by an appropriate training system and not by choosing tricky bits or extra reins, for this might help in the short term for the symptoms, but not the cause.*

19.2. Back problems

Many horses with back problems do not show any form of lameness. They become difficult to ride or bend, refuse jumps, or show impaired performance weaknesses, even though there is no clinically measurable difference in limb testing for lameness.

The primary feature in the so-called "sore-backed" or "back-lame" horse is the lack of ride-ability and work ethic in the forefront. Diagnosing the ride-ability of these horses is difficult. Therefore, it is important to speak the same language using hippological terminology, so one is capable of speaking about the problem and the far-reaching impacts it can have.

Besides varying sensitivity to pressure on the back, most horses have temporary loss of rhythm through the corners and in extensions without actually going lame. So it is of great value and inevitable to observe the horse being ridden under saddle. Astute owners will frequently notice unusual behavior, for example, biting when saddled or pinning the ears when they see the saddle or bridle. Acts of insubordination can manifest in unusual behavior including rearing, napping and bucking, or putting the rider in dangerous situations.

Depending on the horse's temperament and the strength of character, the problem zones will be manifested in different ways. Differences between the breeds should not be underestimated; for example, a Haflinger will react slower and will be more tolerant to palpation pressure than a fully trained English Thoroughbred that is more sensitive by nature. Palpation diagnostics require an experienced examiner. Noticeably hard and tense longissimus muscles sometimes do not allow the functional tests of mobility and provoke a predictable resistance and defensive reaction from the horse.

> **In Practice:** *The therapist should increase the pressure gradually during the examination to get a good first reaction. Repeated "testing" a painful spot is neither useful nor pleasant for the horse and should be omitted.*

When painful areas of the back are palpated, the saddle and bridle should be inspected to get a complete overview of the situation.

A further diagnostic tool would be a thermo-graphic screening of the spinal cord, as one can find "hot spots" in the muscles in this way. Investigations from Von Schweinitz[25] have shown that there is a large correlation between thermography and other imaging diagnostic processes like x-rays, ultrasound and MRI, justifying the meaningfulness of all of these methods.

When a thermography result is positive, the neck and back vertebrae should be x-rayed. When a justified reason for pain exists, the area can also be anesthetized.

Patients with this problem should undergo an osteopathic examination as well, since many clinical cases are diagnosed with unsatisfactory pictures for the therapist, but the patient cannot be used for riding.

19.2.1. General treatment proposals

Depending on the method of therapy—if it is an osteopathic treatment, or a conventional back treatment—different variations should be considered for follow-up treatment.

If the horse must first be treated with osteopathy, a one day rest period, followed by 3-4 days of walk should suffice to allow the horse to experience difference of leg length, the new posture of his axial skeleton, and the recovered movement possibilities after treatment. During this phase, it is important that the horse not get any anti-inflammatory drugs or infiltration. Drugs can mask the "blue prints" of the movements provoked by the relieving posture, and the horse can fall into the same habit of incorrect movement again after treatment. Homeopathy and acupuncture can support the self-healing of the body on different levels.

> **Note:** *In the primary phase after an osteopathic treatment, anti-inflammatory drugs are contraindicated.*

When a horse gets infiltration and anti-inflammatory drugs for treatment of localized muscular problems, one can, in most cases, see an improvement when they are not caused by osteopathic lesions. The horse

---

25 Dietrich Von Schweinitz grew up on a family farm in the USA and qualified as a veterinary surgeon at the University of Georgia in 1982. He practiced in Maryland at a referral equine hospital before moving to the UK in 1986. During his time in the USA he studied acupuncture and gained the IVAS (International Veterinary Acupuncture Society) Certificate in Veterinary Acupuncture. He was also President of the Association of British Veterinary Acupuncturists and is currently on the Board of Directors for the International Veterinary Acupuncture Society. His pioneering research into acupuncture and thermography has been published widely (Acupuncture in Medicine, Veterinary Clinics of North America: Equine Practice). He lectures internationally in veterinary acupuncture and pain management and he visits Fitzpatrick Referrals on a weekly basis to offer acupuncture to our patients. Acupuncture is performed in conjunction with physiotherapy and hydrotherapy to assist in pain management and post-operative recovery.

should, as a precaution, not be ridden for a few days afterwards so as not to infect the punctures, and should only be moved in the forward and down stretch on the lunge.

The following singled out treatment proposals should not be seen as dogmatic, but must be matched to each individual patient with respect to his capabilities. Standard recipes for treating physiological movement problems are naturally not possible as the holistic thinking approach is thus lost. Therefore the treatment proposals should only be seen as "proposals."

After thorough examination and treatment with mobilization, acupuncture, infiltration etc, the horse should definitely enter a rehabilitation program, since the shortened muscles caused by the relieving posture can only be corrected with the appropriate exercises such as work in-hand, lunge work and cavaletti training. This period will take at least 3 weeks to reach a sufficient stretch through regular training (30-40 minutes daily).

Depending on the state of training and the physical constitution of the horse, the first step can be lengthened or shortened. Fit horses that are in good condition and have fallen, can, after a short stretching phase of rehabilitation, quickly return to their normal training. Completely tense horses as well as those with a large lower neck muscle development and atrophy in the trapezius and longissimus muscles, must be kept in the rehabilitation phase longer due to their compromised starting situation.

In this context, one must be warned against over training, as most owners see this stretching as light movement on the lunge. These horses can easily be overworked. Resting phases are important in this rehabilitation phase, as is the case with proper training, in order to keep the motivation of the horse and his interest in his work going. Horses that are always pushed to their maximum will loose the joy in their work and become either mad or anxious. This will prevent progress in training, for mental relaxation constitutes the basis of physical relaxation required for proper muscle development.

Regular massage with invigorating liniments (arnica, comfrey) on the large muscles and in the area of the croup can be very useful. One can use big effleurage movements, tapotement and trigger point massage to release tension. The lumbo-sacral area especially can be efficiently supported by this. After every massage and after being under the solarium, horses should be covered with a blanket to avoid disorders of the back (especially in cold weather). Horses should also be allowed to rest for at least one hour after being treated; vasodilation brings with it a deeper relaxation making them tired and lazy when being ridden.

TENS treatment on the major local reaction point can also, by superimposing nervous impulse system, generate analgesia, and thus lead to muscle relaxation by means of a rebound effect. Horses move freer after a 15-

20 minute TENS treatment as long as the cause of the movement disturbance is not due to lameness.

Regular mobilization and stretching also favor the course of healing. The previously described carrot test is the best for this as it is the least risky mobilization test. Stretching the leg forward and back will mobilize shortened flexor groups. Rounding the back as well as light lifting of the topline by pressure on the xyphoid sternum can influence the mobility of the spine before riding and driving, as small blockages can easily be released by themselves through these mobilization techniques.

When horses build too little muscle due to lack of fitness, one should absolutely change the saddle so the muscles can develop under it. Muscle enhancing feed additives can also help in the rehabilitation phase, but all these additives only function when the horse is subjected to daily systematic training.

Lateral movements, especially the shoulder-in, and half turn on the haunches can improve the bend of the haunches and thus the arching of the outside lumbar area. The slow, controlled sideways movement is important in these exercises, so that muscle fibers can become used to stretching during the stance phase. Fast sideways movement is not advised for it will only provoke fixing of the thoracic vertebrae, making meaningful use of the back impossible and will cause damage to the joints.

Basically, as far as the construction of the exercises and the implementation of the exercises go, the aforementioned foundations are applicable in the rehabilitation phase just as meaningful training is only possible in a calm and fully controlled gait. This is the only way that the muscular development can be taken into account in a supportive way and the horse can find his psychological balance again, which he has probably lost through overtaxing his system in training.

Transitions in all gaits will promote the activity of the back and bending of the haunches which, in turn, will strengthen the carrying muscles. The performance of the exact school figures can make a substantial contribution to the gymnastic state of the horse. Riding the corners, voltes etc accurately will teach the less advanced horse how he is expected to move in an orderly and coordinated fashion. The ability for collection can be encouraged with the use of the corners and voltes (6-8 m radius).

During cavaletti training, in which horse has to overcome small gymnastic jumps, the abdominal muscles are strengthened. They are important antagonists for the back muscles. All of these exercises must not repeated too often in a training session. The stimulus for the increase of muscle mass of 5 stimuli per side is sufficient in the beginning. With this reasonable number of repetitions, horses do not get mentally nor physically tired and are able to move through the exercises without becoming tense.

Working the horse in-hand (for instance: crossing the legs, piaffe and Spanish walk) can stimulate specific areas and gives the horse a feeling that he needs in the rehabilitation phase. Skilled trainers can use this to motivate the horse without a rider on his back during the rehabilitation phase. This way of furthering the horse should mostly be done by experienced trainers, since it can have the opposite effect on the horse if incorrectly applied and in this case may actually provoke resistances.

> **Note:** *The often so loved "turn him out in the paddock" is the most useless thing one can do for a horse with muscular problems. Horses on the paddock move very little and normally loose their muscles, especially when they do not get any extra feed.*

This process is already evident after three days in the resting period and is quickly evident in the whole body of the horse.

Being "softer" after being put on the paddock is nothing more than a weakness in the horse's muscles. Weak muscles defend themselves against the weight of the rider. Problems that seem to have been corrected suddenly appear again with intensified training, as the basic problems have not been solved.

19.2.2. Kissing spine syndrome

The often diagnosed kissing spine syndrome (See fig5.15) is often the result of incorrect riding and, in very few cases, is influenced by faulty conformation (sway backed). This response frequently disappears when the horses learn to lift their backs with sensibly constructed training. The space between the vertebrae will automatically become wider.

Vertebrae that have already been ankylosed however, are no longer helped by any kind of therapy. Nevertheless, in such cases, the body parts that are influenced by this process by means of incorrect compensatory loading, for example the sacroiliac joint, hips, thoracic vertebrae, neck vertebra, can all receive mobilization treatment. The surgical dissection of the spinous processes should be critically questioned, for these vertebrae also serve a biomechanical function.

In the first place, the approaching of the spinous processes in the breast and loin vertebrae occur because the horse, through incorrect training, never learned to use his back adequately. Through the contraction of the M. longissimus dorsi, a lordosis is provoked and the spine is thus fixed. This happens when the flexor group of muscles of the spine cannot lift the back sufficiently due to fatigue and loss of tone. The extensor muscles, as the vertebrae stabilizing group, then take over the job of carrying the rider, which is only possible to a limited extent. The extreme contraction of the M. longissimus dorsi, M.iliocostalis as well as the stabilizing back muscles lead to metabolic compromise in the area where oxygen, blood and lactic acid accumulate and produces irritation in the motor end plates. The space between the vertebrae becomes narrower. Periostal reactions can be provoked within 14 days.

This fatigue phenomenon is often overlooked in green horses, which initially may round their backs well under the weight of the rider for a short while, then let it hang down when the muscles are not yet powerful. In such cases, the military service regulation [*H. Dv. 12*, Xenophon Press 2014] stipulates the immediate dismounting of the rider with a break of ten minutes where he just leads the horse by hand, and then rides the horse again after that. An inconsiderate "riding through" this predictable resistance, which is a sign of painful and over-trained muscles, makes useful training difficult, de-motivates the horse and can leave permanent physical and psychological damage.

The movement of the hindquarters will indeed be transferred to the spine, but due to the inelastic mobility of the spine it cannot continue through to the neck and horses look like they have been cut in half. The hindquarters are no longer able to step under the center of gravity of the horse due to the horizontal position, and carrying and rounding becomes impossible. These horses become heavy in the hand and are uncomfortable to sit; most riders try to correct this bad state of affairs by increased hand influence and reach exactly the opposite result. Because the back muscles never get used, the back does not become well muscled, even though it is trained every day. According to this author, the main pain is less from the periostal reactions, but much more from the hardness of the muscles that then influence the corresponding nerve roots due to accumulated lactic acidosis.

Many horses can be taught to use their backs again through an adequate training program on the lunge. With the correct use of their backs, these problems often disappear altogether. Great importance should be given to daily work on the lunge with the modified Pessoa training system, which should be done 6 days a week for 3-4 weeks, for it is possible in this time to stretch the muscles that have been shortened by the relieving posture and return them to their proper utility once again.

The rounding and lifting of the back can clearly improve the mobility of the back and should be done at least 10x per day before riding and also after the lesson has been finished. The supraspinous ligament that is shortened in this disease, should be stretched by consistently riding forward and down with an elastic feel.

Regular acupuncture mobilization of the back and daily lifting of the topline will have a positive influence on the preservation of mobility.

In especially persistent cases it is useful to infiltrate the back with neural therapeutic medication in order to interrupt the pain reflex arc that prevents the forward and down posture. When the muscles must be built from scratch, it can take up to three months, requiring daily and regular training.

As long as the horse does not have a pronounced saddle spot, the back bascule can be carefully built up with work in-hand, for a saddle that does not fit will not aid muscle development, since most saddles are too narrow.

19.2.3 Tension, vertebrae and joint blockage

Definition: *An osteopathic lesion or a blockage is not a luxation or subluxation in the classical sense, but a reversible functional movement restriction of a functional movement segment, consisting of two bones, ligaments/cartilage, tendons, blood vessels and nerve bundles.*

These are always in a physiological area and can therefore be returned to their original mobility through targeted manipulation techniques. Lesions, in the classical sense, like luxation or subluxation are of pathological functioning and are mostly associated with tissue destruction (tear in ligament). These cause not only functional, but also structural damage.

Blockages can be triggered by falls, slipping and other traumatic influences and form the basis for movement restrictions. The muscles in the area develop secondary tension in order to protect the segment where the movement restriction has occurred in an attempt to avoid further damage. Initially this happens unconsciously and through the local malnutrition and poor metabolism of the battered tissue. The tissue seeks a relieving posture while the removal of waste products and oxygen utilization can no longer take place. This will cause more painful reactions, causing an even worse relieving posture and the vicious circle is amplified. Horses do not speak when they are in pain, but can definitely articulate with body language, so observing the horse and his behavior is definitely of value.

These horses refuse to bend, step under their body, refuse jumps, nap, rear and buck in an "unmotivated manner," which can make a dangerous situation for the rider. The relieving posture can lead to sudden painful sensations, making horses react in panic.

The touchy, oversensitive behavior of a mare can come from a blockage, which can influence the body via the viscerocutaneous reflexes. This is one of the stones on which acupuncture rests, and also a reason why many autonomic organic disturbances can be regulated by osteopathic manipulation.

Blockage of the neck vertebrae, especially the atlas, causes many problems, such as leaning on the bit, heavy contact and poor bend, and the horse develops problems in being maneuvered. Differential diagnosis should exclude wobbler, ataxia and neck vertebrae fissures through allopathic medicine, since manipulation of previously damaged neck vertebrae can cause greater damage.

Horses that have problems in rounding or lifting their backs should always be accurately examined in the thoracic and loin vertebrae as well as in the rib joints. One can often find osteopathic lesions in these horses which will make their training difficult. The rider is frequently pushed over to one side in his seat and the horse finds it very difficult to move straight.

Blockage of the sacroiliac joint is very common, as this vulnerable joint is the only articulated connection between the hindquarters and the spinal cord. It is very mobile and therefore, very prone to blockages and crookedness of the pelvis after falls or accidents.

Due to the crooked transmission of the forward impulsion on the spinal column, one frequently finds secondary lesions on the atlanto-occpital intersection. This can be explained first by the function of the long back muscle which connects the pelvis with the head and secondly, through the connection via the meninges of the Cavums cranii to the sacrum.

These horses avoid collection and prefer to move somewhat sideways, rather than stepping straight under their center of gravity. When this prevails for a longer period of time, one can notice an obvious asymmetry of the croup muscles and the Tuber sacralia are irregularly prominent.

Horses often remain asymmetrical after being manipulated, even though functional health has been re-established, which can be explained as follows: ultrasound studies of the ligaments of the sacroiliac joint have shown of up to 1.5cm deviation in size and prominence between the two sides of the back without showing clinically relevant lameness or functional restriction. This difference can be seen as the cause of the seat bones being asymmetrical.

Nevertheless, a functionality test should always be made to determine the lesion, so the osteopathic lesions in this area can give no reason for compensatory overuse on the diagonal front legs.

Osteopathic manipulation should only be performed by appropriately qualified persons, otherwise there could be serious structural damage caused. In this context, the combined acupuncture-mobilization therapy is recommended, whereby acupuncture can significantly increase the relaxation of the disturbed meridian and thus the tense muscles. Every osteopathic treatment should be followed by a day of rest to get the horse accustomed to the changes in his skeleton. The different lengths in the bones must be balanced by the adjustment of the proprioceptors. After every treatment the controlled movement on the lunge or under saddle is important, depending on the muscular state of the horse, to show the horse his newly found freedom of movement. Once the horse is capable of stretching forward and down, the steps of the training scale should be followed to ensure long term therapeutic success.

19.3. Head shaking

Scholars have wracked their brains for centuries over uncontrollable, reflex-type shaking of the head, and up to this date there are only inadequate diagnostic and therapy possibilities available.

Commonly, one starts with the conventional diagnostic exclusion processes to investigate the different causes that can trigger this disease. Apart from allergic illnesses, UV sensitivity, teeth problems, trigeminal neuralgia and disorders of serration balance can all be potential causes. Faulty hands when ridden and intolerance to metal. For example a nickel allergy, and a badly fitting saddle can all be possible causes. When a horse cannot tolerate a certain alloy in a bit, careful testing should be able to eliminate this disruptive factor.

Horses with osteopathic lesions in the neck vertebrae and wither area show a predisposition for this symptom, especially when the saddle is too narrow and puts pressure on the trapezius muscles. Often, one can recreate head shaking when one pushes on the sensitive area of the withers with the hands. In such a cases the saddle should be made wider and adjusted according to the angle of the shoulder blade, to minimize the development of pressure in this area. Horses with osteopathic lesions in the neck vertebrae should be restored with suitable manipulation by a qualified veterinarian.

Unfortunately, not all head-shakers are so easy to explain. With photosensitive horses, implanting UV impermeable contact lenses has been successful. Anesthesia of the N. infraorbitalis can be successful in some patients and a neurectomy of the nerve branch can lead to a temporary improvement of this syndrome. Carbamazepine and Cyproheptadine can be used as medicinal support and can deliver varied results.

The teeth and temporomandibler joint must also be checked, since sharp edges on the teeth can often be the cause of headshaking, especially when the reins are taken up they push painfully against the mucous membranes of the cheeks. In this case, a dental renovation is recommended. The so-called "bit seats" can in some cases work wonders. A slight bevelling of the P1 in the upper and lower jaw, will prevent the pinching and bruising of the sensitive mucous membranes between the nose-band and P1, which can also lead to a similar defense reaction such as head-shaking. When the bit is too big, has sharp edges on the rings or the horse does not tolerate the metal, one must find a suitable alternative bit for the horse. Bit-less bridles can work wonders in this case when the problem lies with the bit.

19.4 Tendon damage

Tendon damage as a form of lameness that has its own special place, for tendons have a bad regeneration tendency due to their morphological and physiological characteristics. Tendons are generally insufficiently supplied with circulation. Tendon injuries often occur on uneven terrain and due to fatigue.

As a result of loss of tension in the muscles that attach to the tendon due to fatigue, the overload can lead to partial or complete tearing of the fibers. An ultrasound examination can show if a central or marginal lesion has occurred. Due to the loss of structure by tearing, tissue fluid will spontaneously run out, which will cause expansion of the lesion.

Tendons are the continuation of their muscular origin, therefore effective tendon therapy must include the muscle as well. Tension and shortening of the muscle is accompanied by loss of elasticity and a reduction of nutrient supply.

Therefore, it is important to apply passive mobilization of the extensors and flexors. This can release the fibrin adhesions and improve the gliding of the tendon again. Crosswise friction is also helpful for partial and specific mobilization of the injured tendon, to loosen localized adhesions and re-establish the functional integrity.

When a tear of this structure is brought on by overloading, further tension on the tendon will lead to further splicing up to the point of a complete breaking of the damaged structure. It is for this reason that controlled movement at the walk is important in the rehabilitation phase, for it is only through movement that blood flow can be increased. Dr. Dominique Giniaux [*Healing Hands* and *Equine Osteopathy*, Xenophon Press] has estimated the movement quota for a horse with tendon lameness to be 700 km of walk on a hard surface, and has thus given an objective and measurable count for the regeneration phase.

In the acute phase, the tendon should be cooled several times a day with ice water or cooling bandages to curb the swelling. Laser and magnetic field therapy can be used in conjunction with anti-inflammatory medication. The goal of these initial measures is to avoid adhesions as much as possible, so that functional movement restriction does not develop later in therapy.

In order to avoid overtaxing the other leg, it should also always be bandaged.

An essential therapeutic agent is time. Due to the fact that the tendon has poor circulation, it can take 6 months to one year to heal. When a horse is worked too early, even when he does not show lameness, it can lead to chronic tendinitis, which can reduce his suitability as a sport-horse to zero.

When the acute phase is concluded, the local region must be warmed. One can then make use of laser, magnetic field or ultrasound therapy. Shock waves also have good success when used in combination with physiotherapeutic after care. Activating injections can loosen adhesions locally and can clearly improve the future usefulness of the horse.

Activating injection in the tendon of Müller-Wohlfart[26] mixtures can serve in the secondary phase because of the stimulating action on the blood flow. The main factor for regeneration, besides the resting phase (3-12 months, depending on the damage) is the restoration of a resilient tendon structure through the stimulation of blood flow in the damaged area.

Local blistering or rubs that increase the blood flow to the area can also be used, although this is not recommended from the viewpoint of animal welfare due to the irritation caused to the skin. Only Heparin liniments or DMSO-mixtures, which penetrate the skin readily, can be used. All other blistering agents do not have sufficient penetration properties to actually reach the damaged area and will only have a limited impact.

Lymphatic drainage and mobilizing cross friction massage techniques can loosen adhesions in the area and can re-establish normal mobility.

In Practice: *Stretching the tendon is possible with the following procedure: one puts the damaged leg of the horse on a wooden wedge, and by developing pressure on the wither, try to load it increasingly. Once the horse is used to this feeling, the opposite leg can be lifted to increase the effect. This position should be sustained for 10-20 seconds to stimulate the golgi-apparatus. This can be repeated up to 10x daily to stretch the muscle and its tendon. When the horse shows resistance, one should return to cross friction massage technique and then wither pressure once more.*

Nutritional support can be provided with MSM preparations which give an internal impetus for regeneration of the torn sulfur bridge, making the

---

26   Hans-Wilhelm Müller-Wohlfahrt (born 12 August 1942 in Leerhafe) is the club doctor at Bayern Munich and is a world leader in the treatment of sports injuries. Many of the German doctor's treatments are controversial, including using injections of a substance called Hyalart, extracted from the crest of cockerels, which is claimed to help lubricate knee injuries and take away the pain. He has also injected honey or Actovegin into patients. Müller-Wohlfahrt's use of homeopathic medicine to treat human athletes is somewhat controversial.

final outcome of scar tissue significantly better and more resilient.

Controlled movement on hard surfaces and exercises that stretch the muscle of the tendon are indispensable to avoiding muscle shortening and faulty loading.

Corrective shoeing or setting the heels higher with damage of the deep digital flexor tendon is being controversially discussed, for the height of the heels will automatically bring a different pull on the tendon and the shortening of the muscle is thus promoted. The apparent relieving effect is therefore brought into a dubious light. In the view of several American authors, normal shoes should be used to help with regeneration.

19.5. Arthritis

Arthritis is wide spread among sport horses today due to high demands. The bones, although they are very adaptable structures which are constant remodeling, react to pull and pressure stimuli. These changes can be seen on x-rays as seemingly benign outgrowth of bone. These marginal ridge formations and hardening of tissues is frequently an effort of the body to strengthen the sensitive joints of the legs. Faulty conformation and insufficient training regimes, especially in the younger years, can all have a negative influence on the arthritic evolution.

Often the young horse of 2-2.5 years will have his growing skeleton lunged intensively, ridden at 3 years of age so they can be more "profitable" and especially for the purpose of being sold sooner. This will quickly cause overloading. In the sport of racing one often sees the phenomenon of bucked shins, a painful thickening of the cannon bones as a result of micro fissures of the periosteum. These growths are caused by too much training, but rest and anti-inflammatory medication can cause them to subside somewhat.

Apart from the hereditary joint problems such as OCD[27], arthritis also includes chronic degenerative joint diseases like podotrochlosis and bone spavin in horses. Both diseases have a progressive pathophysiology, whereby the spavin comes to a rest due to its etiology and all the involved joint gaps have been ankylosed. The change in the navicular bone is often more difficult to classify, for other structures can also be involved, thus making a diagnosis very challenging.

---

27 Osteochondritis dissecans (OCD) is a condition that develops in joints, most often in young animals. It occurs when a small segment of bone begins to separate from its surrounding region due to a lack of blood supply. As a result, the small piece of bone and the cartilage covering it begin to crack and loosen.

Primarily the basic illness must be cured, which is today, possible with suitable hyaluronic acid, glycosamine and bisphosphonate[28] therapies. The new bisphosphonates that come from human medicine can bring good success to podothrochlose patients and bone spavin, and horses can be used for longer in sports and remain pain free.

After an exact diagnosis is found, therapy should be matched to it. An important point in arthritic patients is the treatment of secondary tension that would result in partially relieving posture(s) or faulty loading.

Muscle spasms reduce blood flow, which further inhibit regeneration and even cause additional pain.

When it is not possible to do mobilization or passive movement therapy due to mechanical factors, it is up to therapist to treat the consequences. Bone spavin patients often have irritations in the knee and secondary tension in the hamstrings and loin area. These can be treated very effectively with acupuncture, mobilization techniques, and TENS therapy.

The process of bony changes can locally be supported by magnetic field therapy around the tarsal joint. Warming bandages and rugs in winter can have a positive effect, along with solarium or horse sauna in the cold winter months.

In bone spavin, which is a slow bony-changing process, it is only the actual active changes that are painful. This makes correct pain management inevitable, otherwise it will lead to relieving postures and muscle atrophy which can burden the horse even more and further the course of the disease. Local joint infiltration, anti-inflammatory, phosphastes[29], hyaloronic acid or devil's claw can be efficacious in treatment.

It is important that the horses have peace after treatment, are blanketed and not exposed to drafts, otherwise the state might worsen.

> **Note:** *Regular movement and an adequate warm-up phase of at least 15 minutes should always be considered with arthritis patients.*

Horses with spavin should be moved much more calmly. Standing for long periods or being in the paddock for long periods does not help the arthritis patient, quite the opposite—they become even stiffer and will figuratively "rust." They need much longer warm-ups— in order to become flexible—than horses that can follow an individually adapted training program. Frequent lungeing should be omitted as should riding on tight turns, especially during

---

28 A class of drugs that prevent the loss of bone mass, used to treat osteoporosis and similar diseases

29 Any of several classes of esterases of varying specificity that catalyze the hydrolysis of phosphoric esters

an acute stage—due to the increased torque in the tarso-metatarsal joint.

Mobilization of the hock and its joints are contra-indicated due to the progressive process of the disease. Mobilization can massively negatively influence the course of the disease and it can increase the painful phase.

Shoes with a square or rolled toe can assist the horse in break-over. Natural balance shoes on the hind foot can also be of help if the horse can tolerate them.

Putting a pad on one foot only, as was the case earlier with spavin horses, cannot be justified from a biomechanical perspective. Even though it can indeed relieve the hock joint, it will, at the same time, put more strain on the knee joint, potentially causing secondary lesions. Apart from a higher load on the knee joints and an extreme strain on the suspensory ligaments—shoeing both feet with the help of a pad will not bring more benefits and can potentially bring more damage.

19.6. Orthopedic shoeing

In this Chapter, the necessity of a correctly trimmed hoof will be discussed. According to the established rules, the hoof should have a flat contact with the ground, without any broken axis, otherwise it will have undesirable biomechanical action that will delay therapeutic success or compromise it.

The supreme principle is that the hoof must fit the angle of the fetlock and the horse must be able to move without problems. Many of the "magic shoes" have no use since the horse cannot move with them.

Whether a special shoe must be fitted depends on the indications and the conformation of the hoof. Hot or cold shoeing should also not become a question of belief. The art of correct shoeing lies in the proper trimming of the hoof and not in the ingenious techniques of inventors of new methods.

The best case is if the horse were able to go barefoot, where the hoof mechanism can develop its best possible implementation, as long as the footing is adequate. This should mean that dressage horses that normally work in a covered or open school can work barefoot without problems when they have normal, healthy hooves. For a carriage horse, however, it is unthinkable, regardless of the quality of the hoof, to work on asphalt roads due to high abrasion without shoes.

In the rehabilitation phase, the natural balance shoe (NBS) when fitted correctly, help to improve freedom of the shoulder, but only with an acute angled hoof with under-run heels. This will cause an improved break-over and a relief on the deep digital tendon and the navicular bone. In this way the problems in this area can be successfully supported in therapy.

When the posterior portion is also used to carry or when pressure is put on them, egg bar shoes can be used. This is also used in laminitis as it provides relief to the deep digital tendon.

The so-called heart bar shoe can improve the hoof mechanics in horses with narrow heels, since the stalk-like part of the shoe gives positive support to the frog every time the horse steps. One should be extra careful when affixing this shoe, for an even pressure distribution is necessary, so as not to cause extra pressure points. Narrow heels can also be corrected with shoes that have a slight flare to the outside, so the hoof wall can widen with every step by sliding to the outside of the shoe and, in this way, open the heels. Narrow heels will impede the proper function of the pumping mechanism, and the movement will travel up the joints unchecked. This will cause more wear on the joint and ossification of the cartilage. The absent elasticity of the hoof and, commonly, shoes that are too small or too narrow will result in increased tension on the hoof wall, often causing it to tear, or crack.

Synthetic shoes and especially glue-on shoes are often used in rehabilitation, but are not recommended due to the strong decelerating action they have. Every horse makes a rotation movement when he lifts his foot, and the synthetic shoe will brake this to a greater or lesser extent. This can cause very high stress loading of the taut distal tendon.

Putting the foot at an angle by inserting a wedge should only be used with deep digital flexor lesions, for this can then be relieved during the phase of healing (at least according to some sources). Nevertheless, the necessity of placing the heel high should be carefully considered, for the muscular part of the deep digital flexor will shorten through a reflex action. This "artificial" relief of tendons should also be questioned because it inevitably leads to increased pull on the suspensory ligament which will become overloaded. The foot should be shod with normal shoes, for a permanent slanted position will affect the supportive and knee ligaments since they become overloaded when the horse has to stand on a permanent slant.

Studs should not be used during the rehabilitation phase. They compromise the rotation movement of the hoof or even stop it completely and will cause rotation blockages in the taut tendons. This can cause arthritic processes to flare up.

In order to prevent slipping, stud nails are suitable. They provide enough traction without overly influencing the mechanics of the hoof.

A regular massage, once or twice per week, with laurel oil on the coronet band, will keep the wall of the hoof elastic, will stimulate hoof growth and all the pathological processes in the hoof itself can be improved while the circulation is increased.

Washing and drying the hoof will improve the hoof mechanism. Hours of standing in moist places will only favor mud fever and eczema and will likely damage the quality of the hoof. Moisture policies should be kept to a sensible level.

Horses with extremely dry, small hooves (Spain, Portugal, Arabia) that tend to have contracted heels should be treated with water and coronary massage for as long as it takes until the hoof regains its physiological form and performs its work in an elastic and effective manner (hoof pump).

In practice: *Imbalance in the hoof can be verified with thermo-graphic pictures, and an owner will also be able to distinguish differences once improved circulation is achieved after one corrective treatment.*

In closing....

I hope that the system I have presented will aid riders to help their horses improve in wellness and further progress their training. It is completely possible for horse and rider, during their movements, to become a "work of art in the moment"—similar to classical music. In my experience, this synergy creates a consuming atmosphere of love and passion in the rider's heart. The technique I have presented should improve horses' nature by restoring lightness and balance under the foreign weight of the rider. If followed correctly, the method prevents tension and easily resolves stiffness through my holistic approach of mobilization work based on Baucher's flexions and the osteopathic method of my teacher, Dominque Giniaux D.V.M., author of *Healing Hands* and *Equine Osteopathy: What the horses have told me*, both also Xenophon Press titles.

Finally, I hope that we have presented very powerful tools for maintaining your horse's health and developing his desire to work.

The "equestrian art in lightness" is the only way to maintain and improve your horse's abilities by transforming him into a willing partner. I sincerely hope that many horses will benefit from this training system.

Dr. Robert Stodulka

Lightning Source UK Ltd.
Milton Keynes UK
UKHW051026060223
416527UK00005B/96